Introduction to Radiobiology

Introduction to Radiobiology

by
M. Tubiana, J. Dutreix
Institute Gustave-Roussy, Paris, France

and
A. Wambersie
Unite de Radiotherapie, Brussels, Belgium

translated by
D. K. Bewley
MRC Cyclotron Unit, London, UK

Taylor & Francis
London • New York • Philadelphia
1990

UK   Taylor & Francis Ltd, 4 John St., London WC1N 2ET

USA   Taylor & Francis Inc., 1900 Frost Rd., Suite 101, Bristol, PA 19007

The original edition was published in France under the title *Radiobiologie* by HERMANN, publishers of sciences and arts, Paris.

British Library Cataloguing in Publication Data
Tubiana, Maurice
  Introduction to radiobiology
  1. Radiobiology
  I. Title.   II. Dutreix, Jean
  III. Wambersie, André
  574.1915

  ISBN 0-85066-745-3
  ISBN 0-85066-763-1 (soft)

Library of Congress Cataloging-in-Publication Data
Tubiana, Maurice, 1920–
  Introduction to radiobiology/Maurice Tubiana, Jean
  Dutreix, André Wambersie; translated by David Bewley
  p. cm.
  1. Radiobiology. I. Dutreix, J. II. Wambersie, A. II. Title.
  [DNLM: 1. Radiobiology. WN 610 T885i]
  QH652.T83   1990
  574. 19'15—dc20
  DNLM/DLC
  for Library of Congress   90-10748 CIP

Typeset in 10/12 Century School Book by Chapterhouse, The Cloisters, Formby

Printed in Great Britain by Burgess Science Press, Basingstoke on paper which has a specified pH value on final paper manufacture of not less than 7.5 and is therefore 'acid free'.

Contents

Preface

The present book is both a translation and an update of the French book 'Radiobiologie' published in 1986. Many new developments have occurred during the intervening four years and the three authors and the translator have taken the opportunity to modernize the text and to include newer references. The structure of the book, however, remains the same.

The subject matter is primarily human radiobiology. The main emphasis of the book is the biological, physical and chemical basis of radiotherapy. An important section is concerned with the biological basis of radiation protection and the action to be taken in the event of a radiation accident.

Despite new developments in the treatment of cancer by surgery and chemotherapy, radiotherapy has not lost its importance and is used at some stage in about half of all cases. The new methods, such as the use of new drugs and immunotherapy, have not replaced the use of radiation; rather, they are combined with radiation to provide a more comprehensive means of attack.

Molecular biology has brought new insights towards understanding the principal mechanisms underlying cell death and loss of reproductive integrity following irradiation. In this respect the importance of repair of radiation-induced damage such as lesions has become increasingly evident.

Radiation protection is a subject of increasing importance. There is greater understanding of the damaging effects of irradiation than of the effects of any other noxious influence in the environment. Consequently the regulations controlling exposure to radiation have served as a model for other noxious agents. Medical use of radiation, mainly in diagnostic radiology, represents the principal contribution to the irradiation of the human population from artificial sources and is comparable in magnitude to that from natural background radiation. Nuclear methods of generating electricity have assumed an increasing share of the total during the last few decades but have added very little to the radiation received by the general population. Atmospheric pollution and fear of increasing global temperatures due to the burning of fossil fuels, together with lack of discernible progress towards the economic use of nuclear fusion, are arguments supporting the further development of reactors based on fission. At present this is held back mainly by fears of accidents such as that at Chernobyl. The gross disproportion between the anxiety felt by the population of Western Europe after Chernobyl and the reality of the hazard demonstrates the need for improved education of the public and of bodies responsible for public health and protection of the environment. The same was true, to perhaps a greater extent, for the population of the USA after the accident at Three Mile Island.

The aim of this book is to provide information to those concerned with the relevant fields of knowledge. We hope it will be of value particularly to trainees in radiology, radiation oncology and nuclear medicine and to scientists concerned with cancer or radiation. We hope it will also be valuable in general medical education and in the wider sphere of public administration in relation to the advantages and disadvantages of ionizing radiation in all areas of human activity.

We would like to record our thanks to all those who have given us advice on the content of this book. The list would be too long but we wish to thank especially G. Adams, M. Bertin, D. Chassagne, Ch. Chevalier, S. Field, J. Guelette, G. Hahn, H. Jammet, L. Lallemand, F. Laval, A. Léonard, E. Malaise, A. Michalowski, J. Ninane, N. Parmentier, P. Pellerin, and F. Zampetti-Bosseler.

Chapter 1.
Initial physical effects of irradiation: dosimetry — microdosimetry

The biological effects of irradiation are the end product of a long series of phenomena which are set in motion by the passage of radiation through the medium. The initial events are ionizations and excitations of atoms and molecules of the medium along the tracks of the ionizing particles. These physical perturbations lead to physico-chemical reactions, then chemical reactions and finally the biological effect. The sequence of these stages is represented schematically in Table 1.1.

Here we recall briefly the changes of energy in ionizations and excitations, the mechanisms which are at their origin and the dosimetric expressions which characterize their spatial distribution.

1.1 Slowing down of charged particles

Ionization — excitation

In matter the electrons have regular places in the structure of atoms, molecules or ions. To detach an electron, i.e. to produce ionization, it is necessary to supply a quantity of energy (symbolized by W) which represents its binding energy. Some examples of binding energies in atoms are given in Table 1.2. In the ground state the electron occupies the available places in the most strongly bound positions. The binding energy of the outermost electron which corresponds to the first ionization potential is of the order of 10 eV ($W=13\cdot6$ eV for the atom hydrogen).

An electron can be carried into a more external orbit, normally empty, which constitutes an *atomic excitation*, e.g. in an atom of hydrogen the electron can be carried from the K shell into the L shell by giving it an energy of $10\cdot2$ eV. In molecules the energy needed to extract one of the outermost electrons (first molecular ionization potential) is of the order of 10 eV as for atoms. Rather lower energies may be able to produce excited molecular states.

It must be emphasized that the ionization energy is considerably greater than the energy of intramolecular binding, i.e. the chemical energy, which is, for example, $4\cdot9$ eV for the bond C=C and $5\cdot16$ eV for the bond H–OH. The ionized

1

Table 1.1. Chronology of events.

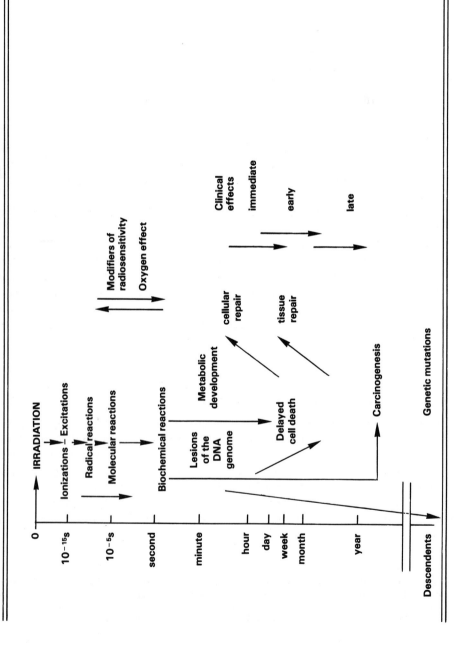

Table 1.2. Binding energy of electrons (eV).

		Atoms			
			Shell[†]		
Atom	Z	K	L	M	N
H	1	13·6‡	(3·4)	(1·5)	
C	6	284	11·2		
O	8	532	13·6		
P	15	2142	128	10·9	
Ca	20	4038	346	47	6·1

	Molecules	
	H_2	15·6
	O_2	12·5
	H_2O	12·6
	NO_2	11·0
	CO_2	14·4

† For the L, M, N...shells only the lowest binding energy is given.
‡ The underlined figures represent the binding energies of the most weakly bound electrons (the first ionization potential).

molecule has an excess of internal energy equal to the energy of electronic binding supplied to provoke ionization, which is therefore more than enough to produce dissociation of the molecule. Molecular excitation can have the same consequence.

Ionizations and excitations are created in the medium when it is traversed by fast *charged particles* as a result of interactions with the electrons which are located close to their tracks. The radiation incident on the medium is classified as *directly ionizing* if it is composed of charged particles, e.g. electrons, protons, deuterons, heavy ions, etc. The radiations which are composed of uncharged corpuscles, photons and neutrons, produce ionization through the charged particles which they set in motion in the medium—secondary electrons in the case of photons and secondary protons in the case of neutrons (see later in this chapter); they are called *indirectly ionizing* radiations.

General mechanism of the interaction between moving charged particles and the electrons of the medium

The interactions between a charged particle and the electrons of the medium which it is traversing are the essential cause of the slowing down of the particles.† In addition, they are the origin of the absorption of energy by the medium and of the effects which result. The mechanism of interaction is common to all the charged particles and is shown in Figure 1.1.

The Coulomb force (of attraction or repulsion) which exists between the two electric charges during the brief passage of the particle close to the electron,

---

†Another cause of slowing down of charged particles is interaction with nuclei which results in the appearance of *bremsstrahlung*; this mechanism has a very important application, namely the production of X-rays by fast electrons bombarding a target of high Z. In biological media the slowing down of electrons or other charged particles by nuclear interactions is of very minor importance.

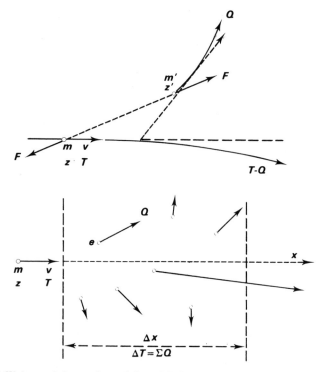

Figure1.1. Collisions of charged particles with the electrons of the medium. The Coulomb force acting between the incident particle (an electron in the case illustrated) and an electron of the medium involves the transfer to the latter of energy Q which is drawn from the energy T of the incident particle. Over a distance Δx the particle loses energy ΔT (the sum of transfers Q resulting from collisions occurring over this distance). The stopping power is defined by $S=\Delta T/\Delta x$; it depends (as does Q) on the speed and charge of the incident particle and on the number of electrons per unit volume of the medium.

gives an impulse to the electron; as a result there is a transfer to the electron of an energy Q which is derived from the kinetic energy T of the incident particle. The transfer of energy has a maximum value, Q_{max}, in the case of a head-on collision, the electron being exactly on the track of the incident particle.

Q_{max} depends on the mass of the particle:

(i)   if this is an electron $Q_{max}=T$ (because the two electrons cannot be distinguished, it is convenient to consider the secondary electron as the one with the lower energy, which implies that $Q_{max}=T/2$);

(ii) for a particle of mass M very much greater than the mass m of the electron, $Q_{max}=4Tm/M$: for example, a proton cannot transfer to an electron more than $0\cdot2\%$ of its kinetic energy.

For distant collisions the transfer Q depends on the distance h between the electron and the trajectory of the particles, on the speed v and on the charge z of the latter:

$$Q=K\frac{1}{h^2}\frac{z^2}{v^2}$$

The transfer Q diminishes quickly as h increases; for example, a fast electron of 1 MeV transfers to an electron of the medium $Q=1\,\text{keV}$ for $h=10^{-6}\mu m$ and $Q=10\,\text{eV}$ for $h=10^{-5}\,\mu m$. (One should note in this example what is represented by the distance h for collisions called 'distant' with small transfer of energy.)

For a given distance h, the transfer Q becomes greater as the speed of the particle becomes less because the impulse communicated increases with the duration of the interaction; for example, Q is 10 times greater for an electron of 10 keV ($v=6\cdot10^9\,\text{m s}^{-1}=0\cdot2\,c$, where c is the speed of light) than it is for an electron of 1 MeV (velocity approximately equal to c). A proton of 20 MeV has the same speed as an electron of 10 keV and produces the same transfer of energy Q. The transfer increases with the charge z of the particle proportionally to z^2; for example, for an α-particle ($z=2$) of 80 MeV, Q is four times greater than for a proton having the same velocity, i.e. an energy of 20 MeV.

Slowing down of charged particles — stopping power — trajectory and range

When a particle traverses a small segment Δx of its trajectory it suffers numerous collisions with electrons located at various distances from the track, corresponding to various transfers Q. The sum of all these transfers Q represents the energy ΔT lost by the particle over the distance Δx.

The ratio $S=\Delta T/\Delta X$ defines the *stopping power* (by collision) of the particle in the medium. S depends on the speed v and the charge z of the particle. If one considers as a first approximation that for each of these collisions the transfer Q is proportional to z^2/v^2, ΔT and hence S are equally proportional to z^2/v^2. A more exact formula established by Bethe takes account of 'close collisions' and of the role played by the binding of the electron to the atom.

At a given speed — the corresponding kinetic energy being proportional to the mass — all particles carrying a single charge (electron, proton, deuteron, meson) have the same stopping power. For protons of energy Tp, the stopping power is the same as that of electrons of energy $Te=Tp/1830$ and of deuterons of energy $Td=2Tp$; for an α-particle ($z=2$) of the same velocity and of energy $T\alpha=4Tp$, it is four times greater. We will see (Chapter 11) that these differences in stopping power which depend on the speed and nature of the particles have radiobiological consequences.

A particle of initial energy T_0 traversing a medium progressively loses its energy over a distance R which represents its *range* (Table 1.3). For a heavy

Table 1.3. Heavy charged particles. Relation between the range (R) in water and the initial kinetic energy (T_0).

Particle			Range R (cm)		
Name	Symbol	Mass	5	10	15
			Kinetic energy T_0 (MeV)		
Proton	H$^+$	1	79	117	145
Deuteron	^{2}H$^+$	2	108	159	199
Helium ion (α-particle)	He^{2+}	4	297	464	584
Carbon ion	C^{6+}	12	1752	2620	3332
Neon ion	Ne^{10+}	20	3420	5918	7575

particle deviations caused by collisions are very small; the track is straight and its length does not vary between one particle and another. For an electron, distant collisions cause only very small deviations, but the rare close collisions involve large deviations: the track is composed of straight segments with sharp changes of direction; the end of the track is very convoluted. Close collisions involve large losses of energy which vary from one electron to another and the length of the track shows important fluctuations.

Effects of collisions on the medium

For the medium the effects of a collision depend on the energy Q transferred to the electron.

1. If Q is a little lower than the binding energy W (i.e. about 10 eV), the electron is not detached from the atomic or molecular structure to which it belongs. It can be taken to a higher energy level (*excitation*). Transfers of energy which are even lower are finally communicated to the molecule to increase its energy of translation, rotation or vibration, representing thermal forms of energy.
2. If Q is greater than W an *ionization* takes place. The electron carries off a kinetic energy $Q-W$ which is subsequently transferred to the medium to produce further ionizations, excitations and thermal transfers.‡ If Q does not exceed a few hundred electronvolts, the kinetic energy of the electron is absorbed in the immediate vicinity of its point of origin and a cluster of ionizations (and excitations) is produced. If Q is greater, the electron has a track distinct from that of the primary particle. It is then called a *δ-ray; δ-rays* are defined as secondary electrons set in motion by incident charged particles (which may themselves be electrons) whose kinetic energy is greater than a conventional value generally taken as 100 eV.

We have seen above that the transfer Q depends on the distance h of the electron from the track of the incident particle. As the electrons are dispersed at random in the medium, distant electrons are more numerous than those which are close and collisions with small transfers Q are more numerous than collisions with large transfers.

On the assumption that the electrons are free, it can be shown that the probability of a transfer Q is proportional to $1/Q^2$, e.g. the incident particle loses twice as much energy in collisions with Q between 50 and 51 eV as in collisions with Q between 100 and 101 eV. When the energy given to the electron is very small, its binding energy to the atom or molecule cannot be neglected; the momentum is then transmitted to the whole structure and on account of its large mass the transfer of energy Q is to all intents and purposes, zero.§

The distribution of energy lost by the particle as a function of the transfer Q is

---

‡A moving electron is called a sub-excitation electron when its kinetic energy is reduced to a level below the first excitation potential (6·6 eV for water) and it is called thermal when its energy is reduced to about 0·02 eV; the time required for thermalization is less than 10^{-12}s.

§The collision gives to the target particle an impulse or momentum $p=mv$ where m is the mass of the target particle and v the speed which is given to it. The corresponding kinetic energy is $mv^2/2=p^2/2m$; this is small if m is large.

shown schematically in Figure 1.2. It shows that the energy $\epsilon=\Delta t$ lost by the particle traversing a small segment Δx of its track is divided more or less as follows:

(i)   40% in transfers $Q > 100$ eV (δ-electrons);
(ii) 30% in transfers $100 > Q > 10$ eV (ionizations);
(iii) 30% in transfers $Q < 10$ eV (excitations and thermal transfers).

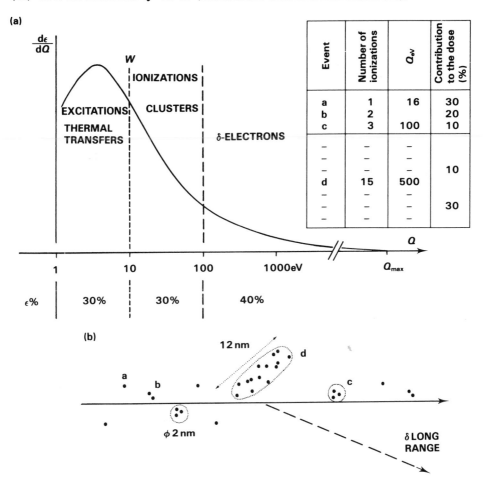

Figure 1.2. Distribution of energy lost by an incident particle as a function of the size of individual energy transfers.
(a) Along a small segment of its track, a particle loses an energy ϵ, the sum of individual transfers Q produced by its collisions (Figure 1.1). $d\epsilon(Q)$ represents the energy lost in transfers between Q and $Q+dQ$. The distribution is represented schematically in the figure (actually there are some variations depending on the nature and energy of the particle and on the medium). Depending on its size, a transfer Q above the binding energy W (taken here as equal to 10 eV) results in an ionization, a group of ionizations or a δ-electron (if $Q > 100$ eV); a transfer Q a little below W causes an excitation.
(b) Depending on the size of the transfer Q resulting from a collision, $1, 2 \ldots n = Q/\overline{W}$ ionizations are produced in the medium. The different types of event are shown in the figure as well as their relative contributions to the production of ionizations, i.e. to the dose. The diagram does not indicate the proportion of different types of event (a is three times more frequent than b and 10 times more frequent than c, etc.). The mean separation of events depends on the LET: when the LET is 25 keV μm^{-1} (1 MeV protons) the groups of diameter 2 nm are contiguous.

This distribution is essentially linked to the relative frequency of close and distant collisions, which is fixed by the random spatial distribution of electrons in the medium. It depends to only a small extent on the speed of the particle or on its charge and so on its stopping power. We have seen above that the transfers Q are individually proportional to the stopping power but their relative frequency, if one takes into account distant collisions with Q very much smaller than Q_{max}, is constant.

This distribution remains constant along the whole length of the track of the particle. It is also constant along the track of the δ-rays, the δ-rays of the second generation which they produce, and so on. Finally, after degradation of all the δ-rays, the energy deposited in the medium is divided *almost equally* between ionization on the one hand and excitation and thermal transfers on the other.

Thus, in the case of electrons, for one ionization produced in water (or in a biological medium) which requires a mean energy of 16 eV the energy absorbed by the medium is $\overline{W}=32\,\text{eV}$, where $\overline{W}$ is the *mean energy per ionization*. It depends very little on the speed or the charge of the particle. One can calculate in this way that a particle of 1 MeV completely absorbed produces along its track and along the tracks of δ-rays $10^6/32=3\times10^4$ ionizations. The linear density of ionization, at a point on the track, is $S/\overline{W}$; an electron of 1 MeV loses along 1 mm of its track an energy of 200 keV and creates 6000 ionizations (6 ionizations μm^{-1}).

1.2 Absorbed dose

The absorbed dose *at a point in the medium* is the quantity of energy deposited close to that point when the radiation passes through the medium. The dose is defined by $D=\Delta\epsilon/\Delta m$ where $\Delta\epsilon$ is the *mean energy transferred* by the radiation to a mass Δm of the medium (Report 33 of the International Commission on Radiation Units and Measurements (ICRU) explains the concept and gives a detailed definition of the dose and of the other quantities concerned in the metrology of ionizing radiation). In practice $\Delta\epsilon$ represents the energy which appears in the form of ionization, excitation and thermal transfers produced in Δm.

The *dose* at a point represents the density of energy absorbed at that point:

$$D=\Delta\epsilon/\Delta m$$

Because of the discontinuous nature of the events which lead to the absorption of energy, dose is meaningful only when the mass Δm is great enough that there is neither an appreciable statistical fluctuation in the number of particles traversing such a mass during the irradiation nor in the energy which they deposit.

The unit of dose is the gray (Gy): $1\,\text{Gy}=1\,\text{J}\,\text{kg}^{-1}$. (An old unit, the rad, is $10^{-2}\,\text{Gy}=1\,\text{cGy}$.) The dose also represents the density $\Delta n/\Delta m$ of ionizations produced at the point considered.

$$\Delta n/\Delta m=(\Delta\epsilon/\overline{W})\times1/\Delta m$$

In water ($\overline{W}=32$ eV) a dose of 1 Gy ($=0\cdot6\times10^{19}$ eV kg^{-1}) corresponds to a density of ionizations equal to 2×10^{17} ionizations kg^{-1}, i.e. 2×10^5 ionizations for a cell of mass 10^{-9} g.

The measurement of dose is not considered here. We recall only that the normal method is to use an ionization chamber: the principle is to measure the density of ionization in a small volume of air placed at the point considered and to deduce the density of ionization or the energy absorbed in the dense medium.

The dose is a quantitative expression of the physical effect produced by the radiation at a point in the irradiated medium. It has biological interest because the biological effect is related to it. The distribution of dose in a region of the body exposed to a particular radiation gives a representation of the biological effect produced at each point and for equal doses the biological effect is the same for a given radiation. However, the relation between the biological effect and the dose depends on the nature of the radiation; the quantitative character attached to the notion of dose must be complemented by its qualitative character which is studied in Section 1.4.

1.3 Dose distributions from beams of radiation

We limit ourselves in this work to the general characteristics of the variation with depth of the dose delivered by beams of radiation currently in use in radiobiology and radiotherapy. We also consider the characteristics (nature and energy) of the ionizing particles set in motion in the irradiated medium and their variation with depth; these characteristics are of radiobiological importance because they govern the distribution on a microscopic scale of the absorbed energy (Section 1.4) and the biological effectiveness of the radiation (Chapter 11).

Beams of heavy charged particles

The heavy charged particles are atomic nuclei. We have seen above that their tracks are straight and that they have a definite range depending on their nature and on their kinetic energy (Table 1.3).

The velocity of these particles diminishes steadily with depth resulting in an increase in the stopping power and at the same time an increase in dose. All beams of monoenergetic heavy charged particles produce a characteristic form of dose distribution (Bragg curve) with a sharp peak close to the end of the range (Figure 1.3). As the Bragg peak is very narrow the dose distribution produced by monoenergetic particles is not usually suitable for radiotherapy. To deliver a uniform dose over a greater thickness, the energy of the particles must be modulated during the irradiation in order to shift the peak; in this way the peak is widened at the cost of a reduction in its height.

Heavy charged particles for external beam radiotherapy are produced by powerful accelerators (cyclotrons or synchrotrons) which provide the large kinetic energy required to attain the necessary depth (Table 1.3). For protons the range exceeds 5 cm when the energy is above 80 MeV. At these energies the stopping power (or the linear density of ionizations) is low at the entry surface of the medium. It increases slowly at first in the course of slowing down of the

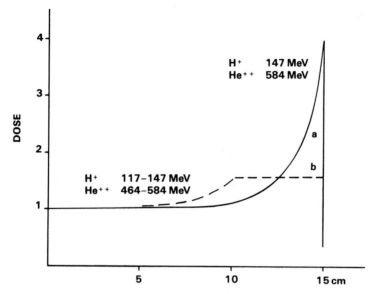

Figure 1.3. Distribution of dose with depth in a beam of heavy charged particles — Bragg curve. For monoenergetic particles the distribution of dose has a characteristic shape with a sharp peak at the end of the range (curve a). The depth of the peak depends on the energy and nature of the particles. By varying the particle energy during the irradiation, the peak can be moved between two depths to give the type of distribution represented by curve b.

protons and more rapidly as their energy become less than about 10 MeV (Table 1.4), i.e. in the last few millimetres of the range which corresponds to the Bragg peak.

Helium ions (α-particles), for an equal range, must have an energy four times greater than that of protons and at all depths their stopping power is four times greater. Stopping power becomes much greater for the particles having a higher charge (C^{6+}, Ne^{10+}, etc.).

In summary, if we consider particles with energy sufficient for a range of around 10 cm: protons are particles with low linear density of ionization over almost the whole of their range; the density of ionization is rather greater for helium ions and much greater for the heavier particles.

We must also consider heavy particles with shorter ranges. Alpha-particles emitted in the course of radioactive disintegrations have energies of a few MeV (the α-particles emitted by polonium have an energy of 5·3 MeV and a range in water of about 50 μm): these are particles with a high density of ionization along the whole length of their very short tracks. The situation is the same for the protons of a few MeV set in motion by neutrons (see later in this chapter).

Table 1.4. Protons. Range (R) and stopping power (S_o) in water as a function of the initial kinetic energy (T_o).

T_o (MeV)	1	5	10	50	100	150
S_o† (keV μm^{-1})	26·8	8·0	4·6	1·3	0·74	0·55
R (cm)	—	0·034	0·12	2·13	7·64	15·6

† S_o represents the stopping power of protons with the energy T_o indicated; it increases with depth as the particle energy diminishes.

Beams of electrons

The distribution of dose as a function of depth for a beam of electrons has the form represented in Figure 1.4. The maximum depth (R) reached by the electrons is proportional to their energy (T):

$$R \text{ (cm of water)} \approx T \text{ (MeV)}/2$$

The large fluctuations in the range of electrons (see earlier) explains the shape of the last third of the curves. The stopping power of electrons is almost constant over a very wide range of energy (Table 1.5). It increases only towards the end of the track when the energy is reduced to a very small value (of the order of 10 keV corresponding to a residual range of a few μm). Owing to the fluctuation in range the track ends are dispersed and at all points in the medium their contribution to the dose is relatively small.

The energy of the electrons falls with depth but, in practice, in the whole of the irradiated volume it remains high enough that the stopping power does not show significant variation (about $0 \cdot 2$ keV μm^{-1}). The linear density of ionization is low in the whole of the irradiated volume.

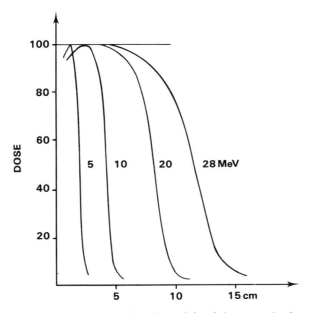

Figure 1.4. Distribution of dose as a function of depth in water for beams of electrons.

Table 1.5. Electrons. Range (R) and stopping power (S_o) in water as a function of the initial kinetic energy (T_o).

T_o	keV	10	30	50	100	MeV	0·5	1	5	10
S_o† (keV μm^{-1})		2·3	0·99	0·67	0·42		0·20	0·19	0·19	0·19
R‡	μm:	5	20	50	150	cm:	0·2	0·5	2·5	5

† The stopping power S_o represents the mean value of the rate of loss of energy which in fact shows statistical fluctuations.
‡ The indicated range R is calculated from the stopping power: it represents schematically the mean length of the track.

Beams of photons (X- and γ-rays)

The dose is delivered by secondary electrons set in motion by the photons. It diminishes with depth (Figure 1.5) due to the progressive disappearance of the photons; the diminution is slower the higher the energy of the photons (in the medium and for the energy range which is of interest to us). With high energy photons there is an initial increase of dose below the entry surface; this is due to the accumulation of secondary electrons over a distance equal to their ranges which is several mm for the γ-rays of ^{60}Co and several cm for X-rays of 20 MeV.

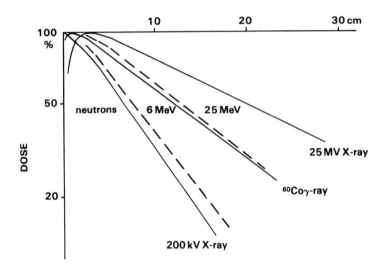

Figure 1.5. **Distribution of dose as a function of depth for beams of photons (X-rays and γ-rays) and neutrons.**

In biological media the secondary electrons derive essentially from the Compton effect, the principal type of interaction between X- and γ-rays and media of low atomic number. The Compton electrons have energy spectra which depend on the energy of the incident photons (Table 1.6).

Secondary electrons are generated at all depths by the photons in the vicinity. As the spectrum of photons shows only a small change with depth (mainly due to the growing contribution of scattered photons) the spectrum of the secondary electrons remains almost constant at all points in the medium traversed by the beam.

When the energy of the photons is greater than a few hundred KeV the energies of the electrons over nearly the whole spectrum are in a region where the stopping power has a constant and low value ($0\cdot2$ keV μm^{-1}); when the

Table 1.6. **Energy of Compton electrons set in motion by photons of energy E.**

	keV		MeV	
E	50	100	1	10
T_{max}[†]	8	28	$0\cdot8$	$9\cdot75$
T[‡]	5	14	$0\cdot44$	$6\cdot8$

† Maximum energy of Compton electrons.
‡ Mean energy of Compton electrons.

energy of the photons is below 100 keV the energies of the electrons are very low and their stopping power is relatively high (Table 1.5). In this way high energy photons for which there is a low linear density of ionization can be distinguished from photons of low energy (X-rays of 200 kV or less) for which the linear density of ionization is noticeably greater.

Fast neutrons

Fast neutrons with kinetic energy between a few and several tens of MeV are slowed down in biological media mainly by elastic collisions with hydrogen nuclei. These, projected in the form of *secondary protons*, are the origin of the production of ionization (to which there is also a small contribution due to other charged secondary particles arising from other types of interaction, in particular α-particles). The dose diminishes with depth due to the progressive disappearance of the neutrons and the dose distribution has a form comparable to that seen with photons (Figure 1.5).

The energy of the secondary protons produced in the course of collisions with neutrons of energy T_n can have any value betwen 0 and T_n with a mean value of $T_n/2$. For the usual energy of neutrons (for the beams of neutrons used in radiotherapy the mean energy is from 6 to 20 MeV) the secondary protons have a high stopping power, i.e. a large density of ionization along the whole of their short tracks (Table 1.4).

Negative pi mesons

Pi⁻ mesons are particles carrying a negative charge with a mass 1/15th of the mass of a proton. Like the other charged particles they lose their energy in the course of electronic collisions and have a finite range (10 cm of water for an energy of 55 MeV). At a given range their stopping power is intermediate between that of electrons and protons. At the end of the range they are captured by an atomic nucleus which then disintegrates; the fragments which are emitted in the form of charged particles show a high stopping power.

Pi⁻ mesons are directly ionizing particles with a relatively low density of ionization along the major part of their track. In the Bragg peak they become also indirectly ionizing with a high density of ionization due to the secondary particles produced.

1.4 Distribution of dose on a microscopic scale

Limit of significance of dose at the microscopic level

Dose represents the density of energy absorbed per unit mass at a point in the medium. On a very small scale of the order of μm the absorbed energy is not distributed in a uniform way because, on the one hand, it is localized close to the tracks of the ionizing particles and, on the other, the transfer of energy takes place in a discontinuous manner, in discrete amounts, during the course of random collisions between the ionizing particles and the electrons of the medium. Dose is a statistical quantity and does not express these character-

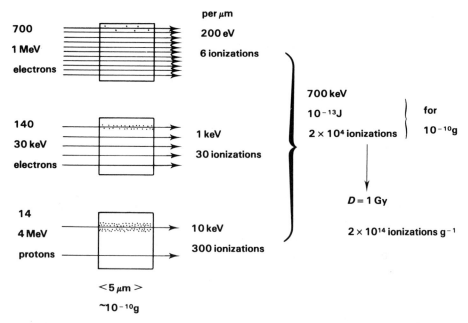

Figure 1.6. Distribution of absorbed energy and ionization on a microscopic scale. Diagram to illustrate the distribution of ionizations in a mass 10^{-10} g (the order of magnitude of a cell nucleus) receiving a dose of 1 Gy corresponding to 2×10^{14} ions g^{-1}, i.e. 20 000 ionizations in 10^{-10} g. These ionizations are distributed along the tracks of the ionizing particles crossing the volume and their distribution depends on the nature and energy of the particles.

A total of 20 000 ionizations can be created by 700 electrons of 1 MeV which lose 200 eV μm^{-1} (in water) in crossing the volume and produce six ionizations each per μm; the same total number of ionizations can be created by 140 electrons of 30 keV or 14 protons of 4 MeV, for which the stopping powers are, respectively, 5 and 50 times greater than that of 1 MeV electrons. In the three cases the mean density of ionizations per unit mass (2×10^4 ions g^{-1}) and the dose (1 Gy) are the same, but the distribution of ionizations, spread respectively along 700, 140 and 14 tracks, is different. Experiment shows that the biological effect is different.

istics. It gives a global value determined in a mass of matter sufficiently large that the statistical fluctuation is insignificant.

In fact the biological effect results from the absorption of energy by cellular structures of very small dimensions for which the non-uniform and discontinuous absorption of energy is important. Experiments show that at a given dose the biological effect depends on this distribution at a microscopic level, i.e. on the nature and energy of the ionizing particles (Figure 1.6). In order to specify the irradiation it is therefore necessary to add an indication of the microscopic distribution of ionizations or of the absorbed energy. We will discuss two modes of representation which are different in principle; the linear energy transfer (LET) and microdosimetry.

LET: distribution of dose as a function of LET

The linear energy transfer (LET) at a point on the track of an ionizing particle represents the energy absorbed by the medium per unit length of track: it is usually expressed in keV μm^{-1}.

A first approximation is to equate the LET to the stopping power S (see Section 1.1); it is then symbolized as LET_∞ (which is justified later).

As a rule the radiation at a point in the medium is composed of particles with various energies (and sometimes different natures), for which the LET has different values L. The contributions to the dose of the different types of particle can be considered separately in order to determine the distribution of dose as a function of LET. It is usually represented as a 'cumulative dose' corresponding at each value of L to the fraction of the absorbed dose (D_c) with an LET lower than L (Figure 1.7).

A more detailed treatment separates the contribution of the δ-rays, considered as independent of the particles from which they arose. The energy deposited in the medium close to the tracks is defined by the energy transfers Q which are below a value Δ, transfers $Q > \Delta$ being considered as imparted to δ-electrons. The energy lost by the particle in transfers $Q < \Delta$ per unit length at a point on the track defines the linear energy transfer (LET_Δ) corresponding to the cut-off value Δ whose choice is to some extent arbitrary. For the most commonly adopted value, $\Delta = 100\ eV$, we have seen above that about 40% of the energy lost by the particle is transferred to δ-electrons and we therefore have $LET_{100\ eV} = 0\cdot6\ S$.

The stopping power S can be considered as the LET without limitation of Q which justifies the symbol LET_∞:

$$S = LET_\infty$$

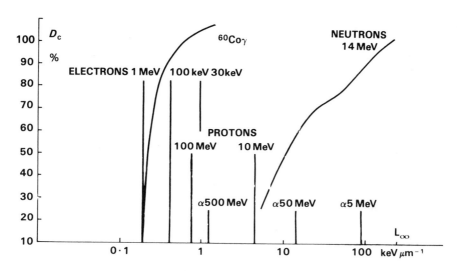

Figure 1.7. **Distribution of dose as a function of LET for different radiations.** For monoenergetic charged particles LET_∞ (=stopping power) has a single value. At a point in a medium irradiated with photons there are secondary electrons with a range of energies. Each component of the spectrum of electrons contributes to the dose at an LET corresponding to the energy of the electron considered. For neutrons, most of the ionizing particles are secondary protons with a smaller contribution from α-particles. The ordinate represents the cumulative dose, i.e. the fraction of the dose with LET below the value indicated on the abscissa. For charged particles there is a unique value whereas for photons and neutrons the curve extends between the minimum and maximum values of LET ∞ of the secondary ionizing particles.

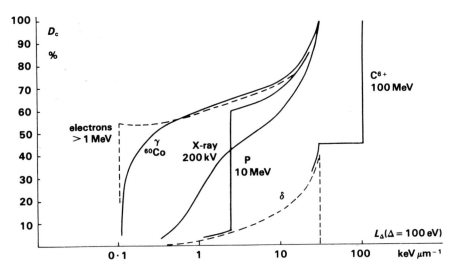

Figure 1.8. Distribution of dose as a function of LET$_\Delta$ (cut-off energyΔ=100 eV). The curves have the same meaning as in Figure 1.7 but the δ-electrons are considered as independent of the ionizing particles which gave birth to them. Their contribution to the dose is about 40% for all the radiations. The spectrum of LET$_\Delta$ which corresponds to them is represented by the dashed lines.
After ICRU Report 16.

For example, for electrons of 1 MeV, LET$_\infty$=S=0·2 keV μm^{-1} and for Δ=100 eV, LET$_\Delta$=0·12 keV μm^{-1}. At a point in the medium where there are electrons of 1 MeV, 60% of the dose is delivered close to the tracks with this LET$_\Delta$, and the δ-rays contribute 40% of the dose with their own value of LET.

The δ-rays passing a point P originate in a very small neighbouring volume because the range of nearly all the δ-rays is very short. The energy of each depends on its initial energy and on the energy lost between its point of origin and P; their energy distribution at P represents the *equilibrium spectrum* of δ-rays. It is the same at all points in the irradiated volume and, for the reasons given in section 1.1, it depends very little on the energy or the nature of the primary ionizing particles; the same is therefore true for the distribution of the dose in LET which they deliver.

The distribution of dose delivered by δ-rays as a function of LET is represented in Figure 1.8. The upper limit, LET=30 keV μm^{-1}, corresponds to T=100 eV; the lower practical limit is LET=1 keV μm^{-1} corresponding to T=30 keV because the contribution of the exceptional δ-rays of higher energy is negligible. Figure 1.8 also represents the distribution of dose as a function of LET (with Δ=100 eV) for different radiations.

From the distribution of dose as a function of LET (L_∞ or L_Δ) one can obtain a mean value of LET ($\bar{L}_\infty$ or $\bar{L}_\Delta$) which is sufficient for a schematic classification of different radiations (Table 1.7), but which may conceal important differences in the *distribution of LET*. The specification of radiation quality in terms of LET (or the distribution of dose as a function of LET) is valuable but may not be enough.

It is satisfactory to consider the density of deposited energy along the *individual tracks* of particles because, for the dose rates normally encountered, the tracks are too well separated in time or space for the radicals formed to be able to interact between one track and the next during their short existence. Interaction only becomes appreciable when the dose rate is $>10^{10}$ Gy s^{-1} which occurs only in exceptional circumstances. However, this may not be true of the δ-rays because a fraction of their energy is deposited close to the track of the particle which gave birth to them.

LET cannot be measured but only calculated; this requires an accurate determination of the spectrum of the particles which is usually difficult to establish. LET depends on the stopping power and, like it, represents a *statistical quantity* which does not take account of the discontinuous character of energy transfers. To overcome the inadequacies of LET another method was introduced by Rossi under the name of *microdosimetry*.

Table 1.7. Mean value of LET$_\Delta$ (Δ = 100 eV) (calculated taking account of the contribution to the dose of each section of the LET spectrum).

Radiation	LET$_\Delta$ (keV μm^{-1})
Electrons of 1 MeV	6
^{60}Coγ-ray	6
X-ray 200 kV	9·5
X-ray 50 kV	13
Protons of 1 MeV	15
Protons of 0·5 MeV	21
α-particles of 5 MeV	34
C^{6+} of 100 MeV	64

Microdosimetry

Microdosimetry is based on the principle that the biological effect is connected with the quantity of energy deposited in an elementary structure of very small size or, which is equivalent, in a volume of very small radius around a point. (The two considerations correspond to different theories of the biological effect but lead to the same physical and mathematical representations.)

An event, i.e. the passage of a particle, involves a deposition of energy ϵ in this small volume. The event can have various aspects as shown schematically in Figure 1.9. The energy ϵ which is a stochastic quantity has different values from one event to another and the distribution of events as a function of ϵ provides a representation of the physical effect at a point in the medium, taking account of all the random phenomena which result from the transfers of energy at a point and the shapes of the particle tracks.

The quantity ϵ is accessible to measurement. This can be done in a small cavity filled with a gas of the same atomic composition as the biological medium under consideration but of greatly reduced density. The depositions of energy corresponding to a given event have the same value in a sphere of gas of diameter d_g as in a sphere of the dense medium of diameter d_s if the diameters are in the inverse ratio of the mass densities, e.g. if the gas (under reduced pressure) is 10^{-4} times less dense than the medium ($d_g = 10^{-4}d_s$), a cavity of gas of diameter 1 cm simulates a volume of the dense medium of diameter 10^{-4} cm (1 μm).

Measurement of the number n of ionizations produced in the cavity by an

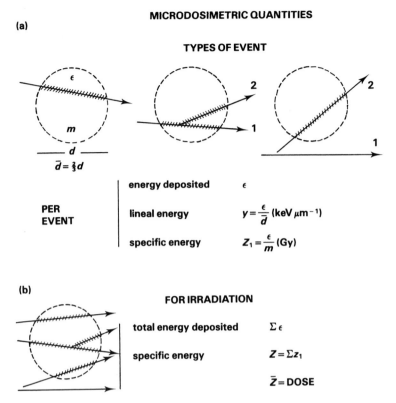

Figure 1.9. Basic concepts of microdosimetry. (a) The biological effect is related to the event produced during the passage of a particle, in a small volume of diameter d. The event is expressed by the energy deposited by the primary particle (1) or by the δ-rays (2) to which they give birth. The lineal energy is defined by $y = \epsilon/d$ where $\bar{d}$ is the mean length of the particle track in the volume. (b) The biological effect produced by a dose D depends on the total energy deposited in this volume (of mass m) by the different events produced in the course of the irradiation. This quantity shows a statistical fluctuation; its mean value corresponds to the dose D.

event enables ϵ to be determined: $\epsilon = n\bar{W}$, where $\bar{W}$ is the mean energy per ionization. The number of ionizations produced by an event is very small but can be measured by an electronic method: the cavity, equipped with two electrodes, functions as a proportional counter.¶ The measuring chamber is irradiated at a low dose rate in order to separate the individual events; in this way ϵ can be measured for a large number of individual events.

The value of ϵ depends on the reference volume which is generally considered to be a sphere having a diameter d, whose choice is arbitrary because the mechanism of radiation action is insufficiently known. The reference volume can be based on the diameter of the nucleus, a chromosome or a gene, respectively, to values of d of the order of μm, tenths of μm, or a few nm.

¶An ionization chamber functions as a proportional counter when the voltage applied to the electrodes is sufficiently great that the ions produced are strongly accelerated towards the electrodes and produce new ionizations by collisions with the gas molecules. In this way the collected charge is considerably amplified and is proportional to the number of ionizations initially produced by the radiation.

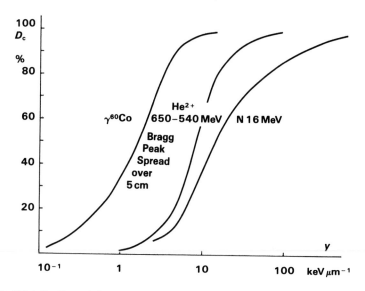

Figure 1.10. Distribution of dose as a function of lineal energy y (Figure 1.9) for different radiations. The ordinate represents the cumulative dose as in Figures 1.7 and 1.8. The proportional counter simulates a sphere of diameter 1 μm in biological tissue.

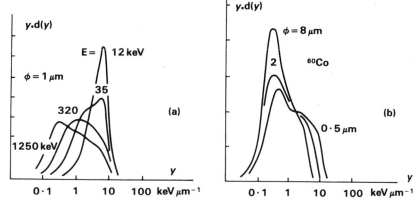

Figure 1.11. Spectra of y. d (y) represents the contribution to the dose of the events for which y has the value shown on the abscissa. (a) Spectra for photons of various energies E, measured in a cavity simulating a sphere of tissue 1 μm diameter. (b) Spectra for ⁶⁰Co γ-rays for different values of the simulated diameter.
(After Kliauga and Dvorak, Radiat. Res., 1978, 73:1).

For these reasons, instead of a deposition of energy, Rossi suggested a quantity $y = \epsilon/\bar{d}$ which has been called lineal energy, where $\bar{d}$ represents the mean chord length (in the case of a sphere of diameter d, $\bar{d} = 2/3 \times d$). This concept does not imply that ϵ must be proportional to d for an individual event but one can expect, and experiment confirms it, that the distribution of lineal energy (y) changes only slowly with variation of d. Thus the distribution of y has a more general significance than the distribution of ϵ and this, to some extent, overcomes the uncertainty in the proper value of d. Spectra of y for various radiations are shown in Figures. 1.10 and 1.11.

The lineal energy y is analogous to LET: it has the same dimension and is expressed in the same units, e.g. in keV μm^{-1}, but while LET is a *statistical quantity* (characterized by the nature and energy of the particle), y is a *stochastic quantity* which depends on each individual event and takes account of the random and discontinuous nature of energy transfers.

Rossi has defined a second microdosimetric quantity, the specific energy $z_1 = \epsilon/m$, the ratio of the energy ϵ deposited by the passage of a particle in the reference volume to the mass m of medium contained in this volume; z_1 represents a density of energy absorbed and has for unit the gray. The mean value of z_1 weighted by the contribution of each event to the absorbed dose is an important parameter of the theory of dual radiation action (see Section 4.3).

The quantities ϵ, y and z_1 depend on the deposition of energy during the passage of a *single particle*. The effect produced on the medium depends on the addition of these depositions of energy in the course of the irradiation.

The sum (Z) of the individual values of z_1 delivered to the reference volume during the irradiation represents the mean density of energy absorbed. From one point to another of the irradiated medium it shows a statistical fluctuation which becomes smaller as the reference volume is made larger and as the number of events in it is increased. Its mean value $(\bar{Z})$ represents the dose.

Knowing the relative frequency of the different values of ϵ, calculations taking account of the random character of the events make it possible to determine the probability of different values of Z for an irradiation delivering a given dose, or the distribution $P(Z)$ of the quantity Z.

The distribution $P(Z)$ depends on the dose D; the dispersion around the mean value (which represents the dose: $\bar{Z} = D$) is large for small doses and diminishes as the dose is increased. It depends also on the diameter d of the reference volume and, at a given dose, the dispersion diminishes as d is increased. Finally it depends on the nature of the radiation, the dispersion at a given dose being greater when the stopping power of the particles is greater.

Experimental evidence has demonstrated the role played in the biological effect by the distribution of dose on the microscopic scale. The parameter LET or the microdosimetric quantities used to represent this distribution make it possible to characterize the physical effects produced by the various types of irradiation and to describe the differences between them.

Representations based on LET permit only a classification of the different radiations. The microdosimetric quantities are closer to the fundamental mechanisms of biological action because they make it possible to understand the physical events and their connection with the biological structures concerned. A theory developed by Kellerer and Rossi (1972) has established relationships between these quantities and the biological effect, and accounts for the experimental results concerning the biological effectiveness of radiation and its variation with dose and with the nature of the radiation.

Bibliography

F. H. Attix, W. C. Roesch, E. Tochilin. *Radiation dosimetry*, 3 vols. Academic Press, New York, 1968.

P. P. Dendy, B. Heaton. *Physics for Radiologists*, Blackwell, Oxford, 1988.

International Commission on Radiation Units and Measurements (ICRU), Bethesda, Maryland:

Report 106 (1964). *Physical aspects of irradiation.*

Report 16 (1970). *Linear energy transfer.*

Report 21 (1972). *Radiation dosimetry: electrons with initial energy between 1 and 50 MeV.*

Report 28 (1978). *Basic aspects of high energy particles interactions and radiation dosimetry.*

Report 33 (1980). *Radiation quantities and units*

Report 36 (1983). *Microdosimetry.*

Report 37 (1984). *Stopping power for electrons and positrons.*

Report 45 (1990) *Clinical neutron dosimetry I: determination of absorbed dose in a patient treated by external beams of fast neutrons.*

H. E. Johns, J. R. Cunningham. *The physics of radiology.* 4th edn. Charles C. Thomas, Springfield, Ill, 1983.

K. R. Kase, B. E. Bjarngard, F. H. Attix, *The dosimetry of ionizing radiation*, vol I, Academic Press, New York, 1985.

K. R. Kase, B. E. Bjarngard, F. H. Attix, *The dosimetry of ionizing radiation*, vol II, Academic Press, New York, 1987.

A. M. Kellerer, H. H. Rossi. RBE and the primary mechanism of radiation action. *Radiat. Res.*, 1971, **47**: 15–34.

A. M. Kellerer, H. H. Rossi. The theory of dual radiation action. *Curr. Topics Rad. Res.*, 1972, **8**: 85–158.

J. L. Magee, A. Chatterjee. Radiation chemistry of heavy particle tracks. *J. Phys. Chem.*, 1981, **84**: 3529–3537.

M. R. Raju. *Heavy particle radiotherapy.* Academic Press, New York, 1980.

H. H. Rossi. *Microscopic energy distribution in irradiated matter*, in: *Radiation dosimetry*, vol. I (F. H. Attix, W. C. Roesch, eds.), pp. 43–92. Academic Press, New York, 1968.

Chapter 2.
Radiation chemistry

The effects of radiation on living matter are the final result of the initial physical events which occur during interactions between the radiation and the medium. It is at once clear that there is a great difference between the number of these events (ionizations and excitations), or the energy which they represent, and the biological effect: a dose of 10 Gy which kills almost all mammalian cells corresponds to an absorption of energy of 10^{-2} J g^{-1} of tissue (equivalent to a rise in temperature of $0 \cdot 002\,°C$) or a density of ionization of $1 \cdot 95 \times 10^{15}$ ionizations g^{-1}, i.e. about 2×10^6 ionizations per cell (of mass 10^{-9} g). As a cell contains about 10^{13} molecules of water and 10^8 larger molecules, the proportion of molecules which suffer an ionization is very small; it is enough, however, to result in the production of significant lesions.

The final biological effect is the result of a chain of physical events and chemical transformations which are initiated by the ionizations and ultimately damage the large molecules which are essential for the life of the cell.

We will begin by a study of these reactions which are the subject matter of *radiation chemistry*. We will then look at their consequences at the level of the principal cellular structures (DNA, chromosomes) (Chapter 3), at the level of the cell (Chapter 4), then at the level of populations of cells making up a tissue or organ (Chapter 5).

2.1 Initial physical events

The interactions of ionizing particles in biological media are essentially collisions with the electrons of the medium. Depending on the energy given to the electron, the molecule to which it belongs either suffers an ionization or an electronic excitation or gains some additional thermal energy. Transfers of thermal energy are without consequence. It is necessary to deliver much larger doses (10^4 Gy) before the rise in temperature of the medium reaches a few degrees and becomes great enough to affect the cellular biochemistry. A rise in temperature of one degree corresponds to an increase in the energy of vibration, rotation or translation (forms of thermal energy) which is, when averaged over all the molecules, about 10^{-4} eV per molecule. During the passage of a charged particle the individual transfers of thermal energy are much greater than this value but they affect only a very small proportion of the molecules and this excess of energy is very quickly dispersed among the neighbouring molecules. On the other hand ionizations and excitations represent a considerable increase in the internal energy of the molecule which compromises its stability.

The physical events produced by a charged particle occur during the very short period of its passage ($<10^{-13}$ s). This physical stage is succeeded by the physico-chemical and chemical phenomena which are the subject matter of *radiation chemistry* itself.

2.2 Radiolysis of water

To a large extent biological effects are mediated through the action of radiation on water which represents about 80% of the weight of living organisms. It has been known since 1901 that radiation is capable of decomposing water; this transformation brings into play complex processes of which we will consider only the principal steps.

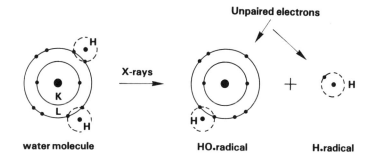

(a) Decomposition of water into radicals due to the action of ionizing radiation.

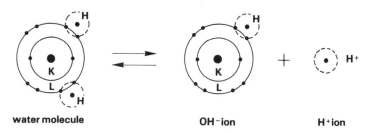

(b) Spontaneous ionic dissociation of water.

Figure 2.1. Radiolysis of water. Schematic representation of a water molecule and its dissociation into two radicals HO. and H. due to the action of radiation.
The term *radical* is used to describe an atom or a group of atoms containing an unpaired electron which results in great chemical reactivity (radicals are represented by adding a . to the chemical symbol). A radical can be neutral or charged (*radical ion*). The radicals HO. and H. which are produced in the course of radiolysis of water (a) are very reactive, a property which distinguishes them from the ions OH⁻ and H⁺ formed in the spontaneous ionic dissociation of water (b); the latter do not have unpaired electrons and are chemically unreactive.
After [8].

Formation of radicals

The initial phenomenon is ionization of water molecules which requires about 13 eV:

$$H_2O \rightarrow H_2O.^+ + e^-$$

It leads to the formation of abnormal ions (*radical ions*) which are extremely unstable (lifetime of radical ions 10^{-10} s) and give birth to neutral radicals which are very reactive (10^{-5} s). $H_2O.^+$ is decomposed as follows:

$$H_2O.^+ \rightarrow H^+ + HO.$$

The hydroxyl radical HO. is a powerful oxidizing agent possessing great chemical reactivity [1] (Figure 2.1).

The electrons detached by ionization have at their origin a kinetic energy which is usually sufficient to enable them to travel a significant distance (for 10 eV the distance is about 15 nm corresponding to about 70 molecules of water), which makes recombination unlikely. They progressively lose their kinetic energy by collisions and, when they have been slowed down enough, are captured by molecules of water (strongly polarized); they are then called *aqueous electrons*† or *solvated electrons*, e^-_{aq}. The aqueous electron is a powerful reducing agent [5, 6].

Some of the water molecules lying close to the aqueous electrons dissociate into H. and OH. radicals. The aqueous electrons can disappear by combining with H^+ ions but in biological systems it is more probable that they will react chemically with dissolved oxygen (see later) or with organic molecules.

The behaviour of excited water molecules H_2O^* is poorly understood. It is theoretically possible that they dissociate into H. and HO. radicals as the energy required to break the bond is 5 eV, but the frequency of such a phenomenon is disputed. We have therefore:

$$H_2O \xrightarrow{X\text{-ray}} H_2O^* \rightarrow HO. + H.$$

where H_2O^* represents an excited water molecule possessing an excess of energy. On the other hand the 'cage effect' makes it likely that the two radicals lying close to one another will recombine. It is, however, possible that certain radicals may possess enough kinetic energy to escape from this cage effect.

The succession of phenomena extending from the ionization of water to the formation of different radicals HO., H. and e^-_{aq} is summarized in Table 2.1. It must be noted that the initial ionization produced by radiation in the water molecule leads to the formation of a radical ion $H_2O.^+$ and an electron which is itself a radical. This ionization is very different from that produced by electrolytic dissociation which leads to two ions (H^+ and OH^-) whose electrons

---

†The existence of aqueous electrons has been demonstrated in pulse radiolysis experiments (absorption bands at about $0.7\mu m$). e^-_{aq} is in fact a free electron captured in a cage of molecules of water. These aqueous electrons are remarkably stable with a lifetime of many microseconds in pure water.

are paired and which are chemically unreactive. The ionic concentration produced in solution by radiation is very small (for 10 Gy it is $1 \cdot 95 \times 10^{15}$ ions g^{-1}, that is $0 \cdot 3 \times 10^{-2}$ mEq l^{-1}) and much smaller than the ionic concentration due to electrolytic dissociation; but the consequences of these two types of ionization are totally different (Figure 2.1).

Table 2.1. Schematic representation of the stages in the radiolysis of water.

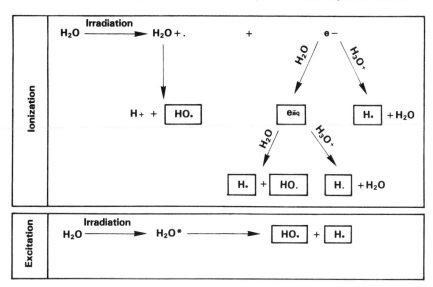

Fate of the radicals and the molecular decomposition of water

The reactions considered above represent the phase of *radical decomposition* of water leading to the formation of highly reactive radicals: oxidizing, HO.; and reducing, H. (atomic hydrogen) and e^-_{aq} (aqueous electrons).

These radicals give rise to a certain number of reactions which occasionally lead to the reconstitution of water but more often to the formation of new molecules and other radicals. This represents the phase of *molecular decomposition* of water. Immediately after the passage of the ionizing particle (10^{-12} s), the radicals are distributed in a very heterogeneous way around the track. This distribution depends on the LET of the particle and varies along the track. The radicals HO. and H. diffuse away from their origin and can react with one another (recombination resulting in formation of H_2O, H_2O_2 and H_2).

Altogether, therefore, at about 10^{-7} s after the passage of the ionizing particle one finds radicals or molecules around the track: H., HO., H_2O_2 and H_2 whose proportion and distribution vary with the type of particle (Table 2.2). The reactions which occur subsequently (between 10^{-7} and 10^{-3} s after the passage of the particle) depend on several factors, such as the LET of the radiation, the purity of the water and above all the presence or absence of dissolved oxygen. The influence of the degree of oxygenation of the solution will be studied later in section 2.4.

The probability that a particular reaction will occur depends on the spatial

Table 2.2. Radiochemical yield *G*, as a function of the LET of the particle, of certain radicals and molecular species formed during the radiolysis of water. The concentration produced by a dose of 1 Gy is $G \times 10^{-8}$ mol l^{-1}.

LET	G						
(keVμm^{-1})	H_2O	e$^-$aq	OH.	H.	H_2	H_2O_2	HO_2.
0·23	4·08	2·63	2·72	0·55	0·45	0·68	0·008
12·3	3·46	1·48	1·78	0·62	0·68	0·84	
61	3·01	0·72	0·91	0·42	0·96	1·00	0·05
108	2·84	0·42	0·54	0·27	1·11	1·08	0·07

After [3].

distribution of the radicals concerned and therefore on the LET. Thus, for example, the probability of the reaction

$$HO. + HO. \rightarrow H_2O_2$$

is small if the ionizations are relatively distant; it is higher at the centre of groups of ionizations and particularly high along the tracks of particles of high LET. The same is true for the reaction

$$H. + H. \rightarrow H_2$$

The influence of the LET of the radiation on the biological effects will be studied in greater detail in Chapter 11.

2.3 Action of radiation on aqueous solutions

To a first approximation a cell can be considered as an aqueous solution. The radiation can have a direct effect on the solute molecules by producing lesions in them or an indirect action due to the interaction between the solute molecules and the products of radiolysis of water (Figure 2.2).

Direct effect

The excited and ionized molecules have an excess of energy and are unstable. This excess of energy can be dissipated either by emission of photons (fluorescence) with return to the initial state or by rupture of a covalent bond and scission of the molecule into two radicals. Scission is more probable after an ionization than after an excitation because the amount of energy received is greater in the first case.

A covalent bond (symbolized by :) is constituted by a pair of electrons whose spins are opposed. When such a bond is broken each fragment carries with it an uncoupled electron (.)

$$R : R' \rightarrow R. + R'.$$

As a result two radicals or molecular fragments are formed, each carrying an

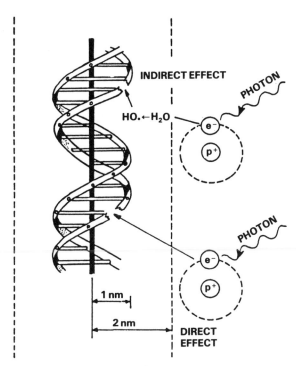

Figure 2.2. Direct and indirect effects of X- and γ-rays. The effect on a molecule of DNA (see Figure 3.2), shown schematically on the left, has been chosen as an example.
Direct effect: interaction between a molecule of DNA and an electron set in motion following the absorption of a photon.
Indirect effect: an electron set in motion following the absorption of a photon interacts with a molecule of water. A radical is produced, e.g. HO., which in its turn produces a lesion on the molecule of DNA. It is estimated that free radicals produced in a cylinder of 2 nm radius with its axis along the molecule of DNA, can attack the latter. The indirect effect is dominant for radiations of low LET.
After [4].

unpaired electron which gives them a high degree of reactivity. The lifespan of these radicals is very short (on average 10^{-5} s).

The breakage of a bond does not require that the initial physical event should take place on the electron of this bond. The energy absorbed can migrate within the molecule (*intramolecular migration*) and the breakage often occurs at the site of the weakest bond. The energy absorbed by a molecule can also be transferred to another molecule (*intermolecular migration*) which thereby suffers the consequence of the attack on the first as though it had itself been directly attacked by the radiation.

Indirect effect

The indirect effect results from the interaction between the products of radiolysis of water and the molecules contained in the aqueous solution. The radicals diffuse in the solution and react with the solute molecules producing chemical modifications. For example, for an organic molecule R : H, one can find (i)　dehydrogenation followed by hydroxylation by HO. radicals

$$R:H+HO.\rightarrow R.+H_2O$$
$$R.+HO.\rightarrow R:OH$$

(ii)　dehydrogenation by H. radicals and the formation of new compounds by addition

$$R:H+H.\rightarrow R.+H_2$$
$$R.+R'.\rightarrow R:R'$$

(iii)　opening of double bonds by aqueous electrons followed by the formation of new compounds by addition.

For the indirect effect produced by X-rays these series of events can be set out as follows:

In the solvent:
absorption of photons,
generation of secondary electrons,
ionization (formation of radical ions) and excitation,
formation of radicals.

Attack on solute molecules:
chemical alterations due to the breakage of bonds,
biochemical reactions,
biological effects.

The time scales of these successive events are very different: thus radical ions have a lifespan of the order of 10^{-10} s and radicals of the order of 10^{-5} s, whereas the various stages between breakage of chemical bonds and their biological expression can extend over days, months or years according to the effects considered (Table 2.3).

Table 2.3. Timescale of radiation chemistry.

Time	Event
10^{-18}	An ionizing particle crosses a molecule
10^{-15}	Time interval between successive ionizations
10^{-14}	Dissociation of electronically excited species. Transfer of energy to vibrational modes (thermal). Start of reactions between ions and molecules
10^{-13}	The electrons are reduced to thermal energies
10^{-12}	The radicals diffuse
10^{-11}	The electrons are solvated in polar media
10^{-10}	Completion of reactions which depend on very rapid diffusion
10^{-8}	Molecular products formed. Radiative decay of singlet excited states
10^{-5}	Capture of radicals by reactive molecules
10^{-3}	Radiative decay of triplet states
1	Most of the chemical reactions are finished. However in certain systems reactions can continue for several days

Radiochemical yield G

Whether the effect be direct or indirect and whatever may be the reaction mechanism, all the molecules in the solution finish by returning to a stable state, but some of them undergo chemical changes [5]. The *radiochemical yield G* for a reaction or chain of reactions is given by the number of molecules damaged or formed per 100 eV of absorbed energy. Table 2.3 presents the radiochemical yield of certain radicals or molecular species formed following the radiolysis of water.

In principle, all the radicals formed from water molecules and which escape recombination, finish by reacting with molecules in solution. In dilute solution the number of molecules transformed therefore does not depend on their initial concentration but only on the number of radicals formed, that is to say on the absorbed dose. However, when the concentration becomes very small the time required for a radical to encounter a molecule becomes longer and the probability of recombination during this interval is greater; under these conditions G diminishes.

Measurement of the number of solute molecules transformed can be used to measure the absorbed dose in the solution. The Fricke dosimeter, based on the oxidation of Fe^{2+} to Fe^{3+} in acid solution (H_2SO_4), is the most frequently used system of chemical dosimetry at the present time (Figure 2.3).

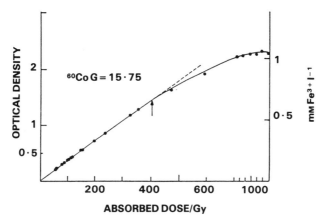

Figure 2.3. **Response of the Fricke dosimeter to radiation. The dosimetric solution contains 1 mM $FeSO_4\,l^{-1}$ in acid solution (H_2SO_4, $0\cdot8$ N). Under irradiation the ferrous ion is oxidized: $Fe^{2+} \rightarrow Fe^{3+}$. The concentration of Fe^{3+} is measured by spectrophotometry (wavelength 304 nm). The relation between the optical density and the absorbed dose in the dosimetric solution is shown and is linear for doses below 400 Gy. The optical density continues to increase at higher doses; the oxidation of ferrous ions is complete at 700 Gy (c. 1 mM $Fe^{3+}\,l^{-1}$).**
After [9].

If we consider a dilute solution containing only one species of molecule A, the number of molecules A' formed, or the radiochemical yield $G(A')$, is almost independent of the initial concentration of molecules A. If a second species of molecule B is present in the solution the attack on molecules A is modified. It is reduced if there is competition between them for capture of the radicals; it can be increased if molecule B increases the activity of the radicals. The action of molecules B can be very important even at a very low concentration if their affinity for the radicals is very high. This is the explanation of the effect of radioprotectors and radiosensitizers.

2.4 *Mechanism of action of chemical modifiers of radiosensitivity*

A certain number of chemical substances can modify the radiosensitivity of biological systems. Some of them act at the level of the initial chemical reactions according to the mechanisms which will be considered in this section. We will return later to their biological effects and their practical use (see Chapter 10).

The oxygen effect

Oxygen is a powerful radiosensitizer: if present at the time of irradiation it increases the effect of the radiation. Thus, for radiations of low LET it is necessary in the absence of oxygen to multiply the dose by a factor of 2·5–3 to obtain the same effect as in the presence of oxygen, and this is almost always true whatever the system (chemical substances in solution or mammalian cells) or the effect considered. The name OER (*Oxygen Enhancement Ratio*) is given to the ratio of doses needed to obtain a given radiochemical or biological effect depending on whether the system is irradiated under anoxic or aerobic conditions (Chapter 7).

Although the mechanism of radiosensitization is not yet entirely understood, oxygen can be considered to contribute to the fixation of radiolesions which would otherwise be reparable. To fulfill this role the oxygen must be present at the time of irradiation (Figure 2.4); partial radiosensitization can, however, be obtained if the oxygen is added a few milliseconds after irradiation.

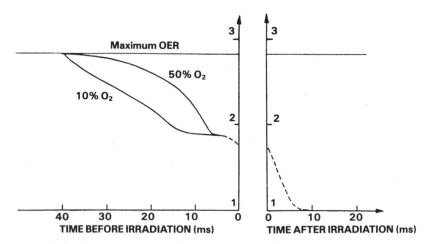

Figure 2.4. Variation of radiosensitivity (expressed in terms of OER) of V79 mammalian cells rendered anoxic *in vitro* as a function of the time *t* separating the injection of oxygen and the irradiation (the technique used is described briefly in the text). Oxygen must be injected 30–40 ms before irradiation to obtain maximum radiosensitivity (an OER close to 3). This interval of time, which varies with the concentration of O_2 (compare the curves for 50% and 10% O_2) corresponds, apparently, to the time necessary for the oxygen to reach the intracellular targets (this time can vary with the biological system). A value of OER close to 2 can be obtained if oxygen is injected only 4 ms before irradiation. On the other hand, when O_2 is injected after irradiation there is still some slight radiosensitization which rapidly disappears when oxygen is injected more than 4 ms later. After [7].

Different types of reaction can take place:
1. Oxygen is a powerful oxidizing agent and its main radiosensitizing effect is probably connected with its affinity for electrons. The oxygen molecule contains two unpaired electrons; it is therefore equivalent to a biradical. Capture of the electron emitted in the course of ionization of a molecule prevents its immediate recombination with the positive ion.
2. A certain number of reactions with the radicals produced in the course of radiolysis of water only occur in oxygenated solution:
   (i) capture of a radical H. by a molecule of O_2:

$$H.+O_2 \rightarrow HO_2.$$

The radical $HO_2.$ is a less powerful oxidizing agent that HO. but it has a longer lifespan and can therefore diffuse further. The following reactions can take place:

$$HO_2.+HO_2. \rightarrow H_2O_2+O_2$$

and

$$HO_2.+H. \rightarrow H_2O_2$$

Moreover the capture of H. radicals increases the number of HO. radicals available by preventing the recombination reaction:

$$H.+HO. \rightarrow H_2O$$

(ii) aqueous electrons can react with dissolved oxygen:

$$e^-+O_2 \rightarrow O_2^-$$

and

$$O_2^-+H_2O \rightarrow HO_2.+OH^-$$

(iii) with dissolved organic radicals chain reactions and formation of peroxides can occur.
Chain reactions:

$$R.+O_2 \rightarrow ROO. \text{(radical peroxide)}$$
$$ROO.+R'H \rightarrow ROOH+R'. \text{(hydroperoxide)}$$
$$R'.+O_2 \rightarrow R'OO. \text{(etc.)}$$

Formation of peroxides:

$$ROO.+R'. \rightarrow ROOR' \text{(peroxide)}$$

Hydroperoxides and peroxides are toxic substances which accumulate in the course of the irradiation and the lesions produced by them are added to those due to the radiation. In living matter an important action of oxygen is peroxidation of unsaturated lipids which results in structural and functional alteration of membranes [2].

Other radiosensitizers and radioprotectors

Substances having a high oxidizing potential have radiosensitizing properties analogous to that of oxygen. The possibility of their use in radiotherapy will be discussed later (see Chapter 10). Radioprotectors are substances which when present during irradiation diminish its effects. They can therefore only have preventive action. The chemical mode of action of these compounds is poorly understood. For example, proteins or peptides with thiol groups (RSH) are excellent donors of H., and can therefore either repair the damage caused by the reactive species (HO., H.) formed from the radiolysis of water or fix it by recombination of radicals. With regard to the mechanism of action of substances RSH in aqueous solutions on lesions in DNA molecules, these depend on the composition of the DNA which has suffered attack (see Section 3.2).

For example, for lesions at the level of deoxyribose, RSH (donor of H.) repairs the damage caused by HO. or H. The repair is effective only under anaerobic conditions:

$$\text{(deoxyribose with H, HO)} \xrightarrow{\text{HO.}} \text{(deoxyribose radical, HO)} \xrightarrow{\text{RSH}} \text{(deoxyribose with H, HO)} + \text{RS.}$$

The radical RS. is not very reactive.

Lesions at the level of pyrimidine bases can also be fixed by RSH:

$$\text{(pyrimidine 5,6)} \xrightarrow{\text{H.}} \text{(C5-H, C6-H.)} \xrightarrow{\text{RSH}} \text{(C5-H, C6-H, H)}$$

$$\text{(pyrimidine 5,6)} \xrightarrow{\text{HO.}} \text{(C5-OH, C6-H.)} \xrightarrow{\text{RSH}} \text{(C5-OH., C6-H, H)}$$

For lesions at the level of purine bases, the mechanisms of action are uncertain.

Reaction kinetics of chemical modifiers

The modifiers of radiosensitivity which operate by competition with free radicals must be present during their brief lifespan which is of the order of a microsecond. They can also interact with the products formed by the reactions of radicals and the duration of their action can extend to 10^{-2} s after irradiation. The kinetics of these reactions can be analyzed by ultra-rapid techniques which consist in exposing biological systems (mammalian cells in culture, bacteria or yeast) to a very short irradiation given at a time t before or after the biological system is mixed with the modifying substance under study (Figure 2.4). In practice, for studies with oxygen a monolayer of cells is placed in an atmosphere of nitrogen; an ultra-rapid valve allows the nitrogen to be instantaneously replaced by an atmosphere of oxygen. An irradiation lasting a few nanoseconds is usually given by means of a beam of electrons produced by a field emission generator.

Figure 2.4 summarizes some results obtained with V79 mammalian cells. When mixing with oxygen precedes the irradiation by more than a few tens of milliseconds a constant survival rate is seen corresponding to full oxygenation of the biological system. The time required for diffusion of O_2 into the cells depends on their thickness: it is 2 ms for Chinese hamster V79 cells whose thickness is $3 \mu m$. When the cells are put in contact with oxygen at a time t after irradiation the surviving fraction S increases with the interval t and approaches a value corresponding to that obtained with cells maintained in an atmosphere of nitrogen. The increase in surviving fraction is very rapid during the first few milliseconds; it continues more slowly for several tens of milliseconds.

These kinetics can be interpreted by considering that the action of O_2 has two components: (i) a rapid phase corresponding to the interaction of O_2 with the radicals which disappear with a half-time of about $0 \cdot 3$ ms; and (ii) a slow phase corresponding to the interaction of O_2 with the initial products formed by the reactions of the radicals which disappear with a half-time of about 4 ms. The respective contributions of these two components in the oxygen effect are about 70% and 30%.

Analogous experiments have been made to study the protective effect of the SH group. They consist in determining the amplitude and kinetics of the O_2 effect on cells pretreated to enrich them in SH groups (glutathione) or to deprive them of SH groups (N-ethylmaleimide fixes SH groups). Other studies have been made to compare the oxygen effect in bacteria and their mutants which are deficient in glutathione.

These studies have demonstrated the very important role of SH groups in the disappearance of free radicals.

References

1. G. E. Adams, J. W. Boag, B. D. Michael. Spectroscopic studies of reactions of the OH radical in aqueous solutions. *Trans. Faraday Soc.*, 1965, **61**: 492–505.
2. J. E. Biaglow. The effects of ionizing radiation on mammalian cells. *J. Chem. Educ.*, 1981, **58**: 144–156.
3. G. V. Buxton. Basic radiation chemistry of liquid water, in: *The study of fast processes and transient species by electron pulse radiolysis* (J. M. Baxendale and F. Busi, eds). D. Reidel, Dordrecht, 1982, 241–260.
4. E. J. Hall, *Radiobiology for the radiologist* (3rd edn). Lippincott, Philadelphia, PA, 1988.
5. International Commission on Radiation Units and Measurements, *The dosimetry of pulsed radiation*, ICRU Report 34, 1982, 7910 Woodmont Avenue, Bethesda, Maryland 20814, USA.
6. J. P. Keene. Optical absorption in irradiated water. *Nature*, 1963, **197**: 47–48.
7. M. A. Shenoy, J. C. Asquith, G. E. Adams, B. D. Michael, M. E. Watts. Time-resolved oxygen effects in irradiated bacteria and mammalian cells: A rapid-mix study. *Radiat. Res.*, 1975, **62**: 498–512.
8. M. Tubiana, J. Dutreix, A. Dutreix, P. Jockey. *Bases physiques de la radiothérapie et de la radiobiologie*. Masson, Paris, 1963.
9. A. Wambersie. Contribution à l'étude de l'efficacité biologique relative des faisceaux de photons et d'électrons de 20 MeV du bétatron. *J. Belge Radiol.*, Monographie No. 1, 1967.

Chapter 3.
Effects of radiation on DNA molecules and chromosomes

The successful functioning of a cell, and the faithful transmission of the genetic information contained in it to its progeny, depend on the maintenance of the structural integrity of each molecule of deoxyribonucleic acid (DNA). Changes in the sequence of nucleotides, or alterations in the structure of the bases or sugars which make up the double helix of DNA, can interfere with the replication or transcription of the cellular genome.

Damage to molecules of DNA is the primary cause of radiobiological effects (cell death, loss of reproductive capacity, mutation). Mechanisms of repair of damaged DNA molecules therefore play an essential role. Repair processes can lead to complete restitution or to misrepair whose practical consequences are liable to be serious (e.g. carcinogenesis).

DNA molecules are the main constituents of chromosomes which are instrumental for transfer of genetic information to the daughter cells. The lesions in chromosomes, or chromosomal aberrations, give a good indication of the lesions in a population of cells and can help in predicting the effects of irradiation.

3.1 DNA molecules and their relationship with chromosomes

Structure of DNA molecules

A DNA strand is composed of a series of links or nucleotides, containing:

(i)   a purine base (adenine, guanine) or a pyrimidine base (cytosine, thymine);
(ii) a molecule of sugar (deoxyribose) connected to the base;
(iii) a molecule of phosphoric acid connected to the sugar.

The nucleotides are joined together by phosphodiester bonds linking the molecules of sugar to those of phosphoric acid. The molecule of DNA is composed of two complementary strands linked by hydrogen bonds between the bases. Opposite thymine (T) on one strand there must be adenine (A) on the other; opposite guanine (G) there must be the complementary base cytosine (C) (Figure 3.1). The molecule is represented diagrammatically in the form of a ladder

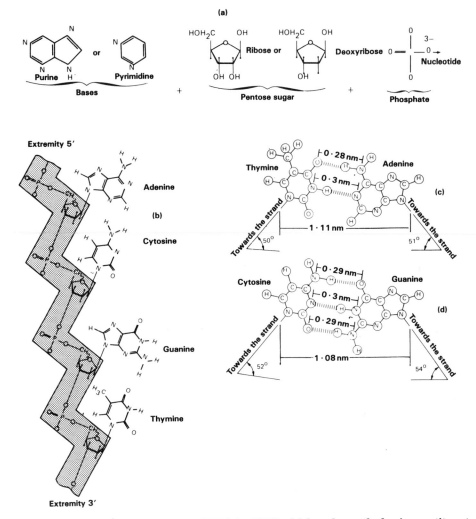

Figure 3.1. (a) The building blocks of DNA (or RNA) which make up the basic constituents (*nucleotides*) of this molecule.
(b) Illustration of the mode of assembly in a strand of DNA: the bases are attached to sugars which are themselves connected by phosphates, the alternation sugar–phosphate forming the backbone of the strand. In the case of RNA the thymine base is replaced by uracil and the deoxyribose sugar is replaced by ribose.
(c) Details of the bonding between strands showing the hydrogen bonds which join complementary bases (here thymine and adenine) and indicating the distances and angles.
(d) As (c) but for cytosine and guanine.
After [18].

whose uprights are composed of the two strands and the treads by the bases joined by hydrogen bonds. The two strands are twisted together to form a double helix. During replication of DNA the two strands separate and each serves as a model for the synthesis of a new complementary strand.

The sequence of nucleotides in DNA is the basis of the genetic information. It codes the sequence of amino acids in the proteins. The DNA of every cell in a single organism normally has the same composition. Moreover, in every

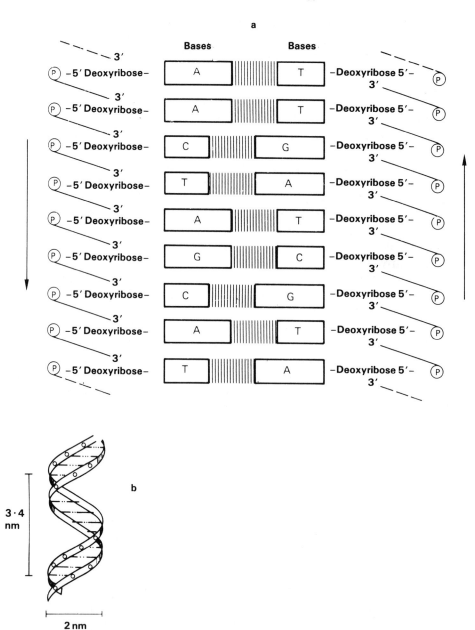

Figure 3.2. (a) Structure of the double helix represented on a single plane. The bases are shown as rectangles of various lengths and the sugars by the word deoxyribose. By convention, reading up and down, the points of attachment of the two phosphates on the pentagonal sugar ring are numbered 3′ and 5′.
(b) The helical structure of the molecule of DNA formed by the assembly of the two strands with the bases (double helix of Watson and Crick).
After [18].

molecule of DNA there must be as many molecules of adenine as of thymine and as many of guanine as of cytosine. Therefore the number of purine bases (A+G) is equal to the number of pyrimidine bases (C+T). In the same way (A+C) equals (G+T) but the ratio (G+C)/(A+T) varies according to the species.

A diagram of the DNA molecule according to the model of Watson and Crick is presented in Figure 3.2. Two sugar-phosphate strands are twisted together and the distance between two successive turns of the spiral is 3·4 nm. One turn contains 10 pairs of bases, the distance separating two neighbouring pairs of bases being 0·34 nm. There are therefore 3×10^6 nucleotides mm^{-1} of the DNA molecule. The molecule is narrow (diameter 2 nm), but its length may reach several centimetres. The interior of the double helix is composed of the paired bases of the two filaments orientated in a plane perpendicular to the axis. Each pair of bases constitutes an ellipse whose axes are about 1·1 and 0·6 nm. These axes make an angle of 36° with the corresponding axes of the base pairs above and below (like the steps of a spiral staircase).

The stability of the double helix is maintained by Van der Waals forces which link each pair of bases to the pairs above and below (in the direction parallel to the axis) and by hydrogen bonds which are responsible for the pairing (in the direction perpendicular to the axis). The molecule of DNA in the form of chromatin presents a series of knots where it is wrapped around histones (*cores*) and zones of linkage (*linkers*). It has the appearance of a pearl necklace the unit of which, *the nucleosome*, contains one core and one linker, the core containing eight histones forming a pearl round which 2·5 turns of DNA are wrapped. There are 150–200 pairs of bases round one pearl and 0–60 pairs of bases between neighbouring pearls (Figure 3.3).

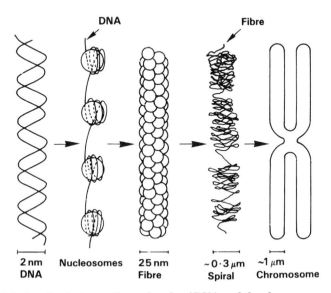

Figure 3.3. Relationship between the molecule of DNA and the chromosome. The DNA double helix is wrapped around histone beads and forms the *nucleosomes* which themselves are piled up to form the *fibres*. These are folded and rolled up in irregular spirals to form the chromosomes which are visible under the microscope. After [26].

The molecular weight of DNA molecules is always very high: 10^6–10^9 for viruses, phages and bacteria, 8×10^{10} for mammalian cells [36]. We now know the complete sequence of a number of nucleic acids. For example, the bacteriophage MS2, a single strand of RNA, contains 3569 nucleotides; the carcinogenic virus of the monkey SV40, a double strand of DNA, contains 5243 pairs of nucleotides.

The nucleus of the human diploid cell contains nearly one metre of DNA, divided among 46 chromosomes, that is to say about 3×10^9 pairs of nucleotides or bases. About 1000 pairs of bases are necessary to code one protein and about 10^5 different proteins are coded in the genome of the mammalian cell [22, 35]. The zones which code for the synthesis of proteins (genes) are not all expressed in a given cell and this selectivity in expression increases with the degree of differentiation of the cell. In general there are not more than about a thousand genes in a cell which are expressed. The other zones which represent about 99% of the DNA probably play a role in the control of genetic expression.

A single molecule of DNA forms the backbone of a chromosome, as shown in Figure 3.3. It extends continuously from one end to the other. The functional integrity of the chromosome depends on the continuity of the DNA molecule. The DNA of viruses and bacteria is often circular with different degrees of twisting in the ring thus formed. In eukaryotes, DNA is anchored at many points in the nuclear matrix and between them there are 'domains' of 20 000–80 000 nucleotides which are twisted to a varying extent.

Replication and transcription

In preparation for each cellular division the DNA dictates a copy of itself in such a way as to give to each of the two daughter cells all of its own genetic information (replication of DNA). The transcription by which DNA expresses its information operates by the formation of messenger RNA (mRNA; Figure 3.4). Of the two functions of DNA, replication and transcription, *replication is the more radiosensitive.*

Replication

Several DNA polymerase enzymes have been identified:

(i)   DNA polymerase α which plays an essential role in the replication of nuclear DNA;
(ii) DNA polymerase β whose role in higher eukaryotic cells is not entirely understood but which plays an important role in the mechanisms of repair;
(iii) DNA polymerase γ which allows replication of mitochondrial DNA;
(iv) DNA polymerase δ.

UNITS OF REPLICATION

Replication does not take place continuously along the whole length of the molecule of DNA, which is composed of a succession of replication units ('replicons'). During replication, *unwinding enzymes* cause the two strands to unwind and separate. This partial unwinding causes supercoiling (hyperhelical structure) in the rest of the molecule or requires rotation of one of the strands round a 'pivot' created by a nuclease.

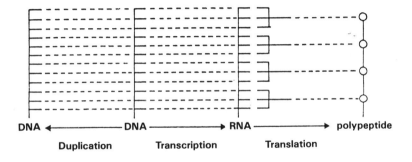

DNA ◄──────── DNA ────────► RNA ────────► polypeptide

    Duplication   Transcription   Translation

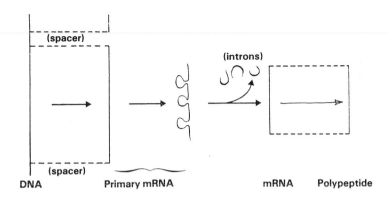

DNA   Primary mRNA   mRNA   Polypeptide

Figure 3.4. Upper diagram to illustrate the relation between *duplication, transcription* and *translation.*
Lower, DNA contains *silent* sequences which are not transcribed. Some (*spacers*) serve to separate the genes from one another. In eukaryotes several sequences of mRNA are excised before translation (*introns*). The parts destined to be expressed (*exons*) are then rejoined end to end apparently in the same order as in the product of the original transcription. In this way there is *colinearity* but with gaps.
After [8].

At the level of each replicon, replication takes place symmetrically in both directions, starting at replication origins located at the same position on both strands (Figure 3.5). Within each replicon, replication always takes place in the direction 5'→3' and progresses in a discontinuous manner by small fragments (named after Okazaki; see later). Replicons replicate themselves independently one from another.

These phenomena, which take place simultaneously on the two strands that have been locally separated by the unwinding, lead to the formation of a *bubble* or *replication space* composed in its medial part by segments of completed double helix and at its extremities by two *replication forks* (Figure 3.6). These advance due to the progressive unwinding of the parental double helix and the synthesis of new fragments of DNA. The opening of DNA (the bubble) is visible under the electron microscope (Figure 3.6). As it becomes larger the inter-replication zone diminishes until the two replicons join together.

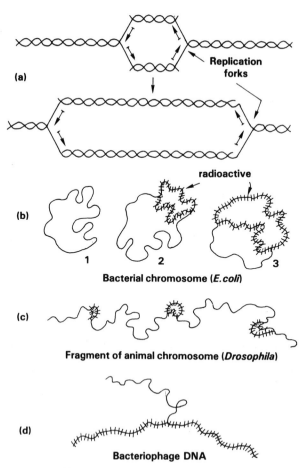

Figure 3.6. (a) Plan of a 'bubble' or 'replication gap' and of its development.
(b) Images of replication bubbles in a bacterial chromosome (*E.coli*). The successive
stages of replication can be seen in the electron microscope. For this purpose the
molecules of DNA are purified, spread on a support and the contrast is increased with
metal shadowing. Complete rings can be seen (1), others contain 'bubbles' of varying sizes
(2 and 3). If the bacteria have been grown in the presence of a radioactive precursor of
DNA, high resolution autoradiography shows that both sides of the 'bubble' are
radioactive and therefore contain newly-formed DNA.
(c) Similar images seen in the much longer molecules of animal DNA (a fragment of a
chromosome of *Drosophila* is shown); there are several replication 'bubbles'.
(d) If the molecules of DNA are single-stranded (e.g. various bacteriophages), simple
replication forks or Y-shaped images can be seen.
After [8].

There is one replicon per chromosome in *Escherichia coli*. There are several
thousand replicons per chromosome in the mouse and the human and about
20 000 base pairs per replicon.

When the parental DNA is circular (e.g. in viruses and bacteria) the two
replication forks finish by joining together. Each of the newly formed strands is
linked up around the parental strands which provided the instructions and two
identical rings are obtained each with a double helix. In the case of phage or
single-stranded viruses, the replication of DNA takes place by the intermediary
of a complementary double helix of which only the newly synthesized half is
recopied (in the complementary form) to produce a number of examples.

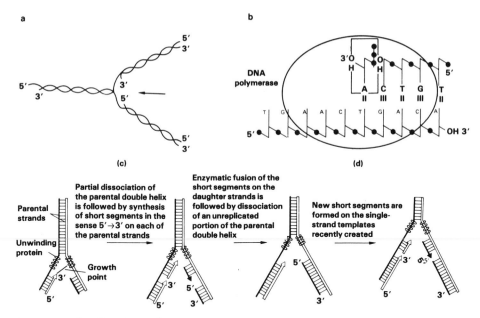

Figure 3.5. Replication of the DNA molecule.
(a) Replication fork where the two daughter strands are synthesized using the parental strands as templates.
(b) Nucleosynthesis in the presence of a molecule of the enzyme DNA polymerase (symbolized by an ellipse).
(c) and (d) Plan of the organization of the replication fork (formation and fusion of Okazaki's fragments).
After [18].

THE FRAGMENTS OF OKAZAKI

DNA polymerase is not capable of synthesizing a new strand right from the beginning; it can only lengthen an already existing strand. It therefore needs a 'primer' which usually consists of a segment of RNA created by RNA polymerase working on particular sequences of DNA called 'promoters of duplication' (Figure 3.7).

After a few dozen nucleotides have been placed in order, the extension of the RNA strand is interrupted, probably by another signal on the DNA, and DNA polymerase is substituted for RNA polymerase. Once started, the elongation of the newly formed DNA strand by DNA polymerase carries on until it meets an obstacle consisting of one of the many primer sites situated along the mother strand. Thus DNA is duplicated in a discontinuous manner by small segments which are called 'Okazaki' segments. These contain 1000–2000 nucleotides in bacteria but only a few hundred in eukaryotes.

The joining together of the fragments of Okazaki requires successively: the copy of the corresponding segments of the model by *DNA polymerase*, the removal of the terminal RNA 5′ primers by *nucleases*, and finally the joining of the extremity of the 3′ of one of the segments to the 5′ phosphate terminal of the other by a *ligase*.

At the end of the replication, the ligases connect the segments together at two levels: first the fragments of Okazaki, then the replicons. Thus the replication of DNA proceeds step by step, by the small fragments of Okazaki, which cannot be demonstrated by autoradiography. The Okazaki fragments are precursors to only half of the daughter strands, those that grow in the direction 3′→5′. Syn-

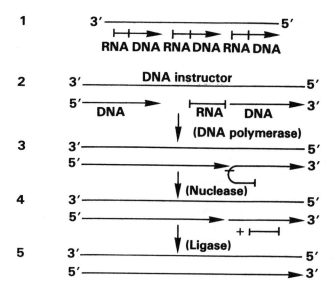

Figure 3.7. Replication of DNA by the synthesis and joining together of Okazaki's fragments (see text).
After [8].

thesis of the strand that grows in the direction $5' \to 3'$ for most part precedes that of the strand appearing to grow $3' \to 5'$ which is therefore called the lagging strand (Figures 3.6 and 3.7).

AVOIDANCE OF ERRORS

The accuracy of DNA replication is achieved by error-avoidance and error-correction mechanisms. If mistakes were as rare as one in a million, 3000 mistakes would be made during each duplication of the genome in a human cell. An organism cannot tolerate such a high rate of error and the actual rate is more like one in 10^9. Three quality control mechanisms ensure such high fidelity.

Errors arising in the course of DNA synthesis can result in non-complementary base pairs or mismatches. The accuracy of replication is due primarily to the effectiveness of the nucleotide selection mechanism. The second process involves proof-reading of the most recently added nucleotide and its expulsion if it is not complementary. The third process takes place after synthesis; it is called mismatch repair. Endonucleases selectively hydrolyze mismatch regions. Polymerases synthesize a new segment in place of the excised one. To be effective the repair mechanisms must distinguish the parental strand from the newly synthesized one and cleave the new one. In higher organisms an alternative possibility is that mismatch repair relies on genetic recombination. The two 'sister chromatids' issuing from the replication fork have homologous nucleotide sequences and so the strands of one chromatid could become templates for reconstructing the other. In this mechanism the repair system does not need to distinguish between the parental and newly synthesized strands. The cleaved strands would interact with the strand in a homologous region of the sister chromatid and the intact sister chromatid strand would direct the repair of the cleaved strand.

A reduction in the efficacy of these control mechanisms would result in a considerable increase in the frequency of mutations (which could be multiplied by as much as 10 000). This is what is meant by the expression 'mutator gene' or 'genetic instability'.

Transcription (gene expression)

The DNA contained in the gene acts as the template for the synthesis of mRNA, thanks to RNA polymerase. Subsequently, the molecules of mRNA serve as matrices to specify the sequence of amino acids during the synthesis of proteins (Figure 3.4). The amino acids (AA) first attach themselves to transfer RNA (tRNA); the combinations AA~tRNA then migrate towards the ribosomes. The mRNA, by moving to the site of a ribosome where protein synthesis occurs, places successive codons in positions which allow the selection of corresponding precursors AA~tRNA. Proteins, in particular enzymes, are necessary for different types of metabolism. Lesions in enzyme molecules can lead to cell death if the stock of this enzyme is exhausted before it can be resynthesized, but it must be presumed that the most serious damage is that occurring on DNA.

Expression of a gene requires a local modification of the folding of the DNA molecule and of the association between DNA and the surrounding protein molecules in the nucleoprotein structure. Thus gene expression modifies the radiosensitivity of this region of the DNA molecule.

The cell cycle

The cell cycle is the name given to the series of events which occur between two mitoses in a proliferating cell. It comprises four phases (Figure 3.8):

1. *Mitosis* or cell division. This takes place in such a way that the two daughter cells receive all the genetic information of the mother cell. Before division the mother cell must therefore have doubled its DNA in such a way that each of the two daughters can receive a complete genome. Just before mitosis, the chromatin condenses into chromosomes each of which divides in two in preparation for its distribution between the daughter cells.
2. G_1 *phase* represents the time between the end of mitosis and the beginning of S phase.
3. *S phase* is the time during which the DNA is duplicated. The cells in S phase have a content of DNA intermediate between those of cells in G_1 and G_2.
4. G_2 *phase* represents the time between the end of S and the next mitosis. It is the phase during which the cell prepares itself for mitosis. The DNA content is double that of cells in G_1.

S phase can be identified by means of specific DNA precursors labelled with a radionuclide, in particular thymidine, labelled with tritium ([³H]thymidine). Thymidine is a precursor of thymidylate (nucleotide) inserted into newly synthesized DNA. As thymine is the only one of the four bases which is not also a component of RNA, during incubation [³H]thymidine is incorporated only into the cells which are synthesizing DNA, that is to say cells in S. Autoradiography

Introduction to radiobiology

then allows those cells to be identified which were in the synthetic phase at the moment of incubation with thymidine (*in vitro*) or administration of thymidine (*in vivo*) and are the only ones to be labelled. The DNA is not modified during the life of the cell — moreover, it is the only molecule which is not renewed in a cell — and it only leaves the cell at the moment of death or of cell division. This makes thymidine the best marker for labelling cells and following their fate.

Cell labelling with [³H]thymidine makes it possible to measure the duration of the four phases of the cell cycle (see Figure 3.8). It is equally possible to measure the percentage of cells in S phase by determining the DNA content of the cells, either by morphometry on histological sections or by flow-cyto-fluorometry. The length of S phase can also be measured by administering bromodeoxyuridine (BrdU), an analogue of thymidine, a few hours before removal of a sample (biopsy) for cytofluorometry [7]. Identification with monoclonal antibodies against BrdU of the cells containing BrdU in the different phases of the cycle makes it possible to measure the cell turnover rate.

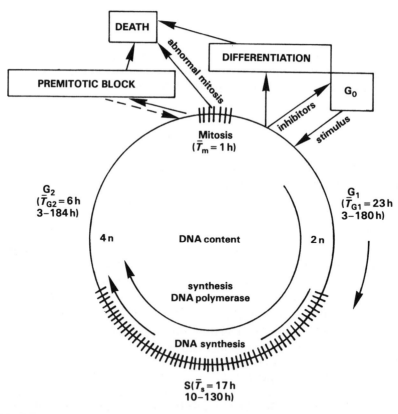

Figure 3.8. Schematic representation of the cell cycle. The average time spent in each phase with 95% confidence limits is indicated for human cells (normal or malignant). The DNA content of a diploid human cell is 2n in G_1 and 4n in G_2; in S it increases progressively from 2n to 4n. Differentiation, or entry into G_0, occurs shortly after mitosis. A block before mitosis has been described in certain tissues (liver). After [34].

3.2 *Lesions produced by radiation in DNA molecules*

The purpose of this chapter is the study of lesions produced by ionizing radiation. However, it is also useful to consider lesions produced by ultraviolet rays (UV) on DNA because they help in understanding certain mechanisms of repair which are important in radiobiology.

Lesions produced by ionizing radiation

Irradiation can result in various types of lesion in DNA molecules, depending on the component which is damaged:

(i)   rupture of the strand, single or double;
(ii) alteration to bases;
(iii) destruction of sugars;
(iv) cross-links and formation of dimers.

Altogether about 100 distinct lesions have been identified, among which breaks predominate both in frequency and importance.

Strand breaks

Strand breaks are the most well known lesions in DNA; they can be demonstrated by ultracentrifugation. This type of lesion is the most frequent *in vitro* (with the highest radiochemical yield). The indirect effect (p. 27) plays a preponderant role in their production.

A *single-strand break* can take place at the level of the phosphate diester bond, between the phosphate and the deoxyribose, or more frequently at the level of the bond between the base and deoxyribose. A large proportion of the single-strand breaks is produced through the action of OH. radicals as has been shown by the use of compounds which specifically trap this radical. The number of single-strand breaks is three or four times greater in well oxygenated mammalian cells than in hypoxic cells.

Following breakage of the phosphodiester bond, the two strands separate like a 'zip-fastener' with penetration of water molecules into the breach and breakage of hydrogen bonds between the bases (Figure 3.9). There seem to be changes in three or four nucleotides close to the break.

A *double-strand break* involves breakage of the two strands of DNA at points less than three nucleotides apart. It can be produced either by a single particle (a localized cluster of ionizations involving an energy transfer of about 300 eV), or by the combination of two single-strand breaks in complementary strands due to two particles traversing the same region before the first break has had time to be repaired. It is homologous if it occurs on the same pair of bases, otherwise it is heterologous. Heterologous double breaks are more frequent.

Owing to the lower molecular weight of the DNA fragments, strand breaks can be studied by means of sedimentation in sucrose gradients. Double-strand breaks can be studied in neutral gradients and single-strand breaks by means of an alkaline gradient which causes the molecule of DNA to open (Figure 3.10). The number of single breaks is directly proportional to dose over a very wide

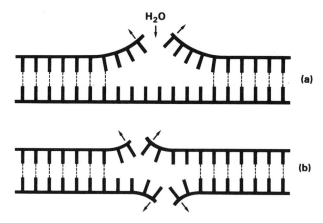

Figure 3.9. Breakage of DNA strands. (a) Single break; (b) double break.

range (0·2–60 000 Gy). The energy required to produce a single-strand break is 10–20 eV. The relationship between dose and the number of double-strand breaks in mammalian cells is a matter of dispute. Some authors find that the relationship is linear but others that it is linear-quadratic (see Section 4.3).

An X-ray dose of 1–1·5 Gy produces about 1000 single breaks and 50–100 double breaks per cell, that is one double break for every 10–20 single breaks. This dose causes the reproductive death of about 50% of mammalian cells. This shows that double-strand breaks are not necessarily lethal and that, in a normal cell, most can be repaired (see Section 3.3). In fact, normal cells repair correctly more than 50% of broken molecules, while cells from a patient with ataxia telangiectasia repair correctly less than 10%. Recently, the number of double-strand breaks has been found to correlate with cell lethality in experimental systems over a wide range of doses [25].

Alteration of bases

The bases can be partially destroyed or chemically modified. Most frequently they suffer hydroxylation (radical HO·) with formation of hydroperoxide in the presence of oxygen. The most important of these reactions is the hydroperoxidation of thymine.

Radicals produced by the indirect effect react with the bases, pyrimidine bases being more radiosensitive than purine bases. They can be placed in the following order of decreasing radiosensitivity:

$$\text{thymine} > \text{cytosine} \gg \text{adenine} > \text{guanine}$$

For each of these bases about 20 modifications of molecular structure have been described and can be identified by chromatography. Two or three of these alterations can be seen for 10 single-strand breaks.

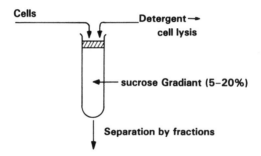

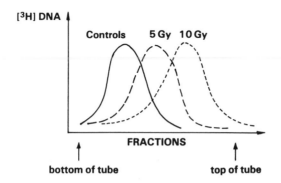

Figure 3.10. Demonstration of the production by radiation of double- and single-strand breaks in DNA molecules. Cells, e.g. human fibroblasts, are incubated in a medium containing [³H] thymidine. After two generations both chains of DNA are labelled with ³H. The cells are then irradiated and immediately placed on the top of a sucrose gradient (e.g. 5–20% sucrose). Addition of a detergent (sarcosyl) causes the cells to lyse. Under centrifugation the cellular contents spread out but are quickly stopped by the sucrose gradient. In the course of centrifugation the DNA molecules or their fragments are distributed according to their size (the large molecules move to the bottom of the tube). After piercing the tube the fractions are collected and their radioactivity is measured (³H being specifically bound to DNA).

For unirradiated cells most of the DNA is concentrated in a well-defined zone whose position depends on the conditions of centrifugation. At an alkaline pH (>11) the double strand of DNA opens by breakage of the hydrogen bonds. After irradiation the sedimentation gradient reveals single breaks (see the figure for the effects of 5 Gy and 10 Gy). With increasing dose the radioactive peak is displaced towards the top of the tube. At a neutral pH the two strands remain linked. After irradiation double-strand breaks can be detected, as the smaller segments of double-strand DNA which are formed float at a higher level than the unirradiated DNA.

Destruction of sugars

Alterations of deoxyribose are rarer and not well understood (0·2–0·3 alterations of sugars per 10 single-strand breaks). They can be measured by chromatography. The sugars are oxidized, then hydrolyzed with liberation of the base, with or without breakage of the phosphodiester bonds.

Other lesions

Among the other possible lesions there are: cross-links in the spiral, intrastrand links (between two parts of a single strand), interstrand links (between the two strands), cross-links between DNA molecules and proteins, and formation of dimers (see later in this section).

Lesions produced by ultraviolet radiation

Absorption of the energy

It is conventional to define three spectral bands of ultraviolet radiation, each with its own biological properties: UVA, 315–400 nm; UVB, 280–315 nm; UVC, 100–280 nm. Most of the studies on DNA and microorganisms have been made with UVC, mainly by means of low pressure mercury-vapour lamps which emit particularly intense radiation at 254 nm [9].

Ultraviolet is a non-ionizing radiation because the quantum energy given by

$$E(\text{eV}) = 1240/\lambda(\text{nm})$$

is below the ionization energy of the atom in biologically important molecules (about 10 eV). Absorption of energy therefore gives rise to excitations and an increase in the energy of rotation and vibration of the molecules. One of the fundamental characteristics of non-ionizing radiation is the selectivity of absorption. The absorption spectrum of a molecular species, which expresses the variation in absorption as a function of wavelength, shows peaks which are characteristic of the molecule (Figures 3.11 and 3.29).

With ultraviolet there is no indirect effect because water does not absorb radiation with wavelengths greater than 185 nm. When a molecule is excited by a UV photon it receives a quantum of energy which is of the same order of magnitude as most of the chemical bonds. The fate of this energy is analogous to that transferred by ionizing radiation (Section 1.1). True photochemical reactions begin when the molecules which are excited (directly or after transfer of energy), or the free radicals, react with neighbouring molecules.

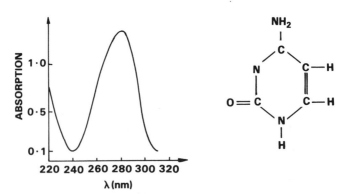

Figure 3.11. UV absorption spectrum of cytosine. Strong absorption bands in the region 200–400 nm are always associated with molecular structures containing conjugated double bonds. Such groups of atoms which selectively absorb certain wavelengths are called *chromophore groups.*

Description of lesions produced by UV

Proteins and nucleic acids are the main chemical structures of biological importance which contain *chromophores*. The effects on nucleic acids are the most important because of their major biological role and their great absorption of UV in the range 200–300 nm (Figures 3.11 and 3.29). Studies have been made principally on isolated DNA *in vitro*. The absorption by DNA of UV at 254 nm depends on the base; the chemical structure of pyrimidine bases are much more sensitive than purines to the action of UV.

Formation of dimers

Under the action of radiation, two adjacent bases of a single strand become joined by covalent bonds with the formation of a cyclobutane ring between them. The formation of these dimers has important consequences because they interrupt the replication of DNA at that point. Thymine dimers (T–T) are the most frequent and are very stable (Figure 3.12). They seem to play an important role in the induction of cutaneous cancers in regions exposed to UV (face, neck, hands). The formation of thymine dimers has also been demonstrated after irradiation with γ-rays [10].

Hydration of pyrimidine bases

Cytosine, for example, is transformed into cytosine hydrate by opening of the 5–6 bond and addition of a molecule of water (Figure 3.12). Pyrimidine hydrates can induce changes of code because it has been shown *in vitro* that cytosine hydrate codes as uracil or thymine.

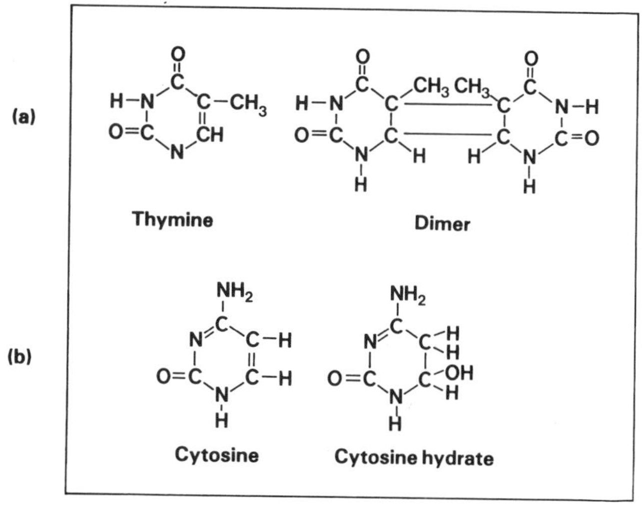

Figure 3.12. (a) Formation of thymine dimers T–T under the action of UV at 254 nm. These dimers are stable and resistant, particularly against acids. Irradiation with UV also produces dimers T–C and C–C between adjacent bases on a single strand. Dimerization C–C is much more difficult to produce than T–T which requires less energy. In order of decreasing frequency one finds T–T > T–C > C–C.
(b) Hydration of cytosine under the action of UV at 254 nm. *In vitro*, cytosine hydrate is formed more readily than thymine hydrate.

Cross-links

In intact cells DNA is associated with basic proteins (in particular histones) and non-basic proteins and is integrated in a nucleoprotein structure (see earlier in this chapter). UV of 254 nm can create stable covalent bonds between the DNA bases as well as between these bases and the amino acids of the polypeptide chains. Cytosine and thymine are easily linked with cystine. Pyrimidine bases become linked with numerous amino acids (such as tryptophan, methionine and phenylalanine).

Other lesions

Other types of lesion have been described: destruction of deoxyribose (sugars show little absorption of 254 nm UV), and lesions of purine bases with dissociation of the pentane nucleus. However, their biological importance is relatively small as the large doses of radiation necessary for these lesions to occur lead to cell death by other mechanisms.

Classification of DNA lesions

Ionizing radiation, UV and some chemical agents produce a number of lesions of varying importance. Ionizing radiation produces mainly single- and double-strand breaks together with lesions of bases, mainly pyrimidine. UV also acts mainly on pyrimidine bases. Deformations of DNA can be classified into various categories.

Negligible deformations of DNA

As an example, 7-alkylguanine is due to a modification of guanine (N_7 of guanine) under the action of an alkylating agent; this molecule is stable. 5-hydroxy-peroxy-methyl-thymine is due to an alteration of thymine produced by ionizing radiation. These two molecules are responsible for modification, without functional repercussion, of the distance between the bases and of their affinities.

Minor deformations of DNA

Alterations of base pairing and of the forces involved in piling up the bases (*stacking*) can break weak hydrogen bonds by causing local separation of the two strands of DNA. A typical example is represented by hydrates of thymine or cytosine induced by UV (Figure 3.12). Moreover, fragmentation of bases under the action of ionizing radiation or UV leads to the formation of sites without purines or pyrimidines. These minor deformations are, however, liable to block replication and transcription; they are highly mutagenic.

Major deformations of DNA

These deformations have important functional consequences. The lesions are *monofunctional* if they affect only one strand and only one function, or they may be *bifunctional*. An example of a major monofunctional alteration is the intercalation of a powerful carcinogenic agent between the two strands, such as acetyl-acetoxy-aminofluorine (AAAF), commonly used in biochemistry. Certain basic dyes (acridine derivatives) have a plane nucleus which intercalates between two pairs of bases; they can give rise to erroneous copies (mutagenic action). Many cytotoxic drugs have similar properties and act by blocking duplication and transcription of DNA (e.g. anthracyclins such as daunorubicin and doxorubicin). Examples of major bifunctional deformations are:

1. Cross-links on a strand induced by UV between pyrimidines (e.g. T–T) and also by alkylating nitrogen mustards or sulphur mustards (yperites). Mustards can also join two guanines and prevent duplication. They were used as cytotoxic drugs for their antimitotic action but have now been replaced by some less toxic analogues.

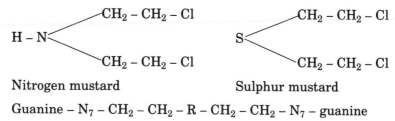

Nitrogen mustard   Sulphur mustard

$$\text{Guanine} - N_7 - CH_2 - CH_2 - R - CH_2 - CH_2 - N_7 - \text{guanine}$$

2. Cross-links between the two strands of DNA.

In the treatment of psoriasis and vitiligo, furocoumarines, natural substances found in essence of bergamot, whose characteristic molecule is psoralen, can be used. The treatment employs the combined action of UV radiation and psoralen (PUVA therapy). UVA of 365 nm is used (the wavelength selectively absorbed by the psoralen molecule). The latter, usually 8-methoxy-psoralen (8-MOP), sometimes 4, 5, 8-trimethoxypsoralen, is given orally (sometimes also applied locally). It has no effect on its own but is activated by the UVA radiation. Psoralen becomes bound to DNA and forms mono- or bifunctional adducts, creating cross-links between the two strands. Activated psoralen reacts by its double bond 3–4 with thymine or cytosine; the double bond 4'–5' can react under the action of a second photon with another thymine, which links the two strands of DNA in a stable manner, inhibiting the synthesis of DNA and so delaying or blocking mitosis.

The lesions induced by ionizing radiation and UV are more frequent in *linkers* than in *cores* where the DNA is better protected. On the other hand, lesions in the region of linkers are repaired more rapidly than those in the cores, in particular excision is more efficient. Differences in DNA structure can therefore have an effect on the radiosensitivity of the cell. Thus differentiation and gene expression may modify the vulnerability or repair capacity of some regions of DNA molecules and therefore alter cellular radiosensitivity. The inability of unstimulated lymphocytes to repair lesions is attributed to this cause. Moreover, the sequence of bases has an effect on the distribution of lesions. As thymine is very radiosensitive, regions rich in thymine–adenine are more easily damaged than regions rich in guanine–cytosine.

DNA repair is more rapid and more efficient in active genes than in inactive ones and in the transcribed strand than in the untranscribed one.

3.3 Repair of DNA lesions

Introduction

The mechanisms of molecular repair eliminate the radiation-induced lesions and reconstitute the original structure of the DNA. At the cellular level this results in restoration of *viability*; the increase in the surviving fraction is often used as a measure of the extent of repair. However, survival does not necessarily imply complete restoration of the DNA because there can be induction of *genetic mutations* or *chromosomal aberrations* compatible with viability. Thus other factors are involved in survival, e.g. tolerance of the lesions.

It is therefore convenient to distinguish:

(i)   *error-free* repair mechanisms (for example excision–resynthesis, transalkylation, photorestoration), which restore the DNA to its original state;

(ii) those repair mechanisms which may involve error (*misrepair*) and so increase the frequency of mutations (e.g. the SOS mechanism in bacteria). These latter mechanisms may be brought into play when the former are saturated, for example when the dose or the dose rate are high (this may explain why the mutagenic effect per unit dose increases with dose or dose rate; see Section 12.3).

Repair at the molecular level takes place under the control of genes which govern repair by the production of *enzymes*. Some mechanisms operate by a single step (e.g. photorestoration and transalkylation). Others take place in several steps and require more than one enzyme (e.g. excision–resynthesis). Some enzymes involved in repair mechanisms are also involved in the *normal biosynthesis* of DNA (e.g. DNA polymerase, ligase).

Among the systems of repair some are *constitutional*: they exist permanently in the cells and continuously control the integrity of DNA (e.g. excision–resynthesis). Others are *inducible*: they do not normally exist in the cell, or are present in low concentration, but appear as a response either to the development of specific lesions (e.g. photolyase in higher plants or the repair system SOS in bacteria) or after treatment with DNA-damaging agents. Photorestoration only occurs after irradiation by UV, whereas excision–resynthesis, post-replicative repair and SOS repair take place after irradiation with UV, ionizing radiation or exposure to chemical agents.

Several techniques make possible precise study of the various types of lesion and modes of repair of DNA molecules. Moreover, there are mutants (microorganisms or cell lines) which are defective for particular repair mechanisms. Radiosensitive mutants and hybrids produced by hybridization of a mutant cell with a normal cell or with a mutant of a different cell line, provide powerful methods of studying repair mechanisms. The radiosensitivity of these mutants is transmissible, but most of the hybrids have normal radiosensitivity; this shows that a large number of genes (10 or more) are involved in the control of radiosensitivity. Mutants have been studied in the cells of many species (bacteria, yeast) and man where various hereditary diseases involve the loss of certain repair mechanisms (see later in this section). Among the many genes which are involved in DNA repair mechanisms in human cells, XRCC1 (X-ray repair cross-complementing) is located on chromosome 19 and XRCC2 on chromosome 7. So far 6 genes for UV repair have been cloned and at least 5 for X-ray repair. These genes are able to repair or complement sensitive cell lines from rodents [30–33].

Repair systems

Excision–resynthesis

Excision–resynthesis is the principal mechanism of repair; it takes place in DNA molecules which are not in the replication phase. A lesion in one strand of the DNA molecule is recognized, excised and the missing segment is synthesized using the intact complementary strand as a template (Figure 3.13). Specific enzymatic mechanisms control the different stages of repair.

For the *excision of certain bases*, altered by X-rays, UV or alkylating agents, the first step is the action of a specific *glycosylase* which cuts the bond between the damaged base and the sugar. The resulting site lacking a purine or a pyrimidine is recognized by a specific *endonuclease* which cuts the phospho-diester strand at the right point. An *exonuclease* excises the segment of the strand containing the lesion and the repair is completed by the action of a *poly-merase* and a *ligase*. In *E. coli*, DNA polymerase 1 acts both as an exonuclease

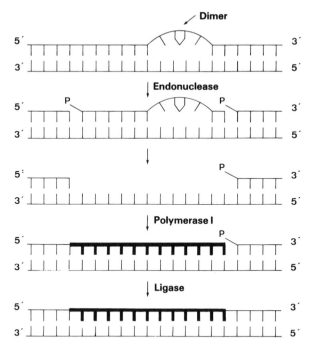

Figure 3.13. Mechanism of repair by excision–resynthesis. An *endonuclease* recognizes the lesion (e.g. in this case a thymidine dimer produced by UV) and cleaves the phosphodiester chain at the right point. The segment containing the lesion is excised. A *DNA polymerase* synthesizes a new segment using the intact complementary chain as a template. Finally, a ligase rejoins the two ends of the strand, completing the repair of the DNA.
After [24].

and a DNA polymerase; it excises the nucleotides at the same time as it synthesizes a new segment of about 20 nucleotides, the intact strand serving as template. Different glycosylases specific for altered bases have been described in mammalian cells.

A different mechanism is involved in the repair of dimers (UV). In this case there is *excision of nucleotides*. In *E. coli*, an endonuclease coded by three different genes (UVRA, UVRB and UVRC) cuts the phosphodiester bonds on both sides of the dimer and eliminates the segment of single-strand DNA containing the dimer. The structure of DNA is then restored by the action of polymerase and ligase (Figure 3.13). A similar mechanism of nucleotide excision has not yet been shown with certainty in mammalian cells, although the study of cells of xeroderma pigmentosum suggests its existence (see later in this section).

Three enzymes are involved in the repair of single-strand breaks: an exonuclease, a polymerase and a ligase. The repair of single-strand breaks in mammalian cells is rapid and decreases exponentially as a function of time; half the single breaks are repaired within 15 min. If there are also lesions in the bases, or gross alterations of the DNA molecule, or if the breach includes more than 30 nucleotides, a mechanism of excision–resynthesis is brought into play but the repair is much slower and takes several hours or even longer.

DNA–DNA cross-links can also be repaired by the mechanism of excision–resynthesis which occurs in the repair of pyrimidine dimers, followed by a recombination step in order to recover the genetic information lost due to the presence of DNA lesions on the two strands of DNA. In cells not in S phase, repair by excision–resynthesis is revealed by DNA synthesis. Incorporation of [^{3}H]thymidine makes it possible to follow this unscheduled DNA synthesis.

A large number of independent genes act in the various mechanisms of excision–resynthesis: at least 15 in *E. coli*, as many in yeast and probably more in human cells. The structure and organization of DNA can influence these repair mechanisms. It is for this reason that there are fewer excisions in unstimulated lymphocytes than in differentiated cells.

Transalkylation

Alkylated sites are simply de-alkylated by an alkyl transferase. *In vitro*, alkyl groups are reduced to alcohol; *in vivo*, their fate is unknown.

Photorestoration

This process of DNA repair is due to an enzyme, *photolyase*, which shows a great affinity for pyrimidine dimers and breaks the bond of the dimer to restore two monomers; its action is activated by visible light. This enzyme has been isolated; its synthesis is governed by a single gene. In bacteria and yeast there are mutants which are defective in this enzyme. In these mutants survival after irradiation with UV is the same whether or not the cells are exposed to visible light. Photolyase is a natural enzyme in bacteria, yeasts and eukaryotes. On the other hand, in higher plants it is not detectable in the dark but appears as soon as the plants are exposed to light. The existence of photorestoration has also been demonstrated in human cells.

Recombination or post-replication repair

Resting cells can repair lesions by the mechanism of excision–resynthesis, but cells which are actively replicating (S phase) have recourse in addition to another mechanism. DNA polymerase can only copy structures which it recognizes. Therefore, when irradiation induces lesions close to the replication fork (e.g. alteration of bases: hydroxypyrimidine, T–T dimers), the daughter strand which is in the process of synthesis contains a gap opposite the lesion because the DNA polymerase does not replicate the lesion and searches further away for another site at which to start the replication of a new segment (Figure 3.14). This produces a lesion in the mother strand, and consequently a gap or a stop in the progression of the fork.

In bacteria this gap is filled by a mechanism of 'genetic recombination'. Segments of DNA are exchanged between the parental strand of the other intact chain and the damaged, newly synthesized strand in order to fill the gap in the new strand. The gap formed in this way in the parental strand is filled by DNA polymerase which uses as a matrix the corresponding new strand. Finally, the residual lesion in the damaged parental strand is repaired by excision–resynthesis.

Repair by recombination requires more enzymes than repair by excision–resynthesis. It has been demonstrated in prokaryotic cells and mammalian cells but in the latter the mechanisms of action are still uncertain. In mammalian cells there is probably a temporary disturbance of DNA replication close to the lesions. Replication then continues and the DNA contains lesions which may or may not have been modified. This makes the lesions more tolerable but no repair has taken place (Figure 3.14).

SOS repair

This mechanism of repair has been revealed by the study of certain viruses (e.g. bacteriophages) which are unable to repair damage caused by UV or γ-rays or to replicate except after infecting a bacterium. If before the infection the bacteria are irradiated with a small dose of X-rays, the survival of irradiated virus is considerably improved but the number of mutants amongst the viruses is increased. This experiment shows that this type of 'repair' prevents death but results in frequent errors.

To study the mechanism involved, bacterial mutants are used which are unable to repair lesions by the methods of excision–resynthesis or post-replication repair described above. In those mutants which enable the damaged virus to be repaired, a protein called 'recA' appears following irradiation (molecular weight about 40 000). This protein can represent up to 1% of the total weight of the proteins. The bacterial mutants which do not synthesize the recA protein (recA$^-$) are not able to reactivate the virus.

The recA protein is synthesized in large quantities when the irradiation has led to accumulation of single-strand DNA fragments originating from the degradation of DNA or from an arrest of replication. Nalidixic acid, an inhibitor of replication, has the same effect as irradiation. The recA protein is endowed with protease activity which prevents repression of at least 20 genes, leading to full depression of all the SOS genes. In *E. coli* a new and less accurate

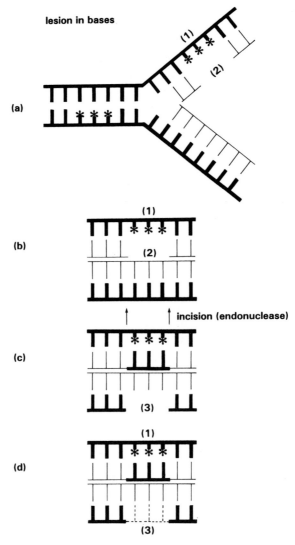

Figure 3.14. Schematic representation of the repair mechanisms by *recombination* or *postreplicative repair* in bacteria close to the replication fork.
(a) Opposite a radiation-induced lesion (1) on the parental strand (thick line), there is a gap (2) in the newly-synthesized strand (thin line).
(b) This gap is filled by transfer of a segment of DNA coming from the intact parental strand of the other chromatid and moving towards the damaged daughter strand to fill the gap in the latter.
(c) This exchange causes a gap (3) in the parental strand.
(d) This gap (3) is filled using the intact daughter strand as a template. The remaining lesion on the other parental strand (1) is then repaired by the mechanism of excision–resynthesis.
After [6].

polymerase is synthesized in the course of the SOS process. This may insert mismatched bases at the level of the lesion and so cause an increase in the frequency of mutations.

The existence of the SOS system has not been proven in mammalian cells although there are indirect arguments suggesting its presence. In particular, after large doses of radiation the appearance of new proteins and enzymes has been shown which intervene in repair. If a mechanism of this type does exist, it probably begins to act with doses which kill about one-third of the cells.

Repair of double-strand breaks

Repair of single-strand breaks is active and fast in mammalian cells; it takes place by excision–resynthesis. Double-strand breaks can be repaired in bacteria, yeast and mammalian cells. A repair mechanism by recombination with the homologous molecule of DNA has been demonstrated in many species and probably exists in mammalian cells. After a double break, a sequence of bases may be missing on both strands, and there may be a lack of continuity between the two free ends of the DNA molecule. A model — which remains hypothetical — is shown in Figure 3.15. After a double-strand break the free ends can rejoin, but the initial sequence of bases is not always re-established and the frequency of error may be high. It is likely that lesions which are too large cannot be repaired correctly. Two factors influence the radiosensitivity of a cell line: the capacity for repair of double-strand breaks and the fidelity of that repair. Rydberg [23] has shown that V79 Chinese hamster cells repair double- (and single-) strand breaks with equal efficiency whether the cells are blocked in mitosis or in the exponential growth phase.

Mechanisms of DNA repair and human diseases

Some congenital diseases are due to malfunction of the enzymatic repair systems described above. We will limit ourselves to three of these which are of particular interest and are clinically important.

Xeroderma pigmentosum (XP)

This is a rare genetic disorder, inherited as an autosomal recessive trait in which the skin changes are first noted during infancy or early childhood. Affected children who are unable to repair DNA damaged by ultraviolet light are sensitive to light in the wavelength range 230–310 nm (UVB) — see below — and develop extensive solar changes in exposed skin. Areas exposed to sunlight such as the face, neck, hands and arms are most severely involved, but lesions may occur at other sites including the scalp.

CLINICAL MANIFESTATIONS

1. *Skin lesions* consist of erythema, scaling, bullae, crusting, ephelides, telangiectasia, keratoses, and skin *cancers* such as basal and squamous cell carcinomas and malignant melanomas.
2. *Ocular manifestations* include photophobia, lacrimation, blepharitis,

symblepharon, keratitis, corneal opacities but also *tumours* of the lids and
sometimes eventual blindness.

3. The *association* of xeroderma pigmentosum with microcephaly, mental
   retardation, dwarfism and hypogonadism is known as *de Sanctis-Eacchione
   syndrome.*
4. Finally, *predisposition* to other forms of *cancer* have been described.

This disease is a serious, mutilating disorder, and the lifespan of the subjects
is often quite short. Affected families should have genetic counselling. Affected
children should be protected from exposure to sunlight; opaque broad-spectrum

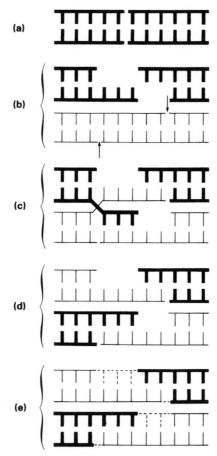

Figure 3.15. Model proposed by Resnick to explain the repair of double-strand breaks.
(a) Double-strand break of the DNA molecule (thick line);
(b) enzymatic excision of a segment of each strand, one on each side of the breakage point;
(c) the terminal unjoined segments of each strand 'interact' with the homologous
segments of the other intact DNA molecule (fine lines) in such a way as to allow repair
according to a mechanism analogous to that described in Figure 3.14 (by recombination
or postreplication). For this purpose the intact double-strand molecule must be cleaved at
two sites by an endonuclease;
(d) reciprocal exchange between the double strands of DNA; two single-strand breaks
remain, together with two gaps;
(e) the breaks are repaired by means of a ligase; the gaps are repaired (dotted lines) by a
mechanism of resynthesis (Figure 3.13).
After [6].

sunscreens should be employed even for mildly affected children. Early detection and removal of malignancies is mandatory. Grafting of skin from areas not exposed to sunlight may be helpful. Prenatal diagnosis is now possible.

STUDIES OF THE MECHANISM OF DNA REPAIR
The cells have normal sensitivity to X-rays but are very sensitive to UV. There is an alteration in the system of excision–resynthesis connected with a deficiency in the system of incision by means of endonuclease cleavage. After irradiation with UV there is a persistence of dimers and a relative absence of unscheduled DNA synthesis.

On the other hand the three enzymes which are involved later in the system of excision–resynthesis function normally. Thus, repair of DNA breaks due to X-rays or incorporation of labelled nucleotides takes place as in normal cells. The addition of purified viral endonuclease to a homogenate of XP cells re-establishes the excision of dimers, proving that the trouble is connected with malfunctioning of endonuclease. For the photoreactivation system the level of enzymes is much lower in XP cells than in normal cells.

In terms of genetics, there are at least eight types of XP. To identify the genes involved one can take skin biopsies from two subjects and obtain two lines of fibroblasts. When cells of the two lines are mixed in the presence of polyethyleneglycol, some will fuse to give hybrid cells. After irradiation with UV there is no unscheduled DNA synthesis when the two lines of fibroblasts are examined separately. If unscheduled DNA synthesis is seen in the hybrid line this indicates that the two subjects have mutations in different genes (the condition is recessive). On the other hand if it is not seen in the hybrid line the same gene must be responsible for the disease in both subjects.

In a variety of xeroderma pigmentosum (variant), equally serious clinically, the mechanism of repair by excision–resynthesis is normal and the failure occurs in the DNA synthesis after irradiation with UV. XP cells show hypermutability (at a given dose, ten times more mutants than in a normal cell line).

Ataxia telangiectasia (AT)

This is a complex disorder in which a specific immunological dysfunction is associated with progressive cerebellar degeneration, telangiectasis of bulbar conjunctiva and skin, and an increased likelihood of malignancy. The condition is transmitted on an autosomal recessive basis.

CLINICAL MANIFESTATIONS
These may be subdivided into those caused by central nervous system dysfunction, skin changes and immunological disorders.

1. *Neurological manifestations* usually begin in infancy. Affected children learn to walk later and their gait is always ataxic. Late in childhood there is progressive dysarthria, nystagmus, intention tremor, and choreoathetosis. The tendon reflexes are diminished or absent. A peculiar abnormality of eye movements is characteristic, the child being unable to move the eyes on command, while involuntary movements are retained.

2. *Skin changes*, usually evident by 5 years of age, consist of telangiectases over the bulbar conjunctiva, along the nasolabial folds, over the external ears and along flexor creases of the extremities.
3. Clinical evidence of *immunological deficiency* is variable. Some children have severe recurrent sinus, ear and pulmonary infections from early childhood, while others never suffer from increased susceptibility to infection. Tonsillar tissue is diminished or absent and there are usually no palpable lymph nodes. Also, as a consequence of immunodeficiency, the incidence of several tumours is increased, especially leukaemias and lymphomas. It should also be stated that due to the DNA repair syndrome present in this disease, both radiotherapy and chemotherapy carry the risk of severe side effects like skin burning, fibrosis of the mucosae and persistent bone-marrow aplasia. It is therefore important that the syndrome should be recognized and the therapy adapted.

The illness is slowly progressive: death usually occurs in late childhood or adolescence as a result of pulmonary failure, severe infection or malignancy.

LABORATORY FINDINGS
These include, in varying combinations, a decrease or absence of serum IgA, IgE, IgG_2 and IgG_4, a decrease in the number of circulating lymphocytes, and a decrease or absence of delayed hypersensitivity reactions to intradermal injections of several antigens like mumps, DNCB (dinitrochlorobenzene), *Candida*, etc. Serum fetoprotein (αFP) is often raised. More specific tests like chromosome breaks and sensitivity to X-rays are given below.

THERAPY
This is limited to the prompt treatment of the associated infection, replacement treatment with intravenous gamma globulins and treatment of malignant diseases.

STUDY OF DNA REPAIR MECHANISMS
Subjects with AT are three or four times more sensitive to ionizing radiation than normal subjects (Figure 3.16). *All* the cell lines derived from these subjects are abnormally radiosensitive, but a defect in DNA repair has only been demonstrated in certain cell lines (e.g. elimination of damaged bases). The cells of these subjects show *systematically* two abnormalities after irradiation:

(i)   lack of delay in DNA synthesis, allowing less time for repair than in normal cells;
(ii) a reduction in mitotic delay in G_2 [28, 30, 31, 37].

These two abnormalities shown by AT cells during their progression through S and G_2 have led Painter and Young [19] to suggest that the absence of mitotic delay may reduce the time available for repair of potentially lethal lesions. This would explain the greater radiosensitivity of the cells and the abnormally high frequency of chromosome aberrations. Recently it has been shown that AT cells repair double-strand breaks poorly and with low fidelity. There is inefficient rejoining of the free ends of the DNA molecule. In contrast with what is

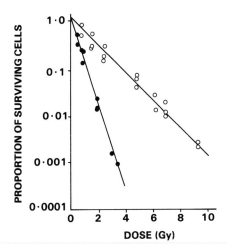

Figure 3.16. Survival curves of human skin fibroblasts irradiated with X-rays; ○, Controls; • subjects with *Ataxia telangiectasia*. After [6].

observed in xeroderma, these cells are hypomutable. This suggests a deficit in genetic recombination.

Fanconi's anaemia (FA)

The constitutional aplastic anaemias, known as Fanconi's anaemia or Fanconi syndrome, are familial disorders inherited on an autosomal recessive basis.

CLINICAL MANIFESTATIONS

1. *Congenital abnormalities* are observed in about half of affected children; especially common are microcephaly, microphthalmia and absence of radii and thumbs; abnormalities of heart and kidney are also relatively common. Some children have no serious anatomical defects, but are short in stature and have a peculiar dark pigmentation of the skin and *café au lait* spots, as do most of those with structural anomalies. Pancytopenia is not usually present at birth or during early infancy. *Bruising*, the first indication of haematological disease, is observed by 3–13 years of age. The consequences of a progressively severe anaemia and leukopenia are noted shortly thereafter.
2. *Laboratory data*: severe *pancytopenia* is evident in peripheral blood. The bone marrow is strikingly hypocellular. Analysis of the haemoglobin reveals an increase in fetal haemoglobin (*HbF*). Serum αFP may be raised. Finally, chromosomal studies reveal an abnormally high percentage of *chromatid breaks* and unusual chromosomal alignments.
3. *Treatment*: when possible, bone marrow transplantation is the treatment of choice. Particular attention should, however, be paid to the dose of cyclophosphamide and total-body irradiation used for preparation for bone marrow transplantation. When a suitable histocompatible bone marrow donor is not available, the treatment is mainly symptomatic and consists of

blood transfusion and antibiotics. However, in some cases therapy with androgenic steroids may be beneficial, at least temporarily. Haemorrhagic cysts of the liver (peliosis hepatis) and malignant hepatomas occur with increased frequency in patients receiving prolonged treatment with large doses of oral synthetic androgens.

4. *Excess of malignancies*: besides hepatomas which are probably due to androgens, an increased incidence of leukaemia has been described in children suffering from Fanconi's anaemia and in their close relatives.

STUDY OF DNA REPAIR MECHANISMS

Cells from FA patients show an increased sensitivity *in vitro* to cross-linking agents (alkylating agents, nitrogen mustard, mitomycin C), to UV potentiated by psoralen and also to ionizing radiation.

The molecular mechanism responsible for this hypersensitivity is not known. In some cell lines it has been shown that there is inability to excise cross-links between the strands. Study of the chromosomes of lymphocytes following treatment with mitomycin has shown that lesions at any point in the cell cycle lead to the maximum frequency of chromosomal *aberrations*, whereas in normal cells lesions at the beginning of G_1 are more easily repaired than at the end of G_1 and at the beginning of S.

3.4 *Effects of radiation on chromosomes*

Introduction

Chromosomes are the support of the genes. The action of radiation on chromosomes is an interesting example of the morphological phenomena produced by irradiation.

In a human cell (except the germinal cells) there are 22 pairs of autosomal chromosomes and 1 pair of sex chromosomes or gonosomes (XX or XY). One chromosome of each pair is of paternal origin and the other maternal. The genes are located along the chromosomes; there are at least 50 000 in a human cell. During interphase the diameter of the chromosomes is of the order of 50 nm. They form long filaments which roll up on themselves at the beginning of mitosis, thereby becoming much thicker. After fixation and appropriate staining at the beginning of metaphase, the chromosomes in the nucleus are visible under the optical microscope.

Among the chromosomal alterations produced by ionizing radiation, abnormalities of number or structure (clastogenic effects) are visible under the microscope. In addition there are changes which cannot be seen microscopically but which can nevertheless have serious functional consequences (*gene mutations*).

In addition to ionizing radiation, a large number of agents in the environment are able to produce chromosomal abnormalities or aberrations. Among the physical agents one can cite non-ionizing electromagnetic radiation (UV, microwaves) and mechanical waves (ultrasound). However, chemical substances appear to constitute the largest potential danger. Their number grows continually as does the risk of human exposure to them.

Methods of chromosome analysis

Theoretically, the karyotype of somatic cells drawn from any tissue can be studied, provided the cells are able to divide *in vitro* in an appropriate nutritive medium. In practice the only techniques available at present are for culture of *lymphocytes* and *fibroblasts* (taken aseptically by cutaneous biopsy) and, in addition, culture of cells from *amniotic fluid* taken for prenatal diagnosis. Studies by direct examination of dividing cells from the bone marrow is done only in cases of *malignant haemolymphopathy*, in most of which the cells concerned show chromosomal abnormalities. Finally, the possibility of studying germinal cells must be mentioned, after biopsy of the gonads, thanks in particular to the association of homologous chromosomes in meiosis.

Among the methods of chromosome analysis, we will study in turn: production of satisfactory *mitoses* and their analysis after *standard staining*, *banding* and *dynamic techniques*. We will focus on the chromosomes of lymphocytes because of their importance in radiation protection.

Mitotic analysis after standard staining

In the case of lymphocytes, interpretable mitoses can be obtained by adding to the cell culture a growth factor such as *phytohaemagglutinin* (or PHA), a mucoprotein which induces a lymphoblastic reaction. Two or three hours before arrest of the cultures, after 48 or 72 h of incubation at 37 °C, *colchicine*, an antimitotic which blocks mitosis in metaphase, is added to the culture, as it inhibits formation of the spindle. Finally, a hypotonic shock is given which causes the cells in division to swell and spreads out the chromosomes, thereby avoiding superposition of images.

The classical method of staining (Giemsa) makes the chromosomes appear as small uniformly-coloured rods and allows them to be classified according to their size and the position of the centromere. In this way it is possible to observe abnormalities of chromosome shape (e.g. dicentric chromosomes, rings and fragments) together with abnormalities in chromosome number. This technique is the conventional method for the study of hereditary diseases associated with chromosomal abnormalities (Figure 3.17).

Banding techniques

In 1970, Caspersson [4], after staining chromosome preparations with a fluorescent dye (quinacrine mustard which is an alkylating agent for DNA) observed with ultraviolet light that the fluorescence emitted was not uniform along the length of the chromosome but was distributed in the form of bands which were alternately strongly and weakly fluorescent. The sequence of fluorescent bands is specific for each pair of chromosomes. This makes it possible to distinguish chromosomes which are almost the same in terms of length and position of the centromere. In addition it demonstrates alterations produced by X-rays or other agents. This is the technique of '*Q-banding*' (quinacrine).

Several techniques demonstrating chromosomal banding have been developed. The first to appear after the technique of Q-banding was that of '*R-*

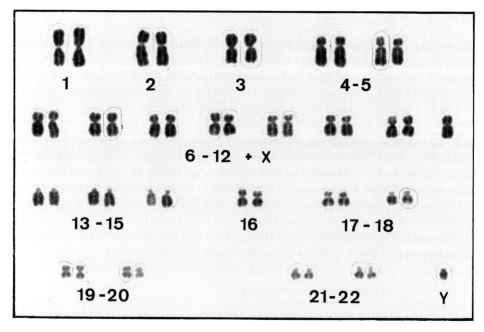

Figure 3.17. **Karyotype of a human lymphocyte after standard staining with Giemsa. For classification the micrographic images of the two chromosomes of each pair have been placed side by side and the pairs ranged according to their size and the position of the centromere. This allows a rough classification but several ambiguities remain (pairs 4 and 5, 13–15, 21 and 22). The numbering system is that of the international nomenclature. By courtesy of A. Leonard.**

banding' (reverse or reciprocal) which was devised by Dutrillaux [11]. After heating the chromosomal preparations (heating probably affects mainly the proteins) they are stained by the method of Giemsa. The bands which appear are reciprocal to those obtained by staining with quinacrine mustard. Another technique involves the action of a proteolytic enzyme, trypsin, on the chromosomal preparations before staining with Giemsa (technique of *G-banding*). This illustrates the important role played by chromosomal proteins in staining. In the G- and Q-banding systems the bands show the same topography, while the R-system is reciprocal (Figure 3.18).

Dynamic techniques: incorporation of BrdU

Use is made of compounds which are incorporated into DNA at replication and whose presence in the chromosome can be detected later. Precursors or analogues of thymine are the most important as thymine is the only specific constituent of DNA; adenine, guanine and cytosine are found also in RNA.

The original method involved the incorporation of [³H] thymidine followed by autoradiography. Nowadays an analogue of thymidine, *bromodeoxyuridine* or BrdU, is usually employed. This substitution leads to a defect in the condensation of the chromosome and an alteration in structure in the region which has incorporated BrdU. To bring out these zones, the preparations are stained either with a fluorescent dye (acridine orange) or, after special treatment, with Giemsa. With acridine orange, the chromosomes normally emit a brilliant green fluorescence; the fluorescence is dark red in the region which has incorporated BrdU. Incorporation of BrdU has largely supplanted autoradiography because of its better resolution and convenience in use. It can be localized at the molecular level by specific antibodies against BrdU.

Incorporation of BrdU during the cell cycle

If BrdU is allowed to be incorporated during the second half of the synthetic phase S, the distribution of fluorescent bands with acridine orange is that of R-banding while the G-bands remain dark. Therefore it is the G-bands which incorporate BrdU during the second half of S phase. This observation shows the relation between chromosome structure and duplication: the G-bands are duplicated late whereas the R-bands remain fluorescent because they completed DNA duplication before being brought into contact with BrdU.

On the other hand if BrdU is added during the first half of S phase the G-bands fluoresce brightly while the R-bands remain dark. Therefore the R-bands correspond with zones which duplicate early. The duplication of DNA requires about 9 h in lymphocytes in culture.

Incorporation of BrdU during several cycles

During S phase the *chromosomes* divide into two daughter *chromatids* which are identical. Each of these contains the same genetic information that was in the original chromosome and which will thus be transmitted to the two daughter cells. During metaphase the two identical daughter chromatids are easily visible in the microscope; they are still attached at the centromere. Thus if BrdU is added during two cell cycles, after staining with acridine orange the chromosomes show one bright fluorescent chromatid and one dark. The bright chromatid has substituted BrdU only on one strand of its DNA molecule whereas both strands of the dark chromatid have been substituted. With Giemsa the staining is weak where the level of incorporation of BrdU is strong. The chromatids containing only one substituted strand of DNA are stained rather less than the normal chromatids, whereas the chromatids both of whose strands of DNA have incorporated BrdU are stained very weakly with Giemsa (Figure 3.19).

This difference in staining between the two sister chromatids allows exchanges between them to be demonstrated. These exchanges seem to take place during or after duplication; they occur spontaneously but their incidence is increased after repair of lesions in the chromosomes. Their frequency is used as a test of mutagenicity, hence their interest. However, all mutagens do not lead to an increase in the frequency of exchanges between sister chromatids.

If BrdU is allowed to be incorporated during three cycles, three-quarters of the chromatids are dark and entirely substituted and one-quarter is bright after staining with acridine orange.

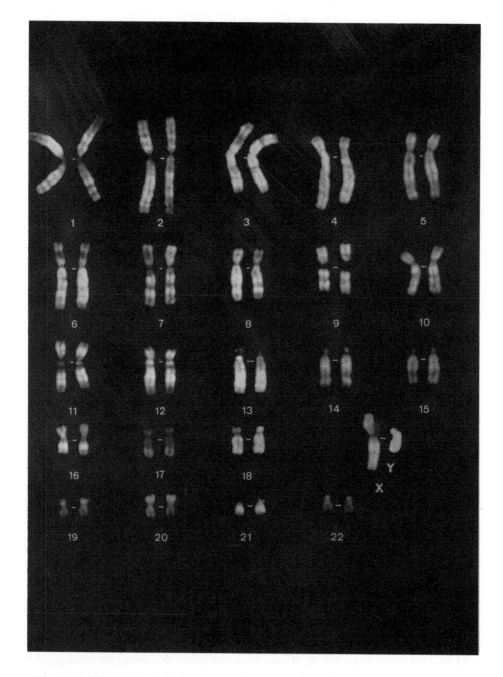

Figure 3.18. Technique of banding.
(a) Karyotype of a human lymphocyte (male) after staining of Q-bands. Note the strong fluorescence of certain heterochromatic regions (the long arm of the Y chromosome in particular).

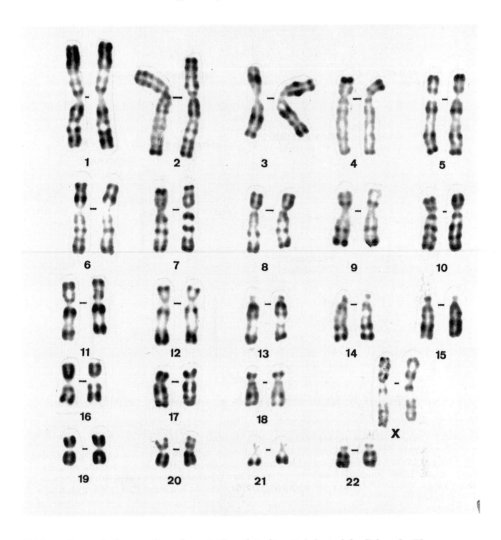

(b) **Karyotype of a human lymphocyte (female) after staining of the R-bands. The topography of the bands obtained is the reciprocal of that of the Q-bands. By courtesy of B. Dutrillaux and J. Couturier.**

High resolution labelling techniques

Finally, the number of identifiable bands can be further increased by analyzing the chromosomes in early metaphase or prometaphase. This technique requires synchronization of the cells. First the synthesis of DNA is inhibited; the block is then lifted and the culture is arrested at the appropriate moment to recover the maximum number of cells in the phase of interest. Banding is obtained by incorporation of BrdU.

Description and classification of chromosome aberrations

A large proportion of the cellular damage produced by radiation has been ascribed to lesions in the chromosomes. It has not been possible to establish a

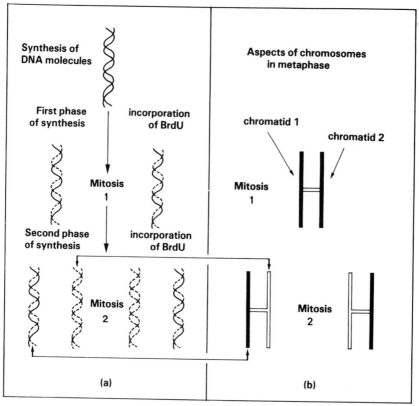

Figure 3.19. Study of chromosome structure by incorporation of BrdU.
(a) Duplication of DNA molecules. At the first mitosis each double helix or daughter DNA molecule contains a single strand which has incorporated BrdU. At the second mitosis one daughter DNA molecule has incorporated BrdU in both strands and the other in only one strand. ——————, a normal strand of DNA; – – – – – –, a strand of DNA which has incorporated BrdU.
(b) Appearance of chromosomes in metaphase. At the first mitosis each chromatid contains one substituted DNA strand and one normal. Both chromatids are therefore stained by Giemsa. At the second mitosis one chromatid is substituted on one strand while the sister chromatid has both strands substituted. The first will be stained with Giemsa (the black strand) and the other not (the white strand).

correlation between dose and anomalies in the *number* of chromosomes because these are rare after irradiation. In practice one can take account only of *structural* abnormalities or chromosome *aberrations*. These are of several types and can be classified according to a number of criteria.

Chromosome and chromatid aberrations

Depending on the position of the cells in the mitotic cycle at the time of irradiation, various types of aberration are observed.

Chromosome aberrations are produced when irradiation is given *before* S phase. If the lesion is not repaired before replication the two daughter chromatids are both damaged.

Chromatid aberrations are produced by irradiation after S phase, i.e. during

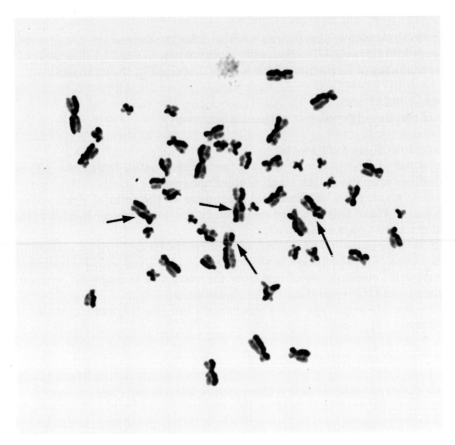

(c) Image of metaphase at the second mitosis after incorporation of BrdU and staining with Giemsa. On each chromosome the chromatids are differentially stained. The chromatids which are well stained with Giemsa contain one strand of DNA not substituted by BrdU whereas the chromatids which are poorly stained contain DNA molecules substituted in both strands. After treatment with acridine orange they would be respectively bright and dark. The arrows indicate exchanges between sister chromatids after irradiation.
By courtesy of A. Leonard.

G_2: only one of the two chromatids is abnormal. If the cells are irradiated *during S phase*, at a time when the chromosomes are only partly duplicated, a mixture of chromosome and chromatid aberrations is produced. Finally, if the cells are exposed to ionizing radiation during prophase, *sub-chromatid* aberrations can be seen involving subunits of the chromatids.

These distinctions only apply in the case of exposure to ionizing radiation. Ultraviolet rays and most chemical mutagens (except 'radiomimetic' substances) only produce chromatid aberrations *after* the cell has passed through a phase of DNA replication. Thus cells exposed to chemical mutagens in G_1 show chromatid aberrations at the following mitosis, whereas cells exposed during G_2 do not show this type of lesion until the second mitosis.

When radiation-induced aberrations are studied in circulating blood lymphocytes, chromosome aberrations are produced because these cells are normally in G_0.

Description of chromosome aberrations

The main chromosome aberrations visible under the microscope are presented in Figure 3.20. This classification, after Buckton and Evans [3], takes account of the mechanisms of formation which will be discussed in the next section.

TERMINAL DELETIONS
Pairs of chromatid fragments without a centromere.

INTRACHROMOSOME EXCHANGES
Interstitial deletions: pairs of very small chromatid fragments without centromeres which look like small coupled spheres.

Acentric rings: pairs of chromatid fragments in the form of rings without centromeres. When they are very small the distinction between these and interstitial deletions becomes arbitrary.

Centric rings: pairs of chromatid fragments in the form of rings and including a centromere. This aberration is accompanied by a pair of acentric fragments.

Paracentric inversion: resulting from the return of a fragment without a centromere and its reinsertion in the chromosome.

Pericentric inversion: the same mechanism but the fragment contains the centromere.

INTERCHROMOSOME EXCHANGES
Reciprocal translocation: between two chromosomes, resulting from exchange of their distal sections. This is a *symmetrical* interchromosome exchange.

Dicentric or *polycentric aberration*: this results from an exchange between two (or more) chromosomes in the course of which the proximal parts (including the centromere) become joined. This abnormality is accompanied by one (or more) acentric fragments. This is an *asymmetrical* interchromosome exchange.

AGGLUTINATION OF CHROMOSOMES
Immediately after *large doses* of ionizing radiation the chromosomes become thicker, forming irregular packets with aggregates of chromatin, apparently more viscous and with excessive adherence. Normal division of the chromosome becomes impossible. These phenomena are probably related to a modification of the structure of the nucleic acids and proteins which constitute the chromosome. They may be reversible and at a given dose are more severe if the dose rate is high. Lesions in the spindle may cause difficulties during separation of the chromosomes.

No differences have been noted between the *nature* of the aberrations produced by the different clastogenic agents. On the other hand the *proportions* of the various types of abnormality depend on the mutagen and, as discussed above, on the moment in the cycle at which the cells are exposed.

Mechanisms involved in the formation of chromosome aberrations

Several mechanisms have been proposed for interpretation of the formation of the chromosome aberrations which are observed [17, 27]. The two principal ones are those of breakage followed by linkage and that of 'exchange'.

CHROMOSOME ABERRATIONS

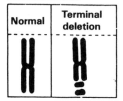

Normal	Terminal deletion

INTRACHROMOSOME EXCHANGES

Normal	Interstitial deletion	Centric ring and fragment	Acentric ring	Pericentric inversion

INTERCHROMOSOME EXCHANGES

Normal	Dicentric and fragment	Symmetrical exchange

CHROMATID ABERRATIONS

Normal	Gap	Fragment
Normal		Exchange

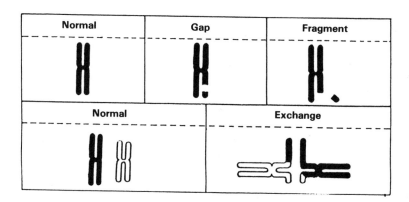

Figure 3.20. Schematic representation of the principal types of chromosomal aberration observed under the microscope.
After [3].

Introduction to radiobiology

The classical theory states that the primary lesions are breaks produced by irradiation in the arms of the chromosomes (or of the chromatids), giving rise to two or more fragments with one or two 'points of breakage'. A proportion, probably the majority, of the breaks are repaired by linkage of the fragments thus restoring the original configuration (*restitutio ad integrum*). When the breaks remain open, they give rise to the formation of fragments (*deletions*).

If there are several breaks (and therefore two or more points of breakage),

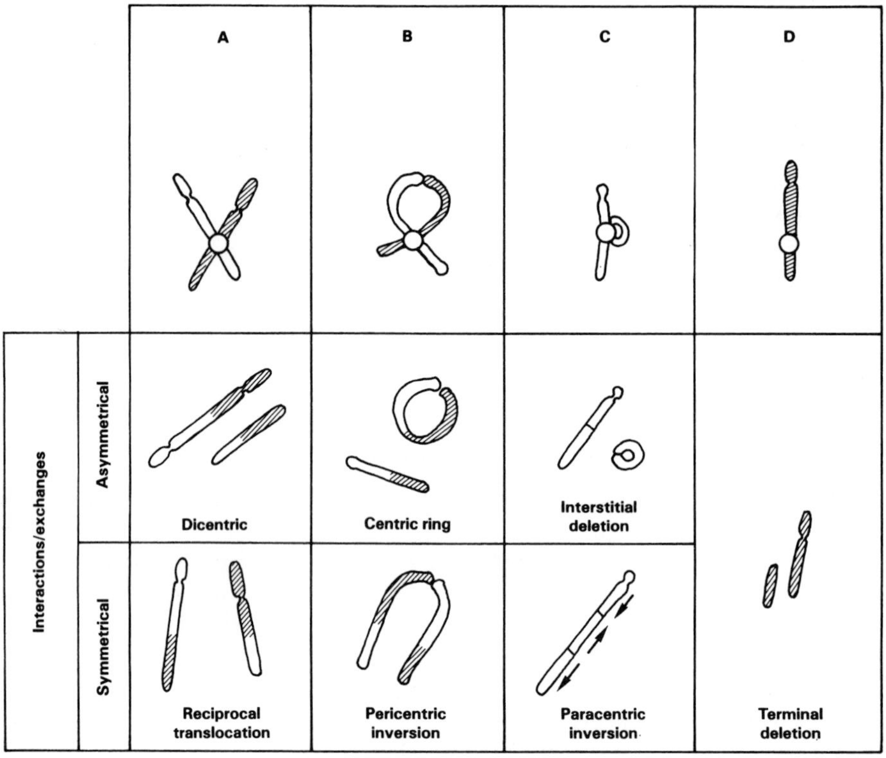

Figure 3.21. **Mechanism of formation of chromosome aberrations: four types of aberration are considered.**
(A) Exchange between two chromosomes. *Two breaks* (discussion in the text) are produced, one in each arm of *two chromosomes*. They can be repaired to restore the original configuration (*restitutio ad integrum*). If the two breaks are sufficiently close in space and time, four fragments are formed which can recombine in different ways leading to exchanges (or aberrations). These exchanges can be symmetrical (leading to a *reciprocal translocation*) or asymmetrical (leading to the formation of a *dicentric chromosome* accompanied by an *asymmetric fragment*). Visualization of the exchanges is facilitated in the figure by shading one of the two chromosomes.
(B) Exchanges between the arms of a single chromosome. *Two breaks* are produced in the two arms of a single chromosome (one arm is clear and one shaded). Following the same reasoning as in (A) this leads to exchanges which result in the formation of a *centric ring* and an *acentric fragment* (asymmetrical exchange) or to a *pericentric inversion* (symmetrical exchange).
(C) Exchanges in an arm of a single chromosome. The two breaks are produced in the *same arm of a single chromosome*. They can lead to an *interstitial deletion* if the fragment of arm produced remains isolated, or to a *paracentric inversion* if the fragment of arm produced is turned round before becoming reinserted in the arm of the chromosome.
(D) *Terminal deletion* following a break in one arm.
After [26].

exchanges can take place leading to the formation of chromosomes which are different from the original chromosome, i.e. to *chromosomal aberrations*.

In 1966, Revel [21] put forward the hypothesis that the primary event was the creation of a localized 'zone of instability' which could react with another primary event of the same type produced at the same moment in its vicinity. This would lead to 'the initiation of an exchange', which in turn might cause an aberration or repair of the damage.

The types of aberration depend on the site where the primary lesions (breaks or zones of instability) are produced and on the way in which the exchanges subsequently take place. In most cases the aberrations can be identified under the optical microscope; some can only be shown by banding techniques. Some of these fragile sites have been mapped and characterized; they can be closely linked to genes which are important for cellular life (proto-oncogenes).

Some mechanisms giving rise to chromosome aberrations are depicted in Figure 3.21. In type A aberrations there is a breakage in two chromosomes. These breaks can either be repaired or, if they are close enough together in space and time, they can give rise to interchromosome exchanges which may be symmetrical or asymmetrical. Type B aberrations result from two breaks in two arms of the same chromosome, followed by exchange. Type C aberrations result from two breaks in the same arm of a chromosome, followed by exchange. Finally, the production of fragments (type D) is the result of a single break.

Relation between the number of aberrations and the radiation dose

After irradiation *in vitro*, chromosome aberrations can be detected after doses as low as $0 \cdot 1$ Gy. Doses of $0 \cdot 5$–2 Gy, according to the type of cell, are necessary to produce an average of one chromosome aberration per cell, a dose which is of the same order as the mean lethal dose for the cells (see Section 4.3). The number of aberrations and the shape of the dose–effect relation depend on several factors.

In general, for low-LET radiation the relationship between the number of chromosome aberrations and the dose is linear–quadratic ($E=\alpha D+\beta D^2$) for aberrations of types A, B and C (Figure 3.21). It is linear for the production of type D aberrations (fragments) seen after a single break. Aberrations of types A, B and C require at least two breakage points sufficiently close in space and time; therefore the number of these aberrations diminishes when the dose rate is reduced or the fractionation increased.

For high-LET radiations, particularly fission neutrons, the dose–effect relation is linear for all the different types of aberration. Moreover, the number of aberrations induced varies more rapidly with LET than does cellular lethality (Figure 3.22).

The relation between the number of dicentrics and dose is presented in Figure 3.23 for X- and γ-rays and fast neutrons. For γ-rays a dose of $0 \cdot 5$ Gy induces two dicentrics per 100 cells and a dose of 2 Gy induces 20.

Chromosome aberrations and biological dosimetry

Analysis of chromosome abnormalities could be made in any tissue whose cells are capable of division (see earlier in this section) but the lymphocytes in

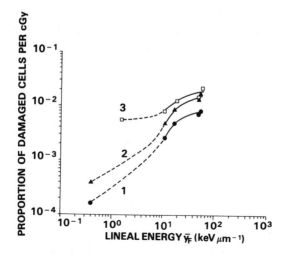

Figure 3.22. Relative effectiveness of different beams of neutrons and photons:
for the production of dicentric chromosomes (curve 1);
for the production of all types of chromosome aberrations (curve 2);
and cellular lethality (curve 3). The relative effectiveness of the beams, evaluated by the
fraction of cells showing aberrations per unit dose, is expressed as a function of the
frequency mean of lineal energy $\bar{y}_F$, a microdosimetric parameter (Section 1.3) directly
linked to the LET of the radiation. The variation of relative effectiveness is seen to be
greater for induction of chromosome aberrations than for cellular lethality.
After [2].

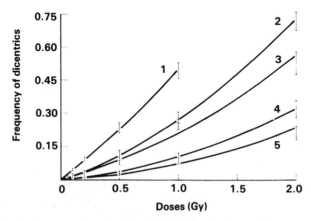

Figure 3.23. Dose–response curves for dicentric induction (dicentrics per cell) by
d(16)+Be (1), d(33)+Be (2), and d(50)+Be (3) neutrons, 250 kV X-rays (4), and ^{60}Co γ-rays (5).
The curves are fitted to the experimental points by using the linear–quadratic
relationship. Poisson errors are represented.
From [13].

After [12].

peripheral blood represent the most useful system. This system can be used in practice as a *biological dosimeter*, to evaluate doses received by workers, particularly after an accidental exposure to radiation (Chapter 12).

Technical aspects

Five to ten ml of blood must be taken from each subject and placed in a heparinized tube. The number of abnormalities observed is influenced by various factors such as temperature and the type of phytohaemagglutinin: it is therefore important to standardize the method. At the present time most laboratories use the technique recommended by the World Health Organization [3].

The culture is arrested after 48 h, i.e. at a time when the majority of the cells are in their first division, because chromosome abnormalities are usually incompatible with the normal completion of mitosis. In fact, it is estimated that the probability of finding a dicentric in the daughter cells is 50% whereas it is 90% for an abnormal monocentric chromosome; 70% of the acentric fragments are lost in the course of the first division.

Usually 200 cells are examined from each subject; if at least one dicentric is observed a total of 500 cells is examined. This allows an approximate estimate of the dose received (Table 3.1). Figure 3.24 shows some examples of metaphases with different types of chromosome aberrations.

Table 3.1. Relation between the frequency of dicentrics and the dose of γ-rays.

Number of dicentrics/ number of cells counted	Estimate of the mean γ-ray dose (cGy)	
0/200	—	(0–47)†
1/200	20	(3–61)
2/200	32	(5–71)
3/200	41	(13–80)
4/200	50	(20–87)
5/200	57	(27–94)
0/500	—	(0–26)
1/500	10	(<2–34)
2/500	17	(2–40)
3/500	22	(6–46)
4/500	27	(10–50)
5/500	32	(14–54)

†95% confidence limits.
After [20].

Relation between the number of dicentric chromosomes and the radiation dose

A calibration curve is needed to estimate the dose received from the observed number of aberrations. It is agreed that radiation has the same effect on lymphocytes whether they are exposed *in vitro* or *in vivo* (in particular the number of dicentrics is the same). Figure 3.23 shows reference curves for different types of radiation. These curves must be established in each laboratory as they depend critically on the techniques used.

As indicated above, the number of dicentrics varies with dose according to a linear-quadratic relation ($E=\alpha D+\beta D^2$), and the ratio α/β is equal to $0\cdot3$ Gy (Section 4.3). Thus, when estimating the dose received by the subjects the linear

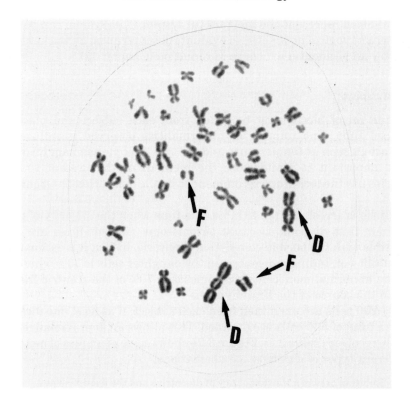

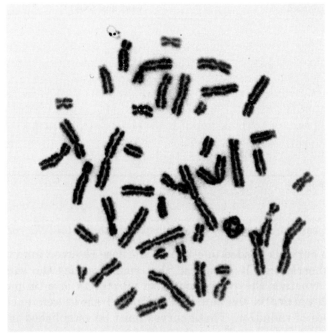

Figure 3.24. Chromosome anomalies in human lymphocytes.
Left, two dicentric chromosomes (D) and two pairs of fragments (F);
right, one ring.
By courtesy of A. Leonard.

term αD is usually predominant and the number of dicentrics observed is almost independent of the distribution of dose as a function of time. Table 3.1 indicates, as a function of the number of dicentrics observed, the integral dose received by the subject as well as its confidence limits. It illustrates in particular the need to examine a large number of cells in metaphase, which lengthens the time required for the analysis. However, it must be noted that the calibration curves are not reliable for doses below 25 cGy or for very low dose rates such as those encountered in radiation protection (except for accidental irradiation).

Importance and limits of the method of biological dosimetry by counting dicentric chromosomes

PERSISTENCE OF RADIATION-INDUCED CHROMOSOME ABERRATIONS: PRACTICAL IMPLICATIONS

Based on observations made on people who have been accidentally irradiated or irradiated for medical reasons, the half-life of the lymphocytes which carry unstable chromosome abnormalities is estimated to be 3 years. Consequently it is not necessary to take the blood sample immediately after irradiation. Also, observation of chromosome aberrations makes it possible to assess the dose accumulated during a fairly long period (with the reservations mentioned above).

PARTIAL-BODY IRRADIATION

Lymphocytes pass quickly from the peripheral blood into a large compartment ('pool') distributed throughout the body. They do not remain for more than 5 min in the peripheral blood; outside the vessels B lymphocytes are transformed into plasmocytes which participate in immunological reactions. If the irradiation is not homogenous, the number of chromosome aberrations does not allow one to estimate the dose at a point, but provides a kind of mean dose integrated over the whole body. In this respect we must emphasize that the majority of the lymphocytes are not to be found in the blood, lymph nodes or bone marrow [12]: for a total body content of 1300 g of lymphocytes, only 3 g is present in the circulating blood, 100 g in lymphoid tissue and 70 g in the marrow.

FACTORS PRODUCING CHROMOSOME ABERRATIONS

The chromosome abnormalities produced by ionizing radiation are not specific and can be produced by various chemical mutagens (in particular tobacco, cytotoxic drugs used in chemotherapy, combustion gases and many chemical pollutants). Thus, if a subject suspected of having been exposed to ionizing radiation shows abnormalities of this type, it is necessary to enquire whether there has been exposure to other mutagenic agents. It is also necessary to take account of age as the frequency of aberrations increases with age.

Conclusion

Biological dosimetry based on the observation of chromosome abnormalities in the lymphocytes of an irradiated person represents an important complement to physical dosimetry. It is based essentially on the counting of *dicentric chromo-somes*, an abnormality which is rare in the absence of irradiation. The number of dicentrics is referred to calibration curves which are only valid in the labor-atory where they have been established and under strict conditions of standard-ization of the examination techniques. It provides an estimate of the average dose and makes it possible in certain cases to demonstrate that a subject has not received any significant exposure. However, its specificity and sensitivity are limited. It is not reliable below 25 cGy or when the dose rate is very low. This method is relatively simple and involves no inconvenience for the subject examined. Its validity and usefulness were demonstrated during the Chernobyl accident. We will return (Chapter 12) to the practical aspects of its use in radiation protection.

3.5 DNA lesions and cell death

Several arguments show that DNA molecules are the main targets for cell death. However, this does not exclude other structures, in particular membranes [1], from being critical for the survival of microorganisms and mammalian cells.

Relative importance of the nucleus and the cytoplasm

It is possible to irradiate selectively either the nucleus or the cytoplasm by means of microbeams of protons or by means of ^{210}Po (this radionuclide emits α-particles whose range in tissue is only 40 μm). Also, with the technique of micro-dissection it is possible to extract the nucleus and irradiate the cytoplasm alone, the nucleus being reimplanted later. Alternatively, an irradiated nucleus can be reimplanted in unirradiated cytoplasm. These different experiments show that to kill a cell the dose which must be given to the nucleus is a 100 times smaller than that which must be given to the cytoplasm.

Other techniques make use of labelled compounds. Compounds labelled with tritium are particularly suitable as this radionuclide emits β-particles of 18 keV whose range in tissue is less than 1 or 2 μm. It is therefore possible to irradiate selectively the structure which has incorporated the compound labelled with tritium. [^{3}H]Thymidine, a specific precursor of DNA, irradiates only the nucleus. On the other hand uridine which is a component of RNA is found both in the nucleus and the cytoplasm. Comparison of the effects of [^{3}H]thymidine and [^{3}H]uridine has clearly shown that irradiation of the nucleus is responsible for cell death.

Similarly, ^{3}H added as tritiated water is 1000 times less effective than [^{3}H]thymidine. Compounds labelled with ^{125}I which are incorporated in DNA are 200–300 times more effective than those which are attached to the cell membrane and irradiate only the cytoplasm.

Role of the chromosomes

The importance of the chromosomes and their relation to radiosensitivity are well established. As long ago as 1949, Latarjet and Ephrussi [16] showed that, for yeast in a haploid or a diploid state, an increase in ploidy increased the radio-resistance. We now know that this is due to the recombination pathway which can repair double-strand breaks only if the cell is diploid.

There is also a correlation between radiosensitivity and factors such as the volume of the nucleus, the quantity of DNA per nucleus and, for a given quantity, the volume of the chromosomes in interphase and their DNA content. These correlations have been shown in cells from different types of organism such as plants, amphibians, insects and mammals (Figures 3.25 and 3.26).

Finally, there is a relation between cellular lethality at the first mitosis and the presence of chromosome aberrations. This relation is seen under different experimental conditions, in particular in different phases of the cycle and also in the presence of radiosensitizing agents.

Administration of [³H]thymidine produces chromosome aberrations, and a relation has been observed between the points of breakage of the chromatids and the regions where [³H]thymidine was incorporated, visualized by autoradiography.

The DNA molecule: the 'target' structure for cellular lethality

Radiosensitivity and DNA content

The first argument is the correlation between the radiosensitivity of different cellular species, from viruses to mammalian cells, and their DNA content, their degree of complexity and the effectiveness of DNA repair mechanisms.

For viruses with a single strand of DNA or RNA, there is a correlation

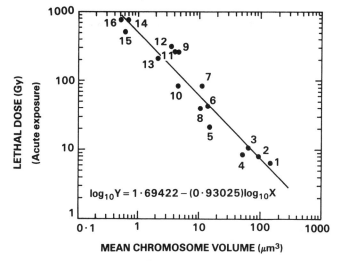

Figure 3.25. Relation between radiosensitivity and chromosome volume for 16 species of plants. Radiosensitivity is measured by the dose needed to inhibit growth of the plant. The mean volume per chromosome is defined as the ratio between the volume of the nucleus in interphase and the number of chromosomes. The relationship on logarithmic coordinates is a straight line of slope close to −1. This shows that the energy absorbed per chromosome to inhibit growth of the plant is practically constant, independent of the dimensions of the target.
After [30].

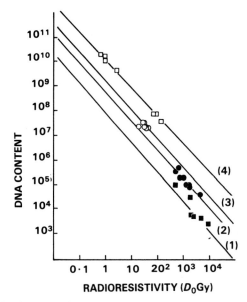

Figure 3.26. Relation between the DNA content (expressed as the number of nucleotides) and radiosensitivity (expressed by the D_0; see Section 4.3) for different types of organism from viruses to mammalian cells. These organisms are subdivided into four classes of radiosensitivity:
(1) viruses consisting of single strand of DNA (or RNA);
(2) viruses consisting of a double strand of DNA;
(3) bacteria and haploid yeasts;
(4) diploid yeasts and cells of birds and mammals.
Within each class there is a relation between the content of DNA (or RNA) and radiosensitivity, indicating that the greater the content of DNA (or RNA) the larger is the 'target' with a greater chance of being damaged, while *within each class* the energy needed for inactivation is relatively constant. The lowest line, which refers to single-strand viruses (DNA or RNA) irradiated under conditions in which the 'indirect effect' (Section 2.3) is reduced to a minimum, corresponds to a *G* value close to unity. Since 100 eV is the order of magnitude of the energy deposited by a primary 'event', *G* can be considered to represent approximately the number of molecules destroyed per primary event. One can therefore deduce that a single primary event taking place at any point in the strand can inactivate these viruses (see text). Apparently the lesions are distributed uniformly along the DNA molecule and there is no region which is particularly vulnerable or preferentially attacked.
After [15].

between radiosensitivity and the amount of nucleic acids, DNA or RNA (Figure 3.26). This suggests that breakage of the strand leads to inactivation of the virus, the energy needed being independent of the length of the molecule. In this case, as the molecule of DNA or RNA constitutes the 'target', the larger it is, the more radiosensitive is the virus.

The radioresistivity of viruses with a double strand of DNA, (normalized per unit mass of DNA) is about 10 times greater. This suggests that inactivation of the virus requires a double-strand break; a single-strand break can be repaired using the intact strand as template. There is one double-strand break for about 10 single-strand breaks (p. 46.)

Experiments using the incorporation of ^{32}P or [^{3}H]thymidine in DNA provide evidence in favour of this interpretation. If a double-strand virus is incubated in

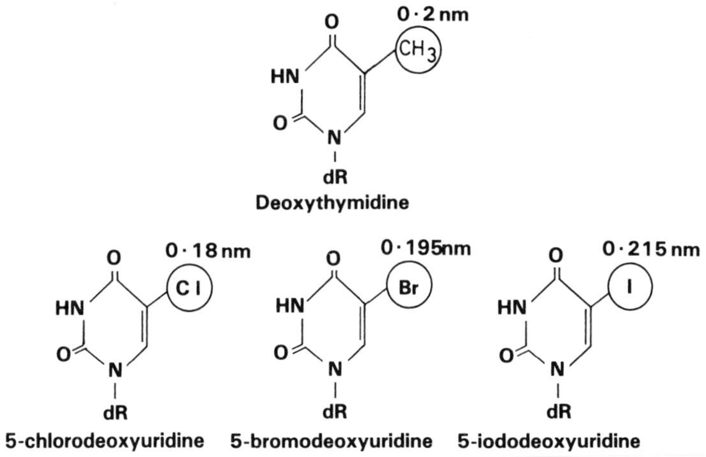

Figure 3.27. The methyl group of thymine shows a Van der Waals radius very similar to that of the halogen atoms, iodine, chlorine or bromine. This explains the possibility of 'metabolic errors' during the synthesis of DNA molecules. After [14].

a medium containing ^{32}P, the molecules of DNA are irradiated selectively during disintegration of the [32]P (suicide effect). Emission of the β-ray seems not to play an important role but the nuclear recoil (which carries an energy of about 80 eV) leads to breakage of the strand in which it is incorporated. In a double-strand virus about one disintegration in ten of ^{32}P produces breakage of both strands and inactivation of the virus. In a single-strand virus each disintegration corresponds to one inactivation.

The greater radioresistivity (for a given DNA content) of bacteria and haploid yeast (Figure 3.26) implies that repair mechanisms are more effective and in particular that double-strand breaks can be repaired. The protein support of the chromosome may help to keep the fragments in position and thus facilitate the mechanisms of repair.

Finally, the relative radioresistivity of diploid yeast and mammalian cells (class 4 in Figure 3.26) can be interpreted partly by more efficient repair mechanisms, but also by the fact that much of the information contained in the DNA molecules is not necessary for survival and proliferation. Ploidy also plays a role in that the information is retained in two chromosomes and the destruction of one of them may have less serious consequences.

Experiments with analogues

If microorganisms or cells are cultivated in the presence of 5-bromodeoxyuridine (5 BrdU), errors of metabolism can be induced and DNA molecules are obtained in which a certain proportion of thymidine is replaced by BrdU. BrdU, like 5-iododeoxyuridine, is an analogue of thymidine; its spatial configuration is similar which explains the possibility of metabolic errors (Figure 3.27). The substitution of thymine by the halogenated analogue leads to a separation of the DNA strands because of the presence of the large atom of bromine, and increases cellular radiosensitivity due to the lability provoked by Br atoms. This increase in radiosensitivity is larger when the level of analogue incorporation is greater (Figure 3.28) (see Chapter 10).

Absorption spectra of nucleic acids

When bacteria are exposed to UV of different wavelengths, a correlation is seen between their effectiveness for killing the bacteria and the absorption spectra of DNA. These observations demonstrate the role of DNA lesions in bacterial death (Figure 3.29).

Mechanisms of repair of DNA lesions

A final argument is provided by the correlation between absence, or alteration, in the mechanisms of DNA repair and increase in radiosensitivity. This correlation has been observed with microorganisms (e.g. mutants) and in humans (p. 59). Repair of double-strand breaks seems to play a crucial role in radiosensitivity.

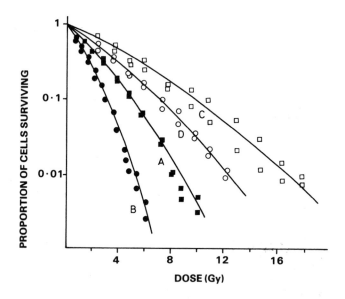

Figure 3.28. Comparison of survival curves of mammalian cells after incorporation of an analogue, BrdU, and administration of a radioprotective agent, dimethyl-sulphoxide (DMSO). Incorporation of the analogue makes the molecule of DNA more fragile and increases the cellular radiosensitivity (curves A and B). On the other hand, administration of DMSO protects both the cells which have incorporated BrdU (D) and those which have not (C). DMSO captures HO. radicals and increases cellular radioresitance, suggesting the role of an 'indirect effect'.
After [5].

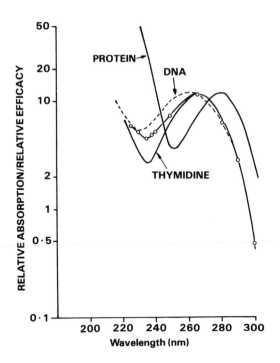

Figure 3.29. Absorption spectra of UV by the DNA molecules of *E.coli*, thymidine and a protein (trypsin). These spectra are compared with the spectrum of UV efficiency for killing *E.coli* (○). The spectrum of effectiveness of UV is similar to the absorption in DNA and thymidine but is different from that of protein.
After [14].

References

1. T. Alper, *Cellular radiobiology*. Cambridge University Press, Cambridge, 1979.
2. G. W. Barendsen. Influence of radiation quality on the effectiveness of small doses for induction of reproductive death and chromosome aberrations in mammalian cells. *Int. J. Radiat. Biol.*,1979, **36**: 49–63.
3. K. E. Buckton, H. J. Evans. Methods for the analysis of human chromosome aberrations. World Health Organization, Geneva, 1973.
4. T. Caspersson, L. Zech, C. Johansson. Differential binding of alkylating fluorochromes in human chromosomes. *Exp. Cell Res.* 1970, **60**: 315–319.
5. J. D. Chapman, in: *Radiation biology in cancer research* (R. E. Meyn and H. R. Withers, eds). Raven Press, New York, 1980.
6. J. E. Coggle. *Biological effects of radiation* (2nd edn). Taylor and Francis, London, 1983.
7. P. N. Dean, F. Dolbeare, H. Gratzner, G. C. Rice, J. W. Gray. Cell-cycle analysis using a monoclonal antibody to BrdU. *Cell Tissue Kinetics*, 1984, **17**: 427–436.
8. Ch. de Duve. *Biochimie médicale*. Univ. Catholique de Louvain, 1985.
9. B. L. Diffey. Ultra-violet radiation in medicine. *Medical Physics Handbooks, 11*. Adam Hilger, Bristol, 1982.
10. M. Dizdaroglu, M. G. Simic. Radiation-induced formation of thymine–thymine crosslink. *Int. J. Radiat. Biol.*, 1984, **46**: 241–246.
11. B. Dutrillaux, J. Lejeune. Sur une nouvelle technique d'analyse du caryotype humain. *C.R. Acad. Sci.* (Paris), 1971, **272**: 2638–2640.
12. H. J. Evans. Use of chromosome aberration frequencies for biological dosimetry in man, in: *Advances in physical and biological radiation detectors*. International Atomic Energy Agency, Vienna, 1971. IAEA-SM-143/77, 593–609.

13. L. Fabry, A. Leonard, A. Wambersie. Induction of chromosome aberrations in G_0 human lymphocytes by low doses of ionizing radiations of different qualities. *Radiat. Res.*, 1985, **103**: 122–134.

14. M. Friedman. *The biological and clinical basis of radiosensitivity*. Charles C. Thomas, Springfield, Ill., 1974.

15. H.S. Kaplan, L.E. Moses, Biological complexity and radiosensitivity. *Science*, 1964, **145**: 21–25.

16. R. Latarjet, B. Ephrussi. Courbes de survie des levures haploides et diploides soumises aux rayons X. *C.R. Acad. Sci.*, Paris, 1949, **229**: 306–308.

17. D.E. Lea, D.G. Catcheside. The mechanism of the induction by radiation of chromosome aberrations in Tradescantia. *J. Genet.*, 1942, **44**: 216–245.

18. E. Moustacchi. Structure et fonctionnement de l'ADN; réparation de l'ADN, in: *Mécanismes de la cancérogénèse; progrès récents et idées nouvelles*. Electricité de France, Paris, 1985, 3–19.

19. R.B. Painter, B.R. Young. Radiosensitivity in ataxia-telangiectasia: A new explanation. *Proc. Natl. Acad. Sci.*, USA, 1980, **77**: 7315–7317.

20. R.J. Purrott, D.C. Lloyd, J.S. Prosser, G.W. Dolphin, P.A. Tipper, E.J. Reeder, C.M. White, S.J. Cooper, B.D. Stephenson. The study of chromosome aberration yield in human lymphocytes as an indicator of radiation dose. IV. A review of cases investigated. Natl. Rad. Protection Board (NRPB) G.B., R 23, 1975.

21. S.H. Revell. Evidence for a dose-squared term in the dose–response curve for real chromatic discontinuities induced by X-rays and some theoretical consequences thereof. *Mutation Res.*, 1966, **3**: 34–53.

22. S. Rose. DNA in medicine. Human perfectibility. *Lancet*, 1984, **2**: 1380–1383.

23. D. Rydberg. Repair of DNA double-strand breaks in colcemid-arrested mitotic Chinese hamster cells. *Int. J. Radiat. Biol.*, 1984, **46**: 299–304.

24. A. Sancar, W.D. Rupp. A novel repair enzyme: UVRABC excision nuclease of *Escherichia coli* cuts a DNA strand on both sides of the damaged region. *Cell*, 1983, **33**: 249–260.

25. N.J. Sargentini, K.C. Smith. Quantitation of the involvement of the *recA, recB, recC, recF, recJ, recN, lexA, radA, radB, uvrD*, and *umuC* genes in the repair of X-ray-induced DNA double-strand breaks in *Escherichia coli. Radiat. Res.*, 1986, **107**: 58–72.

26. J.R.K. Savage. Induction and consequences of structural chromosome aberrations, in: *The biological basis of radiotherapy* (G.G. Steel, G.E. Adams and M.J. Peckham, eds), pp. 93–103. Elsevier, Amsterdam, 1983.

27. K. Sax. Time factor in X-ray production of chromosome aberrations. *Proc. Natl. Acad. Sci.* USA, 1939, **25**: 225–233.

28 D. Scott, F. Zampetti-Bosseler. Cell cycle dependence of mitotic delay in X-irradiated normal and ataxia-telangiectasia fibroblasts. *Int. J. Radiat. Biol.*, 1982, **42**: 679–683.

29. A.H. Sparrow. Research uses of the gamma field and related radiation facilities at Brookhaven National Laboratory. *Radiat. Bot.*, 1966, **6**: 377–405.

30. J. Thacker, R. Wilkinson, A. Ganesh, P. North. Mechanisms of resistance to ionising radiations: genetic and molecular studies on Ataxia-telangiectasia and related radiation-sensitive mutants, in: *DNA repair mechanisms and their biological implications in mammalian cells* (M.W. Lambert, ed), Plenum, New York (in press).

31. J. Thacker. The use of integrating DNA vectors to analyse the molecular defects in ionising radiation-sensitive mutants of mammalian cells including Ataxia-telangiectasia, *Mutation Res.*, 1989, **220**: 187–204.

32. L.H. Thompson, K.W. Brookman, L.E. Dillehay, A.V. Carrano, J.A. Mazrimas, C.L. Mooney, J.L. Minkler. A CHO-cell strain having hypersensitivity to mutagens, a defect in DNA strand-break repair, and an extraordinary baseline frequency of sister-chromatid exchange. *Mutation Res.*, 1982, **95**: 427–440.

33. L.H. Thompson, J.S. Rubin, J.E. Cleaver, G.F. Whitmore, K. Brookman. A screening method for isolating DNA repair-deficient mutants of CHO cells. *Somatic Cell Genet.*, 1980, **6**: 391–405.

34. M. Tubiana. Cinétique de prolifération cellulaire des tumeurs, signification de la période pré-clinique. *Revue du Praticien*, 1980, **30**: 173–186.

35. D.J. Weatherall. DNA in medicine. Implications for medical practice and human biology. *Lancet*, 1984, **2**: 1440–1444.

36. L. Wolpert. DNA and its message. *Lancet*, 1984, **2**: 853–856.

37. F. Zampetti-Bosseler, D. Scott. Cell death, chromosome damage and mitotic delay in normal human, ataxia telangiectasia and retinoblastoma fibroblasts after X-irradiation. *Int. J. Radiat. Biol.*, 1981, **39**: 547–558.

Bibliography

B. Alberts, D. Bray, J. Lewis, M. Raff, K. Roberts, J.D. Watson. *Molecular biology of the cell.* Garland, New York and London, 1983.

K.H. Chadwick, H.P. Leenhouts. *The molecular theory of radiation biology.* Springer, Berlin, 1981.

E.C. Friedberg. *DNA repair,* W.H. Freeman, New York, 1984.

G.G. Steel, G.E. Adams, M.J. Peckham. *The biological basis of radiotherapy.* Elsevier, Amsterdam, 1983.

J.D. Watson, N.H. Hopkins, J.W. Roberts, J.A. Steitz, A.M. Weiner. *Molecular biology of the gene,* vol. 1 (4th edn). Benjamin/Cummings, Menlo Park, Calif., 1987.

Chapter 4.
Cellular effects of ionizing radiation.
Cell survival curves.

A number of effects are produced by the irradiation of cells, among which are the following:

1. Subcellular lesions and particularly chromosome aberrations which have been studied in the preceding chapter.
2. Lengthening of the cell cycle or delay in mitosis which can modify the radiosensitivity of a population of cells (Chapter 5) and which must be taken into account in the study of the kinetics of cell populations (see Section 5.1).
3. Acceleration of processes of differentiation in certain cells which have lost their capacity to divide.
4. Alterations in function, but above all cell death or loss of proliferative capacity. This last effect is the main cause of early and late effects in normal tissues and of tumour sterilization.

   This chapter is concerned essentially with cell death and its relationship with dose and modifying factors. It is therefore necessary to begin by defining the concept of cellular survival and death.

4.1 Cell death

After irradiation with a very large dose, several hundred gray, all cellular functions cease and the cell undergoes cytolysis; this is referred to as immediate cell death or death in interphase. With lower doses of a few gray delivered to cells which are dividing or which are still able to divide (such as cell lines of the bone marrow, skin or intestinal crypts), a proportion of the cells lose their capacity for division or proliferation.† *Cell death* is defined as the *irreversible loss of reproductive capacity* (*reproductive death* which occurs at the next or a subsequent mitosis).

---

†Lymphocytes and oocytes can be killed in interphase (see Section 5.3).

Thus a non-viable damaged cell which morphologically appears intact in tissue may still be able to synthesize proteins or DNA and may even be able to pass through one or a small number of mitoses; this cell is nevertheless killed in the sense defined above if it has lost its capacity to divide more or less indefinitely and if its descendants are doomed to die. On the other hand, a surviving or viable cell is one which has retained its proliferative capacity and therefore is able to give rise to a colony or clone; these cells are called *clonogenic* (Figure 4.1). *In vivo*, in tumours or normal tissues, only a small proportion of the cells is clonogenic; their number is decreased after irradiation (Figure 4.1).

This definition is relevant to radiotherapy because a tumour is locally controlled when all its cells, even those which are still present, have lost their

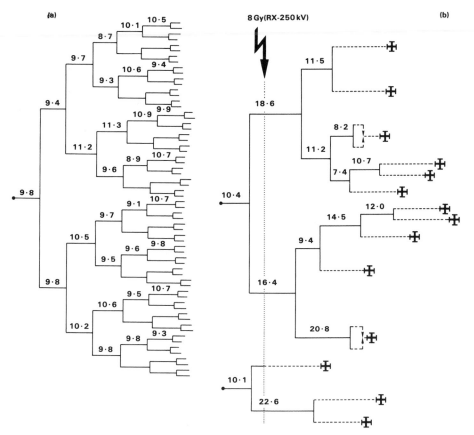

Figure 4.1. **Examples of pedigrees of EMT6 mouse cells.**
(a) In the absence of irradiation, the cell divides giving rise to a clone. The length of each cell cycle is indicated, about 10 h.
(b) After irradiation (in this example: 8 Gy), the cells are killed, that is to say they have lost their reproductive capacity. In certain cases (near the bottom) pyknosis and lysis of the cell occurs at the first mitosis. In other cases (above) the daughter cells are still able to divide a few times before lysis. In a few cases fusion of cells occurs before disintegration ( ). These pedigrees were obtained by microcinematography; the fate and progeny of individual cells can be followed. Microphotographs are taken at regular intervals (e.g. every 4 min) and in this way the length of the cycle of cells of different generations can be measured together with the appearance of pyknosis.
After [16].

power of indefinite proliferation and therefore of local invasion or distant metastasis. In the same way, for normal tissues most of the acute and late effects of radiation are caused by loss of cellular viability.

This definition of cell death is also suitable in radiation protection for interpretation of the acute effects of radiation. When a tissue has been damaged by radiation, its regeneration depends on the number of stem cells which have survived and on the integrity of their capacity for proliferation; it is these surviving cells which, by proliferating rapidly, reconstitute the damaged tissue (Chapter 5).

The concept of reproductive death is clearly not applicable to differentiated cells which are capable of performing a specialized function but which under normal conditions no longer divide, for example, nerve, muscle and secretory cells. These cells are intrinsically very resistant to irradiation but in the tissues to which they belong they can be killed indirectly by damage to interstitial or vascular cells which are essential to their function and survival.

4.2 *Methods of measuring the proportion of surviving cells*

The first survival curves for mammalian cells were obtained by Puck and Marcus [40] whose work marks the beginning of quantitative cellular radiobiology. The curves were obtained by *in vitro* cloning, by techniques similar, though more delicate, to those used in microbiology for measuring the number of bacteria or yeast cells. The practical difficulties have been progressively solved and the techniques are now widely used. The method is relatively simple, rapid, reproducible and not expensive. However, it is difficult to know to what extent the behaviour of the cells cultured *in vitro* is representative of their behaviour *in vivo*.

This question emphasizes the importance of cellular survival curves *in vivo* so that the results obtained *in vitro* and *in vivo* can be compared. Survival curves *in vivo* have been obtained either by cloning *in vivo* or indirectly from observations of tissue reactions or tumour responses. However, these methods have their limitations; they depend on hypotheses which are often difficult to verify and the techniques are generally slow and relatively expensive.

Tests of viability *in vitro*

Irradiation and cloning in vitro

This technique can be applied with varying degrees of difficulty to most cells from animal and human tumours. It can also be applied to certain types of normal cells such as fibroblasts.

A suspension of single cells is cultured under well defined conditions (Figure 4.2). Each viable clonogenic cell, according to the definition given above, is able to multiply and give birth to a colony or clone. The clones are counted; the proportion of seeded cells giving rise to a clone as a function of the dose of radiation is graphically expressed by the cell survival curve. To start with, a sample of tumour is taken from which a suspension of single cells is prepared by trypsinization. This is seeded into culture flasks or Petri dishes. Modern

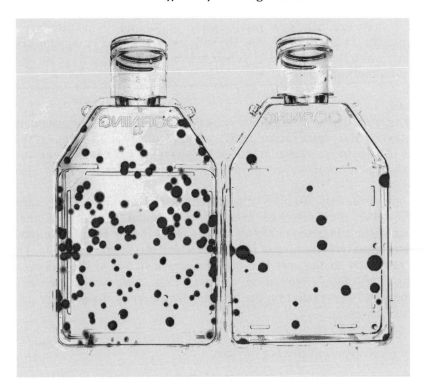

Figure 4.2. Measurement of cell survival curve by cloning *in vitro*. A suitable number of mammalian cells in a single cell suspension is seeded in a culture flask. The conditions of culture are carefully controlled: growth medium, asepsis, temperature and pH. The cells become fixed to the surface of the flask and begin to divide. Each gives rise to a colony or clone which after 1 or 2 weeks contains enough cells to be visible to the naked eye.

A cell is considered to be viable or surviving if it gives rise to a clone containing more than 50 cells. The counting of colonies is easier after staining. In practice the number of visible colonies is always less than the number of cells initially incubated, e.g. 50 instead of 100. The ratio of the number of visible colonies to the number of cells incubated is called the plating efficiency; this varies considerably with the cell line and the experimental conditions.

After irradiation (right) the number of clones is reduced. In practice the dilution is adjusted to give a convenient number of colonies per culture flask whatever the dose of radiation given. The surviving fraction is easy to measure: e.g. if 80 colonies are counted in the absence of irradiation and 8 after a dose of 6 Gy, the surviving fraction S for this dose is 8/80 or 0·10. A number of doses are delivered and the cell survival curve is established in this way point by point.

techniques make it possible to culture most tumour cells for several weeks, after which the cells become exhausted and die.

A small number of cell lines can multiply for a longer time, for several years or even quasi-indefinitely. These cell lines are called established or immortalized and are much used in radiobiological experiments. In order to maintain the cultures, every few days cells must be detached from the surface of the culture bottle by means of trypsin. They are then diluted and a small number reseeded into another flask where they can continue to proliferate.

The population of cells can be irradiated either in *exponential phase* or in *stationary phase*. In the first case a small number of cells is seeded in the culture medium; they are all in a proliferative state and their number grows exponentially. In the second case the culture is allowed to develop without reseeding; when the density of cells becomes very high the cells cease to divide and enter a resting phase.

REMARKS

The test of viability by cloning does not take account of all the consequences of irradiation on the proliferative capacity of the cells [37]. It is known that the number of cells in the clones produced by surviving cells depends on the dose which they have received: the proportion of small clones increases with dose (Section 5.1).

This shows that the kinetics of proliferation are modified in the surviving cells. However, it is not clear from the experimental results whether this functional deficit is irreversible; in certain cases it may be accompanied by a reduction in the total number of mitoses of which the cells are capable. There is also a reduction in the speed of division which is one of the causes of the immediate effects of irradiation on tissue; its repercussion on the final consequences, in particular on the late effects in normal tissues, is probably of little importance.

Irradiation in vivo *and cloning* in vitro

A population of tumour cells can be irradiated *in vivo* under conditions similar to those of radiotherapy; the proportion of viable cells is assayed *in vitro* after preparation of a suspension of single cells from the tumour (Figure 4.3a). This method has practical advantages and is widely used.

In vivo tests of viability

The technique of cloning *in vitro* has several advantages: simplicity, reproducibility and modest expense. However, it is essential to verify to what extent the proportion of surviving cells measured *in vitro* represents the intrinsic characteristics of the cells, since survival can be influenced by the experimental conditions.

The interactions between cells *in vitro* are different from those existing *in vivo*. The importance of intercellular contacts for the repair of lesions is now well recognized. Moreover the *in vitro* technique is delicate and scoring the results is not always simple because the large colonies which are to be included in the count must be distinguished from the small abortive colonies. Finally one must be sure that single cells were seeded and not small groups composed of two or three cells which would vitiate the results.

The viability of malignant cells can be measured *in vivo* by their capacity to induce tumours or to give rise to metastatic colonies. Survival curves of cells from certain normal tissues have also been obtained by *in vivo* cloning. We will describe only the methods used most frequently, namely counting of colonies in the spleen and intestines.

Viability of malignant cells and production of tumours

The first cell survival curve *in vivo* was established by Hewitt and Wilson in 1959 [21]. This was for a spontaneous lymphocytic leukaemia and was measured by the dilution technique. For this technique a suspension of single cells is prepared from the tumour of origin and an increasing number of cells is injected into different groups of animals. To begin with, it is necessary to measure the number of unirradiated cells which must be injected to produce a tumour in 50% of the animals, the TD 50 (Figure 4.3c). TD 50 means 'take dose' 50 — the dose of cells for 50% takes. This number depends on various factors such as the proportion of clonogenic cells and the effectiveness of the immune defences of the recipient animals with regard to the cell line injected. The survival curve of the malignant cells is obtained from the increase in TD 50 with increasing dose delivered to the donor animal immediately before excision of the tumour sample.

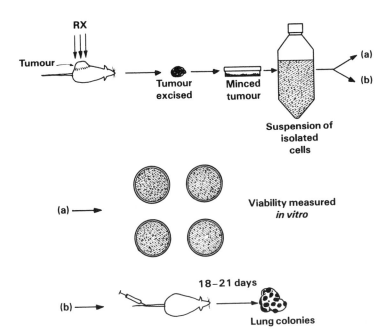

Figure 4.3. (a) Establishment of a cell survival curve combining irradiation *in vivo* and cloning *in vitro*. The solid tumour is irradiated *in vivo*. It is then excised and a suspension of dispersed cells is prepared whose viability is measured by their capacity to form colonies *in vitro*. The advantage of this method is that the irradiation can be given *in vivo* without disturbing cell–cell interactions, the distribution of cells in the cell cycle or the degree of oxygenation; moreover evaluation of the clonogenicity of the cells is easier and less expensive *in vitro* than *in vivo*.
(b) The irradiation is performed *in vivo* as in (a) but the viability of the cells is also measured *in vivo* by their capacity to form colonies in the lung. The cell suspension is prepared as in (a); the cells, after being counted, are injected intravenously into a recipient animal. After about 3 weeks the animal is sacrificed and the number of colonies in the lungs is counted. This number is proportional to the number of viable cells injected. Each colony observed is assumed to result from the proliferation of one injected viable cell. This technique has been used with KHT sarcomas and Lewis lung tumours.
(a) After [2]; (b) after [22].

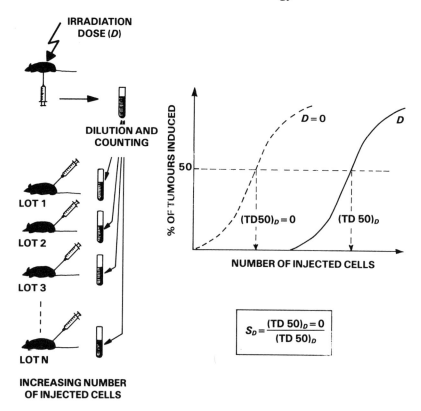

Figure 4.3. (c) Measurement of a cell survival curve *in vivo* for malignant cells by the method of tumour induction [21]. The TD 50 must first be determined (i.e. the number of malignant cells which must be injected to produce a tumour in 50% of the animals) by means of a host/tumour system (a strain of animals which does not reject a particular line of malignant cells). For this purpose, increasing numbers of malignant cells are inoculated into different groups of animals and the TD 50 is deduced from the relation between the percentage of tumour takes and the number of cells injected (dashed line curve). To establish the cell survival curve, this determination of TD 50 is repeated with different doses of radiation (solid curve). For example, if after a given dose the TD 50 observed is 10 times greater than the initial TD 50, 90% of the cells must have been killed in the sense defined above (Section 4.1). Under these conditions the cell survival curve is evaluated from the capacity of the cells to proliferate and produce a tumour. The number of malignant cells to be injected is measured immediately after irradiation of the donor animal: at this time examination under the microscope cannot distinguish between viable and non-viable cells.

Viability of malignant cells and cloning in vivo *by the technique of lung colonies*

The solid tumour is irradiated *in vivo, in situ*. The survival of the cells is assayed by their capacity to give birth to clones in the form of lung colonies in a recipient animal (Figure 4.3b).

Viability of haemopoietic stem cells and counting of spleen colonies

This method was devised by Till and McCulloch [49]. Bone-marrow cells, including haemopoietic stem cells are taken from mice and injected into homologous animals which had previously been irradiated with doses of about

9 Gy, enough to destroy practically all their haemopoietic stem cells but insufficient to kill the animals by the gastrointestinal syndrome. The donor cells injected intravenously become lodged in the haemopoietic sites of the recipient animals, in particular in the spleen where they form nodules. A week later the nodules become visible to the naked eye. Each of these nodules is a colony, or clone, formed by the progeny of one stem cell from the donor animal; their number is therefore proportional to the number of viable stem cells injected (or *colony forming units*, CFU). The survival curve for the stem cells is obtained by irradiating the donor animal (or the suspension of cells to be injected) with increasing doses (Figure 4.4). The spleen nodule technique is also applicable to leukaemia cells.

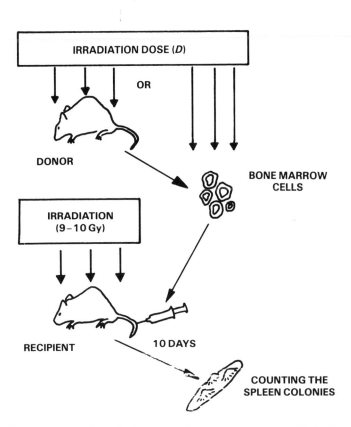

Figure 4.4. Measurement of survival curves of bone marrow stem cells by the spleen colonies method of Till and McCulloch [49]. The bone marrow cells of the donor animal are injected into the previously irradiated recipient (dose of *c* 10 Gy). The recipient is sacrificed after 10 days and the spleen removed. Greyish white nodules are visible and stand out against the dark red background of the spleen. In practice it is possible to count 15–20 colonies per spleen. A large number of cells (average 10^4) must be injected to obtain a nodule as not all stem cells seed in the spleen and only one cell out of several hundred bone marrow cells is a stem cell capable of giving rise to a colony. The stem cells cannot be identified morphologically. To obtain the cell survival curve the bone marrow cells are irradiated with graded doses either in the donor animal or after extraction. The corresponding reduction in the number of spleen colonies is noted. The number of injected cells is adjusted by dilution to obtain a convenient number of colonies to be counted.

In a variant of the method, spleen colonies are counted which arise from proliferation of the stem cells of the irradiated animal itself. This variant does not require injection of cells but the range of doses which can be used (4–8 Gy of γ-rays) is limited if one wishes to obtain a convenient number of nodules for counting [20].

Use can also be made of the diffusion chamber technique. The cells are introduced into the peritoneal cavity of an animal in a chamber which is impermeable to the cells but permeable to biological fluids [3].

Cloning in vivo *of intestinal crypt cells*

In the non-irradiated intestine the stem cells of the intestinal crypts divide and give rise to cells which differentiate and migrate along the villi to replace progressively the cells which die by senescence and are shed into the intestinal lumen (Chapter 5).

A dose of 10–15 Gy, given to mice either total body or to the abdomen alone, kills a large proportion of the crypt cells but has no effect on the differentiated cells of the villi which do not divide. During the days following irradiation the crypts become progressively depleted of cells (Section 5.3).

The method developed by Withers and Elkind [54] to establish a survival curve for intestinal crypt cells in mice consists of irradiating groups of animals with increasing doses and sacrificing them 3·5 days later. At this time the beginning of regeneration can be seen in those crypts in which at least one stem cell has retained its proliferative capacity. These crypts are easy to identify in a histological section and the effect of irradiation is expressed by the number of regenerating crypts per jejunal circumference.

This technique is widely used for studying the effects of fractionation and dose rate and for comparison of radiations of different qualities (relative biological efficiency, RBE). For any modality of irradiation the doses must be adjusted in such a way as to give between 1 and 100 regenerating crypts per circumference, i.e. a single dose of 11–16 Gy of γ-rays.

Cloning in vivo *for other cell lines from normal tissues*

The method of transplantation of single cells as used for haemopoietic stem cells has been adapted to test the viability of cells of the thyroid [5], breast [15] and liver [25].

Methods analogous to that described for the intestine have been developed for the basal cells of skin [53], growth cartilage [32], seminiferous tubules [55] and renal tubules [56]. The principle is to place the stem cells which have survived irradiation in conditions where they can proliferate and give rise to colonies which can then be counted. These techniques can be used only over a limited range of dose, because with doses which are too small the number of colonies is too great (they become confluent) and with doses which are too high there are not enough colonies. The presence of a sub-population of cells which is particularly radiosensitive or radioresistant cannot therefore be demonstrated.

Spheroids: an *in vitro* model of malignant tumours

When mammalian cells are cultured, the cells either become attached to the surface of the vessel or they remain isolated in suspension if the medium is gently agitated. However, certain types of cell behave differently and tend to form clumps or 'spheroids'. In this case, after each division the daughter cells remain attached to one another and give rise to a spherical collection of cells which grows by successive divisions. For example, 5 days after seeding single cells, the spheroids can attain a diameter of about 200 μm and after 15 days a diameter greater than 300 μm [46].

Nutrients, in particular oxygen, diffuse inwards from the surface of the spheroids. Their concentration diminishes progressively with depth, leading to a lack of nutrition at the centre as well as an accumulation of waste products which increases as the diameter increases. Under these conditions, in the middle of the spheroids the cell cycle lengthens and a necrotic region develops at the centre.

In the spheroids the cells are connected together by intercellular junctions as in tissue. The organization of the spheroids thus partially simulates conditions *in vivo*. This cell-to-cell interaction greatly increases the capacity for repair in most cell lines, as shown by modification of the survival curve (Figure 4.5) and by experiments in which the dose is delivered in several fractions [8].

The value of spheroids is that they provide, in a relatively simple and reproducible manner, heterogenous cell populations which simulate the conditions seen in tumours *in vivo*. On the surface of the spheroids there are well-oxygenated cells in normal cell cycle; with increasing depth progressively more of the cells are in resting phase and at the centre the cells are hypoxic. In

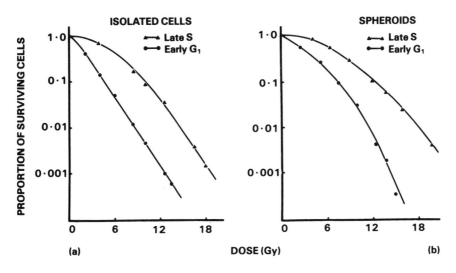

Figure 4.5. Comparison of the effects or irradiation on cells of the same line irradiated in single cell suspension (a), or as spheroids (b). For cells in late S and in early G_1, the modification of the form of the survival curves indicates a greater capacity for accumulation of damage when the cells are irradiated in the form of a spheroid, i.e. linked to neighbouring cells by intercellular junctions.
After [9].

some spheroids with large diameters, up to 20% of the cells are hypoxic as in certain experimental tumours. Spheroids are particularly valuable for studying the actions of sensitizing or cytotoxic drugs (Section 10.1) and their diffusion as well as the effects of hypoxic or quiescent cells.

Other methods

Other methods can be used *in vivo* to obtain cell survival curves or information concerning them. For tumours, the dose required to control 50% (TCD 50) can be determined. This is related to the proportion of surviving cells. Tumour regression or growth delay can also be measured at different dose levels. These end points are affected by the kinetics of cell division in addition to the proportion of surviving cells.

For normal tissues, information can be obtained from studies of macroscopic reactions and in particular isoeffect doses for different schemes of fractionation (Section 8.3). These methods are based on hypotheses which must be established for each particular case as a function of the experimental protocol and the purpose of the experiment.

The results obtained for a given tissue may vary to a considerable extent depending on the method used, partly because different techniques may not give information on exactly the same cells and partly because differences in biological conditions during and after irradiation have a considerable influence on the probability of cell survival [14].

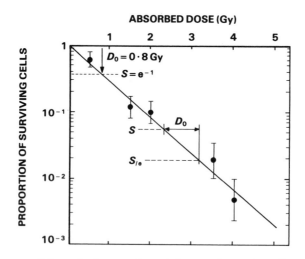

Figure 4.6. Exponential survival curve. In certain experimental studies the curve which best represents the variation of surviving fractions (S) as a function of the dose (D) is an exponential, i.e. a straight line on semi-logarithmic coordinates.

$$S = e^{-D/D_0} \text{ or } \log S = -D/D_0$$

In the case shown in the figure, $D_0 = 0{\cdot}8\,\text{Gy}$; it corresponds to CFUs studied by the technique of spleen colonies (Figure 4.4).

4.3 Cell survival curves

The proportion of surviving cells (S) diminishes as the dose (D) increases. The survival curve is the graphical representation of this relationship; it is obtained by drawing the smooth curve through the experimental points, taking account of the uncertainty of each. It is usually plotted on semi-logarithmic coordinates (log S as a function of D). This type of plot emphasizes the very small values of S at high doses but may make it difficult to appreciate survival after low doses. For comparing curves it is convenient to represent them by mathematical functions. These are based on hypothetical mechanisms of cell lethality, which are usually referred to as models.

The main types of survival curve

Survival curves vary with the biological system studied (bacteria, yeast, mammalian cells), both in terms of their shapes and the absolute value of the surviving fraction at a given dose. Moreover they can be modified by various factors which will be considered below. Some characteristic types can be distinguished. We will consider the most usual survival curves obtained under 'reference' conditions, corresponding to irradiation with X- or γ-rays given as a single dose in a short time and under well-oxygenated conditions.

Exponential survival curves

An exponential relationship (Figure 4.6) between the surviving fraction and the absorbed dose is found for viruses, bacteria and haploid yeasts. For mammalian cells the survival curves usually have a more complex shape but are almost exponential in certain cases:

(i)   certain types of cell (for example, haemopoietic stem cells);
(ii) populations of cells synchronized in M and G_2 (Section 4.4);
(iii) irradiation at high LET (α-particles of several MeV).

The relationship between the surviving fraction S and the dose D is then given by the equation:

$$S=e^{-\alpha D} \tag{1}$$

more commonly represented by

$$S=e^{-D/D_0} \text{ by putting } D_0=1/\alpha$$

where e=base of natural logarithms ≈ 2.7.

The parameter D_0 is called the *mean lethal dose*. D_0 is the dose for which the surviving fraction is equal to $e^{-1}\approx 37\%$, or the additional dose which reduces a surviving fraction S to S/e (this parameter is sometimes denoted by the symbol D_{37}). Equation (1) can also be written

$$\log S=-\alpha D=-D/D_0$$

Table 4.1. Examples of D_0 for various biological species exposed to low LET radiation (photons or electrons).

Species	D_0 (Gy)†
Virus	1500
Bacteria (*E. coli*)	100
Mammalian cells (bone marrow stem cells)	1

†The values indicate orders of magnitude; the survival curves for the cellular species cited are exponential or nearly so. After [20, 27].

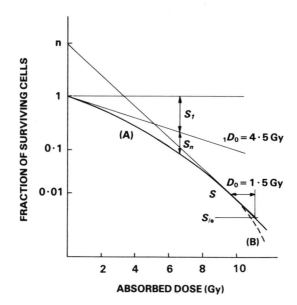

Figure 4.7. Cell survival curves with shoulders. On semi-logarithmic coordinates survival curves of mammalian cells generally show some curvature, usually referred to as a shoulder. Some curves (type A) become straight with larger doses; this part of the curve corresponds to an exponential reduction in surviving fraction and makes it possible to define a value of D_0 which leads to a reduction in the surviving fraction from S to S/e. Extrapolation of the terminal straight line back to the ordinate axis defines the extrapolation number n and the quasi-threshold dose D_q. Other curves (type B, dashed) show continuous curvature over the whole range of doses explored.

In most of the curves of type A and B, the initial slope has a finite value. This slope is defined by the parameter α (or $1/_1D_0$). It can be considered that there are two mechanisms of cell death: (i) due to direct lethal events, leading to a surviving fraction $S_1=e^{-D/_1D_0}$ corresponding to the initial slope; and (ii) due to accumulation of sublethal events leading to a surviving fraction S_n. The total surviving fraction S is equal to the product of the two partial survivals:

$$S = S_1 \times S_n \text{ or } \log S = \log S_1 + \log S_n$$

The survival curve shown in the figure relates to intestinal crypt cells. This curve was obtained from a study of early intestinal tolerance (LD 50) in the mouse [52].

If the cell survival curve is represented by the linear–quadratic relationship, one obtains:

$$\alpha = 0 \cdot 22 \text{ Gy}^{-1}, \text{ and } \beta = 0 \cdot 03 \text{ Gy}^{-2}, \text{ whence } \alpha/\beta = 7 \text{ Gy}$$

With the model of one lethal target and n sublethal targets, the values of the parameters are respectively $_1D_0 = 4 \cdot 50$ Gy, $D_0 = 1 \cdot 5$ Gy and $n = 10$.

With semi-logarithmic coordinates the survival curve is therefore a straight line with slope $-\alpha$ or $-1/D_0$. The value of D_0 shows a wide variation depending on the type of cell (Table 4.1). However, this is reduced if one only considers mammalian cells. It depends on the LET of the radiation (Section 11.1) and can be modified by various other factors.

Survival curves with shoulders

Survival curves for mammalian cells usually show some curvature: the initial part is convex and is called the shoulder (Figure 4.7). Often the distal part tends towards a straight line (curves 2 and 4, Figure 4.8). The parameter D_0 (mean lethal dose) can then be used to characterize the radiosensitivity in this part of the curve. Extrapolation of the terminal straight line (of slope $-1/D_0$) onto the ordinate axis defines a value n, called the extrapolation number. The point at which this line crosses the abscissa for a surviving fraction of 100% is called the quasi-threshold dose D_q.

The two parameters D_0 and n (or D_0 and D_q) define the terminal part of the survival curve but give no information on the initial part (the shoulder) which is, however, the most important in radiotherapy and radiation protection as the doses usually given are found in this area. Measurement of the surviving fraction after small doses requires a high degree of experimental accuracy as the proportion of killed cells is relatively small. When the experiment has sufficient precision it is generally found that the survival curve shows an initial negative slope — the slope of the tangent at the origin — (curves 4 and 5, Figure 4.8).

In certain experimental studies, the survival curves obtained show continuous curvature over the whole region where the surviving fraction has been measured and there is no sign of a straight part in the terminal region (curves 3 and 5, Figure 4.8).

Various mathematical functions have been used to represent these survival curves. They are intended to provide values of the surviving fraction which agree with the experimental values over the range of doses studied, allowing for their statistical precision. The mathematical function depends on the model used.

Mathematical models

Exponential survival curve

This results from simple target theory. Each ionizing particle traversing a cell may produce a lethal event. The production of lethal events is random and the total number of lethal events increases in direct proportion to the dose; the surviving fraction of cells is then an exponential function of dose.

The lethal events produced by a dose D are distributed at random among the cells, various proportions of which suffer 0, 1, 2...n lethal events. A mean number of lethal events per cell (p) can be defined which is equal to the total number of lethal events produced in the cells divided by the total number of cells.

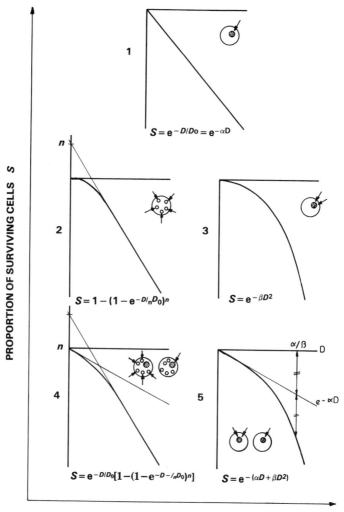

Figure 4.8. Target theory models and cell survival curves.
First model: single hit, single target. Cell death results from damage to a single target by a
lethal event (passage of an ionizing particle). The survival curve is exponential ($S=e^{-D/D_0}$
or $e^{-\alpha D}$) whose slope in semi-logarithmic coordinates is $1/D_0=-\alpha$. D_0 (or $1/\alpha$) is the mean
lethal dose for which the mean number of lethal events per cell is equal to 1. Because of
the random distribution of lethal events in the cells, the proportion of cells surviving a
dose D_0 is e^{-1}, or about $0\cdot37$ (Poisson's law).
Second model: single hit, multi-target. Cell death requires damage to n similar targets
each being inactivated by a single particle. The surviving fraction is given by:

$$S=1-(1-e^{-D/D_0})^n$$

and the survival curve shows a shoulder followed by an exponential part whose slope is
$-1/D_0$. D_0 or the mean lethal dose for each of the n sublethal targets has the same
significance as in the previous model. The extrapolation number n corresponds to the
number of sublethal targets. The tangent at the origin is horizontal.
Third model: two hit, single target (quadratic model). The lethal event for the cells results
from the addition of two independent sublethal events produced by the passage of two
separate particles. The surviving fraction is given by:

$$S=e^{-\beta D^2}$$

The corresponding survival curve shows an initial tangent of zero slope and curves downwards progressively with increasing dose.

Fourth model: single hit, single target, plus single hit, multi-target. Cell death can result from damage to a single lethal target (model 1) or from damage to n sublethal targets (model 2). The surviving fraction is given by:

$$S = e^{-D/_1D_0}(1 - [1 - e^{-D/_nD_0}]^n)$$

The corresponding cell survival curve shows: a tangent at the origin whose slope is given by $-1/_1D_0$; a shoulder; and then tends towards an exponential whose slope is given by:

$$-(1/_1D_0 + 1/_nD_0)$$

The extrapolation number n corresponds to the number of sublethal targets. If one puts

$$1/D_0 = 1/_1D_0 + 1/_nD_0$$

the curve defined by models 2 and 4 are similar for large doses. They differ for small doses, model 4 leading to a tangent at the origin with negative slope.

Fifth model: linear-quadratic. Cell death results either from a single lethal event (linear component model 1) or from the addition of two independent sublethal events (quadratic component model 3). The surviving fraction is given by:

$$S = e^{-(\alpha D + \beta D^2)}$$

It shows a tangent at the origin whose slope is $-\alpha$, followed by progressive downward curvature with increasing dose. Models 4 and 5 both imply the existence of two lethal mechanisms. They lead to a negative slope at the origin but the curve of model 4 tends towards an exponential whereas that of model 5 continues to bend downward with increasing dose.

The statistical law of Poisson indicates that the proportion of cells in which there is no lethal event is equal to e^{-p}; this proportion represents the surviving fraction of cells. By equating the expressions

$$S = e^{-p}$$

and

$$S = e^{-D/D_0} \text{ (or } S = e^{-\alpha D})$$

one sees that $1/D_0$ (or α) is equal to p/D; for a dose D equal to D_0 or $1/\alpha$, the mean number of lethal events per cell is equal to 1.

In biological terms this model signifies that death of the cell is an all or nothing phenomenon; the surviving cell is intact and its radiosensitivity has not been modified. A single hit (damage to the target) is sufficient to kill the cell.

Survival curves with shoulders

In this case the proportion killed by a given increment of dose increases with the dose already given. Two kinds of interpretation are possible:

1. Cell death results from the accumulation of events which individually are incapable of killing the cell but become lethal when added together (target models).

2. Lesions are individually reparable but become irreparable and kill the cell if the efficiency of the enzymatic repair mechanisms diminishes with the number of lesions and therefore with the dose (models based on repair).

Target theory models

Various models have been proposed. We will limit ourselves to those in common usage.

SINGLE HIT MULTI-TARGET MODEL

The cell is supposed to contain n distinct and identical targets which can be individually inactivated by the passage of a charged particle. Inactivation of a target represents a sublethal event and the cell is killed when all n targets have been inactivated. The surviving fraction of cells corresponding to this type of lethality is given by the relation:

$$S = 1 - (1 - e^{-D/D_0})^n \qquad (2)$$

This relationship is based on the hypothesis that damage to the targets is random and that the probability of a target being undamaged is an exponential function of the dose, e^{-D/D_0}.

For a dose equal to D_0 there is on the average one damaging event per target.†

1. The probability that one target is inactivated is

$$1 - e^{-D/D_0}$$

2. The probability that n targets in the same cell are inactivated is $(1 - e^{-D/D_0})^n$; it represents the probability that the cell is killed and the probability of survival is then given by equation (2).

As $D \rightarrow \infty, \; S \rightarrow n e^{-D/D_0}$

This last expression is the exponential equation towards which the survival curve is tending asymptotically; its slope is $-1/D_0$ and it intercepts the ordinate axis at the point n. The dose corresponding to its intersection with the axis of the abscissa is D_q, the quasi-threshold dose. Thus, in this model the parameters D_0 and n (extrapolation number), which define the terminal part of the exponential survival curve, represent respectively the radiosensitivity of the sublethal targets and their number (n) per cell.

QUADRATIC MODEL (TWO HIT, SINGLE TARGET)

Cell lethality results from the addition in a single target of two independent sublethal events, produced by the passage of two separate particles. The mean number of lethal events per cell is then proportional to the square of the dose and the surviving fraction is expressed by the relation:

---

†The ICRU has proposed the symbolism $_nD_0$ to designate the parameter D_0 when there are n targets. $_nD_0$ represents the mean dose for inactivation of the targets.

$$S=e^{-\beta D^2} \tag{3}$$

where β is the parameter relating the dose to the probability of production of a sublethal event.

These two models give a reasonable representation of survival curves for relatively large doses but underestimate the effect of small doses. Equations (2) and (3) produce curves with zero initial slope (i.e. they forecast almost zero mortality for small doses), which is not in agreement with most experimental results; better agreement is obtained with the two-component model discussed below.

TWO-COMPONENT MODEL

According to this model a cell can be killed in two ways, either by a single lethal event or by the accumulation of sublethal events. If these modes of cell death are taken to be independent, the probability of survival (S) is the product of the probabilities of each type of lethal event:

$$S=S_1 S_n$$

where $S_1=e^{-D/_1 D_0}$ (or $e^{-\alpha D}$) is the surviving fraction due to single-hit lethal events, $_1D_0$ is the coefficient relating to the probability of production of directly lethal lesions and S_n is the surviving fraction following the accumulation of sublethal events.

Depending on whether one adopts relation (2) or (3) for S_n, either:

$$S=e^{-D/_1 D_0}[1-(1-e^{-D/_n D_0})^n] \tag{4}$$

where $_nD_0$ is the coefficient for the production of sublethal lesions, or:

$$S=e^{-(\alpha D+\beta D^2)} \tag{5}$$

where $\alpha=1/_1 D_0$. Equation (5) is called the linear–quadratic relationship.

The coefficients α and β relate, respectively, to the two modes of death and their ratio α/β is an index of their relative importance: it is high when the survival curve is almost exponential and small when the shoulder is very wide. When the doses are expressed in Gy, α is expressed in Gy^{-1}, β in Gy^{-2} and α/β in Gy.

The ratio α/β is the dose at which cell death is due equally to irreparable lesions (linear component) and to the accumulation of sublethal lesions (quadratic component); one can then write $\alpha D=\beta D^2$ and $D=\alpha/\beta$ (Figure 4.8). The value of this ratio depends on the type of cell and may be used to characterize the cells from a radiobiological point of view. As we will see (Chapters 5 and 8) it is higher for the cells responsible for early tissue reactions than for those responsible for late effects.

For very high doses equation (4) tends to:

$$S=ne^{-D/_1 D_0} \cdot e^{-D/_n D_0}=ne^{-D/D_0}$$

with $$1/D_0 = 1/_1D_0 + 1/_nD_0$$

Experiments which are limited to large doses give no information about the initial slope and do not make it possible to distinguish between the models represented by equations (4) and (2).

The choice between equations (4) and (5) is difficult as both are usually compatible with the experimental results taking account of their statistical uncertainty (Table 4.2). The second expression (5) has the advantage of needing only two parameters (α and β) instead of three ($_1D_0$, $_nD_0$, n) for the first model. However, for very high doses corresponding to surviving fractions below 1%, the first model usually gives a better fit to the experimental data [1].†

Table 4.2. Radiobiological parameters of some malignant cell lines.

Cell line	Linear–quadratic model			Model with one lethal target and n sublethal targets			
	$\alpha \times 10$ (Gy^{-1})	$\beta \times 100$ (Gy^{-2})	α/β (Gy)	$_1D_0$ (Gy)	D_0 (Gy)	$_1D_0/D_0$	n
T-1	1·8	5·0	3·6	5·6	1·1	5·1	50
R-1	1·8	3·7	4·9	5·5	1·3	4·2	10
RUC-1	1·2	2·3	5·2	8·3	1·5	5·5	20
RUC-2	0·8	1·0	8·0	12·5	2·2	5·7	20
ROS-1	1·8	3·6	5·0	5·5	1·6	3·4	4
RMS-1	2·2	5·4	4·1	4·5	1·1	4·1	10
MLS-1	3·6	2·5	14·5	2·8	1·2	2·3	5

After [1].

Figure 4.7 shows the contributions of the two types of event. The exponential term $S_1 = e^{-D/_1D_0}$ or $e^{-\alpha D}$ represents the initial tangent to the survival curve. For very small doses the surviving fraction S is approximately equal to S_1, i.e. cell death is due almost entirely to direct lethal events. With larger doses the contribution of sublethal events to cell death becomes increasingly important.

According to these models the surviving fraction S_1 depends only on the total dose D and not on its distribution in time. The surviving fraction S_n is given by relations (2) and (3) when the dose is given in a short time (a few minutes), but cell death by the accumulation of sublethal events depends on fractionation and dose rate owing to the phenomenon of *cellular repair*.

REMARKS
These mathematical expressions have practical value and are often used. It is necessary, however, to emphasize the limitations of the concepts on which these models are based. The term 'target' does not imply a cellular structure, damage to which leads to death of the cell, a concept which was at the base of classical target theory. It expresses in pictorial terms the probability that a

---

†Other models have been proposed which lead to mathematical formulae containing a larger number of parameters. They are therefore of no interest if the function is to be used to calculate the surviving fraction, although they may be used to test theories about the physical and biological mechanisms of cell lethality.

certain type of event will lead to cell death. The directly lethal event is not a term of absolute significance. The coefficient which represents it varies with the physical (e.g. temperature; Section 9.2), chemical (e.g. pressure of O_2; Section 7.1) and physiological (e.g. repair; Section 4.5) conditions in which the cells are to be found. In some cases it also varies with the duration of irradiation, i.e. with dose rate.[†]

In a more general symbolism, the most frequently used form of survival curve for a single, short irradiation, can be represented by considering that the probability of a lethal cellular effect is composed of a term proportional to dose and a second term which increases more rapidly than dose. The mean number of lethal events per cell is:

$$p=\alpha D+f(D)[‡]$$

which leads to a surviving fraction $S=e^{-p}$. The value of p depends on the species of cell and can be modified by several factors; it depends also on the nature of the radiation. This general formula has the advantage that it can be applied to models other than the target models described above.

Models based on intracellular repair

In these models, irradiation produces two types of lesion, some of which are directly lethal and others which are potentially lethal but are susceptible to repair. Repair of the latter requires action of an enzymatic system and a suitable time for the enzyme to act. Sublethal damage and potentially lethal damage (see Section 4.5) are taken to be the same and the kinetics of their repair is that of the action of the enzyme. The first mathematical expression of this type of model was that of Orr *et al.* [38]. Numerous versions have appeared subsequently, including those in references [6, 19, 28].

The shoulder on the survival curve arises when the repair system is fully operative, only at low doses. In some theories, this occurs because the repair enzyme becomes saturated as the dose is increased. When the repair system is completely saturated, all the lesions become lethal and the survival curve becomes exponential; its slope then represents the total production of lesions per unit dose (Figure 4.9).

This form of the theory is debatable and it is not necessary to assume

---

[†]According to the definitions given above, directly lethal lesions are those where cell death results from a single event (energy deposition by the passage of an ionizing particle) which causes enough damage to result in the death of the cell; whereas the second lethal mechanism implies the combination of at least two events.

As we will see in connection with the phenomenon of repair (Section 4.5), these lesions may become expressed and lead to the death of the cell or they may be repaired. The probability of these alternatives depends in particular on the environmental conditions after irradiation (repair of potentially lethal lesions). The name 'directly lethal lesions' to define the lethal lesions resulting from a single event is therefore a term which may seem ambiguous. However, like other authors, we will use it in this work to distinguish it from the lethal lesions which result from the accumulation of sublethal lesions, i.e. death caused by the passage of several particles.

[‡]βD^2 is the simplest expression for $f(D)$.

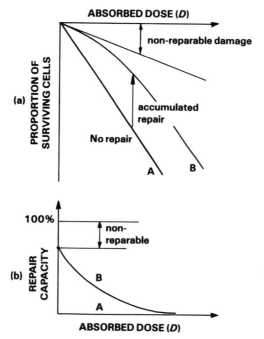

Figure 4.9. Interpretation of survival curves by intracellular repair.
(a) Curve A represents the surviving fraction due to cellular damage in the absence of repair. This is actually observed in mutants whose repair system is deficient, or after inhibition of the repair system by physical or chemical agents. Curve B represents the surviving fraction modified by repair.†
(b) Capacity for repair diminishes as the dose increases.

saturation of the repair enzyme. Some other models do not require this and are based on the kinetics of cellular damage and repair which are partially reversible, but if not repaired eventually lead to cell death.

In the model of Kappos and Pohlit [28], irradiation produces two types of damage: irreparable lesions (state C) which are lethal, and potentially lethal lesions (state B) which can either progress towards an irreparable state (C) or be repaired, restoring the cell to its normal condition (A). Repair occurs if the intracellular conditions are favourable. The shoulder on the survival curve is due to a reduction in the frequency of repair as the dose increases.

Curtis [6] has proposed a unified formulation incorporating major ideas from several models; it is called the LPL model (lethal, potentially lethal). The primary lesions are produced in DNA by the radicals formed along the tracks of charged particles and are potentially lethal. When they are formed very close together, along a single track in a site *c.* 10 nm diameter, they may rapidly (about 1 s) interact to produce lethal lesions. More isolated lesions may be repaired. Alternatively they may combine in pairs and be misrepaired (binary misrepair). These processes are shown schematically in Figure 4.10. The rate of binary misrepair is assumed to depend only on the square of the concentration

---

†The simplest mathematical expression of the mean number of lethal events per cell in the repair model is $p = aD(1 - f(D))$ where $f(D)$ corresponds to the repair capacity which depends on the dose.

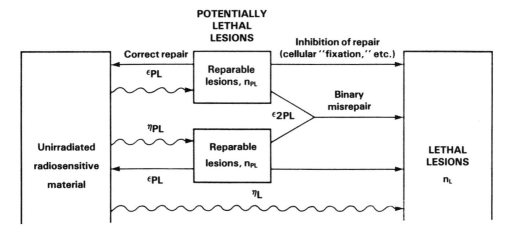

Figure 4.10. Diagrammatic representation of the LPL model and designation of parameters in the biological time frame. The η_L and η_{PL} are the rates per unit absorbed dose for production of the lethal and potentially lethal lesions, respectively. The ϵ_{PL} and ϵ_{2PL} are the rates per unit time of correct repair and binary misrepair, respectively, for the potentially lethal lesions.
After [6].

of potentially lethal lesions present at a given time. The kinetics of repair and fixation of potentially lethal lesions are slow (many minutes) and the same as that of the repair of sublethal and potentially lethal damage (see Section 4.5, which explains the effects of dose rate and fractionation). With a suitable choice of the disposable parameters, this theory can successfully model cell survival curves and their variations with dose rate, fractionation and radiation quality. At low doses, the model leads to a linear–quadratic relationship.

The short-range fast interactions and the longer-range slower interactions can be identified with interactions considered in other models such as the theory of dual radiation action of Rossi and Keller [29, 30].

Biophysical interpretation of the lethal events

In a mammalian cell which has received 1 Gy of X- or γ-rays there are about 1000 breaks of DNA molecules (Section 3.2). A few hours after irradiation, less than 20 breaks remain and despite their presence about half the cells are still viable.

This shows the predominant role of repair mechanisms. It is clear that only a small fraction of the damage in DNA is irreparable or incorrectly repaired. For the same dose, that is to say an equal number of ionizations, high-LET radiations have a much greater effectiveness; moreover there is no initial curvature on the survival curve and therefore no sublethal damage or progressive saturation of the repair system. This shows that among the lesions produced by a large transfer of energy within the DNA molecule, produced by radiations of high LET, the proportion of irreparable lesions is greater than for radiations of low LET, probably because the probability of repair of damage in DNA depends on its severity, i.e. on the quantity of energy that has been transferred at this site.

These large concentrations of energy may be due to:

1. A single particle producing a large density of ionization such as a heavy particle at high LET, an electron at the end of its track or a δ-electron;
2. Addition of the effects of two particles acting on the same target or site. If two events (ionizations) occur within a sufficiently short distance and during a sufficiently short period of time, their effects are additive. If they are situated along the track of a single particle it is called an intratrack effect. If they are situated on the tracks of two different particles it is an intertrack effect.

We will discuss the interpretations offered by the two principal models: that of Rossi and Kellerer in its most recent form [30, 42] and the repair model. They will be studied in the light of experiments which have been made in order to distinguish between them [13].

The model of Rossi and Kellerer has the merit of providing a physical and dosimetric base (microdosimetry) to the study of radiobiological mechanisms. It states that the component βD^2 in the linear–quadratic relation results from the summation of events produced along the tracks of two particles (intertrack effect). Knowing the number of particles traversing the nucleus at a given dose one can calculate the distance between the particles. In order to explain the experimental results it seems that interaction between separate tracks must take place over distances up to $0 \cdot 1$–$1\,\mu$m, although the diameter of a DNA molecule is $3\,$nm.

The model states that the passage of a single particle through a site (target) creates sub-lesions and that two sub-lesions in the same site can combine giving rise to a lethal lesion. Again the interaction may take place over distances from $0 \cdot 1$ to $1\,\mu$m. This is the origin of the term αD.

In addition to the total dose, an irradiation can be characterized by the specific energy (energy divided by the mass) delivered in a certain volume during the passage of a particle. In the symbolism of Rossi, ζ represents the mean specific energy delivered due to the passage of a single particle through the volume considered (site). ζ clearly depends on the size of the volume but also on the LET of the particle; it makes it possible to predict the relative biological efficiency (RBE) of radiations and the variation of RBE with dose.

With small doses mortality is mainly due to events produced by the passage of a single particle (intratrack interaction), whereas at high doses addition of the effects of two particles (intertrack interaction) assumes increasing importance. Mathematical development of the theory indicates that the mean number of lesions per site after a total dose D is $p = k(\zeta D + D^2)$. In this relation the term in D corresponds to intratrack lesions and the term in D^2 to intertrack lesions.

In its initial form [29] this theory stated that two sub-lesions have the same probability of combining whatever their distance from one another, on condition that they are both within the site whose diameter is of the order of $1\,\mu$m. The theory made possible a satisfactory interpretation of numerous biological findings such as the variation of RBE with LET, the role of dose rate and the shapes of cell survival curves. However it did not explain satisfactorily two series of experimental results [13].

Irradiation of cells with pairs of protons whose tracks are about $0 \cdot 1\,\mu m$ apart (associated particle experiment)

This experiment was performed with accelerated ionized hydrogen molecules, H_2^+, as the two protons diverge when the ions enter a condensed medium. The results suggest that their biological effectiveness is greater than that of uncoordinated protons but less than expected on the theory of a high probability of interaction over distances of this length [31]. A high probability of interaction has been deduced for separations much below $0 \cdot 1\,\mu m$, a small probability between $0 \cdot 1$ and $0 \cdot 2\,\mu m$, and finally a very small probability between $0 \cdot 2$ and $4\,\mu m$.

This distribution of probabilities is very different from that which was put forward in the first model of Kellerer and Rossi [29] where the probability was taken as constant within the site and zero beyond.

Irradiation with very low energy X-rays which produce photoelectrons with very low kinetic energy [4, 41]

The photoelectrons from carbon K X-rays have an energy of less than 280 eV and produce about 14 ionizations along their tracks which are 7 nm long. In these circumstances, interactions of two lesions at a distance of $0 \cdot 1$–$1\,\mu m$ can only take place when they are produced by two particles; the term αD should therefore be small. However the effectiveness of these radiations at small doses is in fact high and the initial shoulder is small whereas one would have expected a large shoulder if only the component βD^2 was active. This problem of low energy electrons is important because about a quarter of the energy delivered by cobalt γ-rays is transferred by ionization densities of this order (track ends of the δ-electrons, section 1.4).

Table 4.3. Radiobiological explanations by target models and repair models.

	Interpretation	
Experimental findings	Linear–quadratic model Rossi–Kellerer	Repair model
Initial shoulder on the survival curve	Interaction of sublethal lesions	Impairment of repair capacity
Repair between fractions (Elkind repair)	Repair of sublethal lesions	Recovery of repair capacity
Increase of RBE with LET	Interaction of sub-lesions along the tracks of high-LET particles	Less efficient repair of lesions produced by high-LET particles
Reduction of effectiveness at low dose rate	Repair of sublethal lesions during irradiation. *Prediction*: Survival curve at low dose rate $S = e^{-D}$	Repair system not saturated *Prediction*: Exponential survival curve with slope which may be different from the initial slope of the normal survival curve
Extrapolation to low dose (lethal effect or carcinogensis)	By extrapolation of the linear–quadratic curve	Depends on the mechanisms of repair Possibility of a threshold dose

Based in part on Goodhead [13].

To resolve these difficulties of interpretation, the second version of the Kellerer–Rossi model [30] states that the probability of combination of two sub-lesions depends on the distance separating them and on the biological properties of the cell. A consequence of this is that the parameter ζ which is purely physical and measureable must be replaced by a parameter which integrates the physical and biological characteristics and is not directly measureable. Under these conditions the theory is able to interpret the experimental results but its predictive value is reduced [13].

There are also difficulties with the repair models. In the absence of sufficient experimental results they do not make it possible to formalize the relation between dose and probability of repair and they do not explain satisfactorily certain facts, for example the summation of the effects of the tracks of two protons $1\,\mu$m apart. Table 4.3 shows the explanations given by the two models and the predictions resulting from them. As can be seen, some of these predictions can be submitted to experimental verification.

The mathematical relations based on the various models are in reasonable agreement with the experimental results. In any case, regardless of any hypothesis about the mechanisms of cell death, it is convenient to represent survival curves by a simple expression containing few coefficients and applicable to all the usual survival curves. The linear–quadratic function is satisfactory from this point of view and is very widely used.

4.4 Intrinsic cellular radiosensitivity

Survival curves show large differences depending on the cellular species. They can also be modified by several physical or chemical factors whose action will be studied later. Differences in radiosensitivity connected with the biological characteristics can be appreciated by comparing survival curves obtained with the same radiation under good conditions of oxygenation and nutrition and at normal temperature.

Viruses are very radioresistant biological structures (Table 4.1). The mean lethal dose D_0 is almost inversely proportional to the mass of the virus. This simple relation is at the origin of target theory. Eukaryotic cells† are by comparison very radiosensitive and bacteria show an intermediate radio-sensitivity.

We have seen (Section 3.5) that radiosensitivity increases with the quantity of nucleic acid contained in the biological structure. The shape of the survival curve depends on ploidy: Latarjet has shown with yeast (*Saccharomyces cerevisiae*) that survival curves are exponential for haploid cells but contain a shoulder for diploid or hyperdiploid cells [33]. This can be interpreted by considering that the number of targets which have to be damaged to kill the cell increases with the number of copies of the chromosomes.

The role of repair on survival curves is brought out by bacterial mutants. For a given cellular species (e.g. *E. coli*) mutants deficient in a repair system (rec−)

---

†With a nucleus containing chromosomes.

are more sensitive than the wild type and the survival curve has no shoulder. An analogous phenomenon is seen in man for various hereditary diseases associated with a deficiency in the cellular repair system (Section 3.3). *In vitro* the culture conditions, and in particular the composition of the medium, influence the shape of the survival curve.

Radiosensitivity of different types of mammalian cell

Mammalian cells show considerable differences in radiosensitivity depending on the type of cell but only small variations with the species of animal.

The pluripotent stem cells of the haemopoietic bone marrow (CFUs) and the germinal stem cells of the testis (spermatogonia) are among the most radiosensitive cell lines (Chapter 5). The survival curves of these cells show very small shoulders and are practically exponential up to a dose of 5 Gy; D_0 is about 80 cGy, with a variation of about ±20 cGy depending on the experimental conditions.

For most other cell lines the shoulder of the survival curve is considerably more marked. For the basal cells of the epidermis and mucosa the slope of the terminal part of the curve, or the mean slope for doses of the order of 10 Gy, corresponds to a mean lethal dose D_0 of about $1\cdot3$–$1\cdot5$ Gy. The ratio between the final and initial slopes is close to 3. This ratio is higher, about 5, for other cells such as fibroblasts, cells of the capillary endothelium and glial cells; these cells therefore show a smaller mortality with low doses and a large capacity to accumulate sublethal damage [1]. It has recently been shown that the shape of survival curves of normal cells such as fibroblasts varies from one inividual to another.

In the linear–quadratic model, variations in the shape of the survival curve are expressed by large variations in the ratio α/β (Section 4.3), between values of the order of 30 Gy for curves with very small shoulders and a steep slope (haemopoietic stem cells) and 1 Gy for curves showing a large shoulder and a small initial slope.

The survival curves of malignant cells do not show any systematic differences from those of normal cells, and the parameters which characterize them cover as wide a range as those of normal cells. Table 4.2 shows the characteristics of certain experimental cell lines; variations of the same order occur with human tumour cells (Chapter 6). Differences in the shapes of survival curves (represented by differences in the ratios α/β) depending on the type of cell are at the origin of the differential effect connected with fractionation of dose. This has great importance in radiotherapy (Chapter 8).

Radiosensitivity and phase of the cell cycle

So far we have been considering asynchronous populations of cells, in which the cells are randomly distributed through the different phases of the cell cycle. Variation in radiosensitivity as a function of position in the cell cycle can be studied using synchronized populations of cells. These can be obtained by several techniques of which we shall present only a few examples.

Techniques for obtaining synchronized populations of cells

The technique devised by Terasima and Tolmach [47] is based on collecting the cells in mitosis (taking advantage of the fact that they adhere less well to the surface of the culture vessels). This technique can only be used with cultures whose cells extend in a monolayer on the surface of the vessel. The cells normally adhere to the surface but when they approach mitosis they become rounded and less firmly attached. If the vessel is shaken gently, the mitotic cells become detached and float in the medium. The latter is removed and the cells are reseeded in a new vessel. In this way a population is obtained with almost all the cells in mitosis. If they are maintained at 37°C, they progress together through the successive phases of the mitotic cycle. A synchronized population of cells can be irradiated at any chosen point in the cell cycle by selecting the time of irradiation.

Other techniques of synchronization make use of drugs, among which hydroxyurea has been the most frequently used, both *in vitro* and *in vivo*. Hydroxyurea has two main effects. On the one hand it is incorporated into cells during S phase and kills them, while on the other it blocks entry into S phase. By allowing the hydroxyurea to act during a period equal to the sum of G_2, M and G_1 phases (see figure 3.8), all the viable cells accumulate in a narrow window at the end of G_1. If the action of the drug is stopped at this moment the cohort of synchronized cells begins to progress again through the mitotic cycle. Thus, for example, for Chinese hamster cells (length of mitotic cycle 11 h, Table 4.4), by 5 h after elimination of the drug the cohort of synchronized cells reaches the end of S phase; it reaches mitosis or close to it at 9 h.

Cells in S phase can also be selectively eliminated by incubating them in the presence of a high concentration of [^{3}H] thymidine ('suicide effect', Section 3.5).

Radiation response of synchronized populations of cells

Figure 4.11 shows that Chinese hamster cells are most sensitive in phases M and G_2 and that the corresponding survival curves are practically exponential. The cells are most radioresistant at the end of S phase, a time when the survival curve shows a large shoulder. Cells in G_1 and early S have intermediate radiosensitivity.

Table 4.4. Comparative lengths of different phases of the mitotic cycle of two cell lines frequently used for studies *in vitro*.

Phase	Length of phase (h)	
	V79 cells (Chinese hamster lung fibroblasts)	HeLa cells (human origin)
G_1	1	11
S	6	8
G_2	3	4
Mitosis	1	1
Total	11	24

After [18].

It is interesting to compare these results with those obtained with HeLa cells whose mitotic cycle is longer, essentially due to the length of G_1 (Table 4.4). Altogether, the variation of radiosensitivity among the phases is similar but in addition large variations of radiosensitivity can be seen during G_1. The cells are resistant at the beginning of G_1 whereas at the end of G_1 radiosensitivity is similar to that seen in G_2 and M. Similar variations in radiosensitivity during G_1 may take place in Chinese hamster cells but they are not detectable because of the short duration of this phase of the cycle.

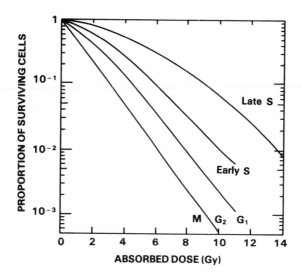

Figure 4.11. Survival curves of Chinese hamster cells irradiated in different phases of the mitotic cycle.
After [43].

Variations of radiosensitivity similar to those found with Chinese hamster and HeLa cells have also been found with other cell lines but not in all. There are important variations in the radiosensitivity during the cell cycle but the technical difficulties connected with cell synchronization must not be underestimated and may lead to erroneous conclusions. Microcinematography (Figure 4.1) can be used to follow the fate of individual cells irradiated in different phases of the cycle, identified by the time separating irradiation from the preceding mitosis. This technique avoids the necessity of using methods of synchronization which are generally not physiological.

4.5 Cell survival and repair: fractionated irradiation and low dose rate

The fraction of surviving cells depends on the distribution of the dose in time, due to the partial repair of damage which can proceed during irradiation or between fractions.

Repair of sublethal damage

Fractionated irradiation: the experiments of Elkind

The response of a population of cells *in vitro* to fractionated irradiation was first studied by Elkind and Sutton in 1959 [10]. Their conclusions were later confirmed *in vivo* as well as *in vitro*. Irradiation in two fractions, separated by an interval of time, produces a smaller degree of cell killing than when the same total dose is delivered in a single fraction (Fig. 4.12). Thus the total dose required to cause a given degree of mortality is greater when the irradiation is given in two fractions than as a single dose.

The second fraction, delivered after an interval of a few hours, gives a cell survival curve which is superimposable on that obtained with a single dose and in particular has the same shoulder. This observation suggests that during the interval between the two fractions the sublethal damage in the surviving cells is repaired, or that the effectiveness of the repair system, which was markedly reduced by the first fraction, has regained its integrity.

The rate of repair of sublethal damage has been studied by measuring the surviving fraction as a function of the interval between the two doses (Figure 4.13). It is generally considered that repair of sublethal damage takes place with a half-time of $0 \cdot 5$–$1 \cdot 5$ h, depending on the type of cell.

The 'fading time' [12] corresponds to the time interval required for the reparable damage to decay to an undetectable level. If two tissues are compared (e.g. an early reacting tissue in which reparable damage represents one fifth of the total, and a late reacting tissue in which it amounts to half of the total damage), even if repair occurs at the same rate in both tissues it will take longer to decay to 5% of the total damage in the tissue in which the reparable damage is large than in the one in which it is small.

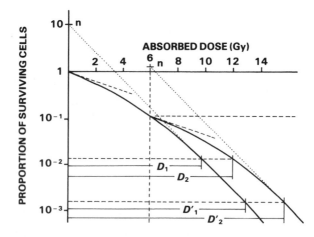

Figure 4.12. Irradiation in two fractions separated by an interval of a few hours produces less cell killing than is obtained when the same total dose is given as a single fraction. The cell survival curve for the second fraction is superimposable on that obtained for the first fraction and in particular has the same initial slope and the same shoulder. The survival curve shown in the figure corresponds to crypt cells of the intestinal mucosa in the mouse.

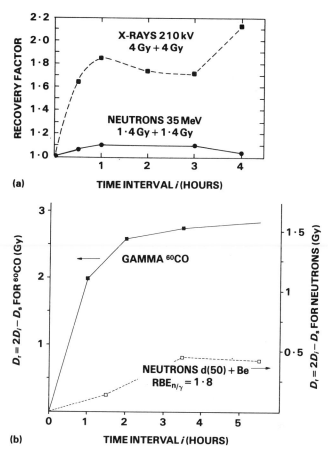

Figure 4.13. Kinetics of repair of sublethal lesions. (a) Studies *in vitro*. Irradiation of Chinese hamster cells by two fractions of 4 Gy of X-rays separated by a variable interval of time *i*. Repair of sublethal lesions is evaluated by the ratio of surviving fractions after fractionated irradiation (2×4 Gy) and after a single dose (8 Gy). In the example shown, repair of sublethal lesions is almost complete after 1 h. The slight reduction in surviving fraction between 1 and 3 h is interpreted as an effect of synchronization of the surviving population, while the increase in surviving fraction after 3 h is due to cellular proliferation (p. 116 in [18]).
(b) Studies *in vivo*. The kinetics of cellular repair can also be studied *in vivo* by making use of effects in tissue. In the example shown in the figure, the biological criterion is intestinal death of mice (LD 50) after single and fractionated irradiations. Repair is estimated from the additional dose (D_r) needed to reach the LD 50 when a single dose (D_s) is replaced by two equal doses (2 D_i) separated by an interval *i* (in hours). When a single dose (of about 10 Gy) is replaced by two doses separated by 3 h it is necessary to increase the total dose by about 3 Gy. For irradiation with fast neutrons, sublethal damage plays a less important role (Section 11.1) and the total dose for a given biological effect is less affected by fractionation.
By courtesy of Gueulette *et al.*

If the half-time of reparable damage is taken to be 1·5 h, calculation shows that the fading time (and therefore the appropriate interval between fractions) would be about 3–4 h for early effects and 5–6 h for late effects. In practice, in multifraction irradiation the fractions should be separated by 6 h or more to permit repair to approach completion in late responding tissues [48, 50].

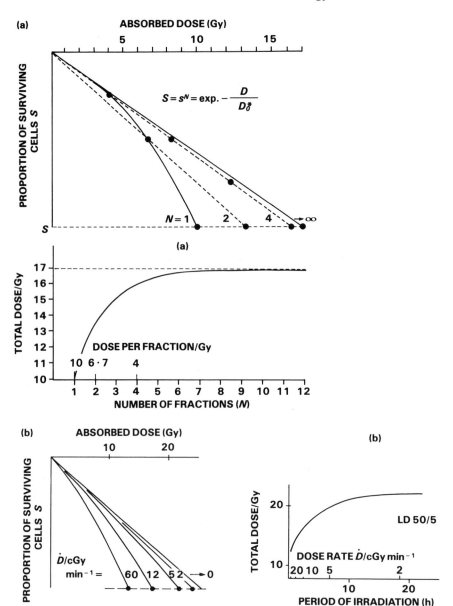

Figure 4.14. Isoeffect curves.
(a) Isoeffect curves as a function of the dose per fraction (or the number of fractions).
When the irradiation is given in N equal fractions (separated by intervals i long enough
for repair of sublethal damage) and assuming that the surviving proportion is the same
after each fraction, the resultant survival curve ($S=s^N$) is exponential with a slope $1/D_0^*$
which becomes smaller as the individual doses per fraction are reduced. The limiting
slope is that of the tangent at the origin ($-1/_1D_0$). From the cell survival curve one can
determine the isoeffect doses corresponding to surviving proportions S (or to given
biological effects) as a function of the number of fractions or of the dose per fraction d.
(b) Isoeffect curves as a function of the length of irradiation (or of the dose rate). In an
analogous way one can deduce the isoeffect doses as a function of dose rate or of the
length of irradiation. The curves shown in the figure correspond to irradiations with dose
rates between 2 and 60 cGy min^{-1}.
(a) and (b) relate to early intestinal tolerance evaluated by the LD 50 in the mouse
(intestinal syndrome) [45].

Additional dose

The importance of cellular repair can be expressed in terms of the increase in surviving fraction, but it is more convenient for many applications to express it in terms of the additional dose needed to obtain a given surviving fraction or, more generally, a given biological effect. The conventional expression is $D_r = D_2 - D_1$. D_r is the difference between the single dose D_1 to produce a given effect and the total dose D_2 given as two equal fractions separated by an interval of several hours. These are the conditions for which the value of D_r is at a maximum.

The additional dose D_r depends on the shape of the survival curve. It is zero for an exponential curve and increases with the size of the shoulder. It also depends on D_1, i.e. on the level of effect; it is small or almost zero with small doses for which sublethal lesions do not contribute to cell killing. It increases with dose and tends towards a maximum value of D_q (Section 4.3) for doses corresponding to the exponential or quasi-exponential part of the cell survival curve.

Fractionated irradiation: isoeffect dose

When the irradiation is given in several fractions, the sublethal damage is repaired during the interval separating the fractions. If the survival s is the same for each fraction d, the total survival S after N fractions is s^N. The resulting survival curve is an exponential passing through the origin, whose slope is reduced as the individual fractions become smaller (Figure 4.14). This slope can be expressed [57] by the coefficient D_0^* (effective D_0):

$$S = s^N = e^{-D/D_0^*}$$

D_0^* increases as the dose per fraction is reduced. In the limit, when the dose per fraction is so small that there are only directly lethal lesions, it is generally agreed that the survival curve has the same slope as the tangent at the origin of the original survival curve, $S = e^{-\alpha D}$ or $e^{-D/_1 D_0}$.

If successive equal fractions kill the same proportion of cells, it implies that the population of cells has a uniform radiosensitivity which does not vary in the course of irradiation. Variation in sensitivity could occur due to redistribution of the surviving cells in the cell cycle (Figure 4.11) or in the capacity for repair [36, 51, 58]. Moreover, cell proliferation which may be stimulated by successive fractions has been neglected, but its role can be considered separately.

From the cell survival curve one can calculate isoeffective doses as a function of the dose per fraction (Figure 4.14). The dose needed to produce a given degree of mortality increases with an increase in the number of fractions N or a reduction in the dose per fraction. It tends towards a plateau which is reached in practice when the dose per fraction is sufficiently low that only directly lethal lesions are involved.

For very small doses per fraction, the number of fractions necessary to obtain a measurable biological effect becomes prohibitive. In order to investigate sparing by fractionation as the dose per fraction is decreased below 2 Gy, the top-up method can be used [7, 39]. In this method, multiple equal fractions of X-rays are given, inflicting damage which, by itself, would be too small to be measured. Graded top-up doses are then added to bring the damage into a measurable range. The value of the top-up dose required to produce the biological effect is related to the damage inflicted by the fractionated irradiation. It is best to use neutrons for the top-up doses as they give nearly linear dose–effect relationships (Chapter 11). The shape of the neutron top-up radiation response must be known from previous experiments. With this method it is possible to measure the sparing effect of X-ray doses per fraction down to $0 \cdot 1$ Gy. At these very low doses per fraction it seems that the damage inflicted may be greater than is indicated by the linear–quadratic relation, perhaps due to failure to 'switch on' repair mechanisms [26].

Cell survival curves deduced from isoeffect curves for tissue reactions

We have seen above how isoeffect curves can be obtained from cell survival curves. Inversely, information on cell survival curves can be obtained from isoeffect curves. In this respect the isoeffect curves obtained for macroscopic reactions of normal tissues are of great practical importance because they provide information on normal tissues which cannot in general be obtained by cloning techniques. For example, the following tissue effects have been particularly well studied:

1. Acute reaction of the haemopoietic system measured by the LD 50 at 30 days (haemopoietic syndrome) after total body irradiation;
2. Acute reaction of the intestinal mucosa evaluated from the LD 50 at 5 days after abdominal irradiation;
3. Acute skin reaction (desquamation) or late reaction (contraction);
4. Late reaction of the lungs, spinal cord, kidney, etc.

From the study of tissue responses, information can be obtained concerning the survival curve of the responsible cells: for example, the haemopoietic stem cells for LD 50 at 30 days, intestinal crypt cells for lethality by the intestinal syndrome, etc. The value of the ratio α/β can be derived from the isoeffect curves without the necessity of measuring the absolute values of α and β (Section 8.3).

It is also possible to construct the cell survival curve from the isoeffect curve on the assumption that a given tissue reaction corresponds to the same proportion of surviving cells whatever the number of dose fractions. However, this is not necessarily true in every case and the conditions of irradiation must be chosen in such a way that the variation of the isoeffect curve is due only to the repair of sublethal damage (Figure 4.15). Repair must therefore be complete during the interval between the fractions. In addition, the influence of other factors such as redistribution in the cell cycle, proliferation of clonogenic cells, and proliferation of cells which have lost their clonogenic power, must be taken to be negligible.

Potentially lethal damage (PLD)

The fraction of surviving cells after irradiation depends on the conditions in which the cells are placed after irradiation. This is attributed to potentially lethal damage (PLD) which can either lead to death of the cell or may be repaired.

The first studies of PLD were made *in vitro*. An increase in the fraction of surviving cells is seen when the cells are incubated for several hours after irradiation in a saline solution which prevents cell division, instead of being immediately cloned in a complete nutritive medium. Another way of allowing repair of PLD *in vitro* is to irradiate a population of cells in stationary phase [24, 34].

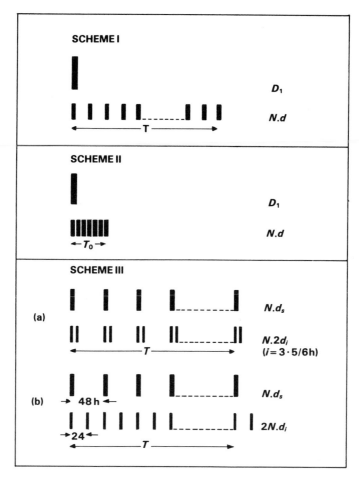

Figure 4.15. Comparison of experimental protocols designed to establish the isoeffect dose for a given response as a function of the number of fractions. *Scheme I*: the dose needed to produce a given effect is determined for a single fraction D_1 and n fractions d, over a period of time T. When T is large the influence of cellular proliferation can no longer be neglected. It is moreover difficult to estimate. *Scheme II*: if the total time T is reduced, the interval separating successive fractions may not be long enough to allow complete repair of the sublethal lesions. In addition a certain degree of synchronization may influence the results. *Scheme III*: the increase in dose required is determined when a fraction d_s is replaced by two equal fractions $2\,d_i$ separated by an interval i long enough to allow repair of the sublethal lesions. To produce the effect required, this irradiation must be repeated a number of times (N) which increases as the dose per fraction (d_s or $2\,d_i$) is reduced. The total time T is kept constant so that one can assume that the rate of repopulation is the same at all times during the two irradiations compared (Nd_s and $2Nd_i$). This does not imply that repopulation must remain constant throughout the fractionated irradiations. In the variant, scheme III(b), a constant interval is maintained between the $2N$ fractions d_i. The influence of cellular redistribution can be evaluated by comparing schemes III(a) and III(b) [52].

If a population of cells is allowed to multiply *in vitro* in a culture flask, after a period of exponential growth the increased number of cells leads to a slowing down of cell multiplication which finally becomes completely inhibited when the cell density is very great. After irradiation in this stationary phase, if the cells are kept under the same conditions for 6 or 12h before testing their viability by cloning, a significant increase in the surviving fraction is seen compared with immediate cloning (Figure 4.16). This suggests that resting cells benefit from sufficient time before dividing to repair damage which would be lethal if it was still present at the time of duplication of the DNA molecules or at the time of mitosis. Stationary culture conditions are probably similar to the situation of cells in many solid tumours.

Repair of PLD has been seen *in vivo* both for normal cells and malignant cells [14, 35]. It is comparable to the repair seen *in vitro* both in terms of its importance and its kinetics.

Continuous irradiation at low dose rate

The response of a population of cells to continuous irradiation at low dose rate is of particular importance both for radiation protection and for interstitial and intracavitary radiotherapy.

A number of experimental studies have been devoted to this subject. Figures 4.17 and 4.18 bring together the results of Hall [17] obtained with HeLa cells. The surviving fraction at a given dose increases as the dose rate is reduced over

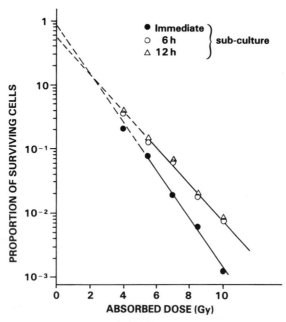

Figure 4.16. **Repair of potentially lethal damage in mammalian cells *in vitro*. Cell survival curves obtained for cells irradiated *in vitro* in stationary phase. The cells are then removed, trypsinized and replaced in culture either immediately or 6 or 12h after irradiation. The surviving fraction is significantly increased when the cells are maintained in the stationary phase which allows repair of potentially lethal damage [34].**

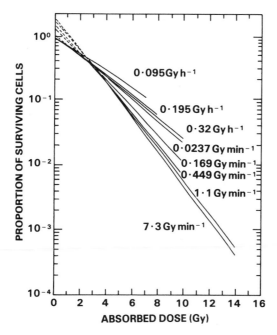

Figure 4.17. **Example of experimental results obtained** *in vitro* **showing the influence of dose rate on cell survival [17]. HeLa cells were irradiated with a large range of dose rates, from 9·5 cGy h⁻¹ to 7·3 Gy min⁻¹, a ratio of 5000. Variation of dose rate has relatively little influence on cell survival at the higher dose rates or the lowest dose rates studied. For the lowest dose rates, the range of doses which can be studied is relatively small due to the total duration of irradiation.**

a range of approximately 1–$0\cdot01\,\mathrm{Gy\,min^{-1}}$. These results can be interpreted according to the models in which cell death is due both to directly lethal events and to accumulation of sublethal lesions. The former are considered to be irreparable and independent of dose rate while the latter can be repaired during irradiation if its duration is long enough. Cell death due to the accumulation of sublethal damage is therefore reduced when the dose rate becomes lower.

For high dose rates (above $1\,\mathrm{Gy\,min^{-1}}$) the length of the irradiation is too short to allow repair of sublethal damage during irradiation†. For very low dose rates (below $1\,\mathrm{Gy\,h^{-1}}$), lethality is due essentially to directly lethal lesions, as in a fractionated irradiation when the dose per fraction is reduced indefinitely. As a result the biological effect no longer varies with the dose rate and the survival curve is a straight line with slope α. The interpretation given by the repair models is not very different. As at low dose rates the repair systems remain fully effective, only the irreparable lesions are lethal; however, in some models

---

†For very high dose rates ($100\,\mathrm{Gy\,min^{-1}}$), Hornsey [23] has seen an increase in the mortality of intestinal crypt cells, suggesting that a part of the repair of sublethal damage may take place very rapidly. With considerably greater dose rates ($10^{10}\,\mathrm{Gy\,min^{-1}}$), the survival curve tends towards that found under anoxic conditions, as the radiation causes an instantaneous reduction in the concentration of oxygen [11]. At even greater dose rates ($10^{12}\,\mathrm{Gy\,min^{-1}}$), interaction between the radicals produced along the tracks of different particles (Section 1.4) becomes significant and leads to an increase in the biological effect.

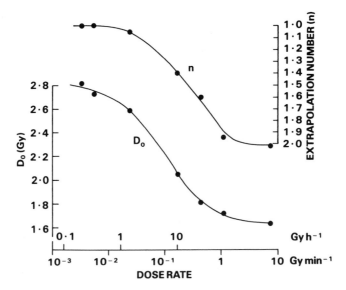

Figure 4.18. This figure, derived from Figure 4.17, shows the variation in *n* and D_0 as a function of dose rate. It shows that dose rate is critical between 0·01 and 1 Gy min⁻¹ (or 1 and 100 Gy h⁻¹); at these dose rates repair and production of sublethal damage are in competition. With lower dose rates the sublethal damage can be repaired as fast as it is produced and the accumulation of sublethal damage never reaches a lethal level. On the other hand, at the highest dose rates there is insufficient time for the sublethal damage to be repaired [17]. It must however be noted that the dose rates at which the values of D_0 and *n* reach their plateau may vary from one cell line to another, depending on their individual capacity to accumulate (and repair) the sublethal damage and on the speed of the repair.

the survival curve does not necessarily have a slope equal to the initial slope of the survival curve at high dose rates.

At low dose rates there are two other factors which must be considered:

1. Increase in the period of irradiation may allow the cells to proliferate during irradiation.
2. The pre-mitotic block (Section 5.1) leads to redistribution of cells in the cell cycle which may increase the effectiveness of the irradiation.

The influence of dose rate varies from one cell line to another, depending on the relative contribution of sublethal damage to cell death. Reduction in dose rate selectively protects the cells whose survival curves show a large shoulder (low ratio α/β), whereas it has little effect on cells for which the shoulder is small.

Recently Steel *et al.* [44] have analyzed the response of 17 human tumour cell lines to variations in dose rate and fractionation of X-rays. Considerable variations were seen both for the absolute sensitivity at high dose rate (1·5 Gy min⁻¹) and for the effect of reducing the dose rate to 0·016 Gy min⁻¹. The dose needed for 1% survival at the two dose rates differed by a factor of 2 for the most radioresistant cell lines but was unchanged (no dose rate effect) for the most radiosensitive lines.

Finally it must be noted that dose rate begins to play a role only when the doses (or the fraction of cells killed) are sufficiently great that sublethal damage contributes significantly to cell killing (Figure 4.14). Thus, under the usual conditions of external radiotherapy with doses of about 2 Gy fraction^{-1}, the dose rate has little importance, at least for those cells whose lethality for a dose of this order is essentially due to directly lethal lesions.

Table 4.3 indicates the interpretation of radiobiological findings according to target and repair models.

References

1. G.W. Barendsen. Dose fractionation, dose rate and iso-effect relationships for normal tissue responses. *Int. J. Radiat. Oncol., Biol. Phys.*, 1982, **8**: 1981–1997.
2. G.W. Barendsen, J.J. Broerse. Experimental radiotherapy of a rat rhabdomyosarcoma with 15 MeV neutrons and 300 kV X-rays. 1. Effects of single exposures. *Eur. J. Cancer*, 1969, **5**: 373–391.
3. H.B. Benestad. Formation of granulocytes and macrophages in diffusion chamber cultures of mouse blood leukocytes. *Scandin. J. Haematology*, 1970, **7**: 279–288.
4. J.J. Brenner, R.P. Bird, M. Zaider, P. Goldhager, P.J. Kliauga, H.H. Rossi. Inactivation of synchronized mammalian cells with low-energy X-rays — results and significance. *Radiat. Res.*, 1987, **110**: 413–427.
5. K.H. Clifton, R.K. De Mott, R.T. Mulcahy, M.N. Gould. Thyroid gland formation from inocula of monodispersed cells: early results on quantitation, function, neoplasia, and radiation effects. *Int. J. Radiat. Oncol. Biol. Phys.*, 1978, **4**: 987–990.
6. S.B. Curtis. Lethal and potentially lethal lesions induced by radiation — a unified repair model. *Radiat. Res.*, 1986, **106**: 252–270.
7. J. Denekamp. Changes in the rate of repopulation during multifraction irradiation of mouse skin. *Br. J. Radiol.*, 1973, **46**: 381.
8. R.E. Durand. Repair during multifraction exposures. Spheroids versus monolayers. *Br. J. Cancer*, 1984, **49**: Suppl. VI, 203–206.
9. R.E. Durand, R.M. Sutherland. Intercellular contacts: its influence on the Dq of mammalian cell survival curve, in: *Cell Survival after Low Doses of Radiation*. (T. Alper, ed), pp. 237–247. John Wiley, Bristol, 1975.
10. M.M. Elkind, H. Sutton. Radiation response of mammalian cells grown in culture. 1. Repair of X-ray damage in surviving Chinese hamster cells. *Radiat. Res.*, 1960, **13**: 556–593.
11. E.R. Epp, H. Weiss, A Santomasso. The oxygen effect in bacterial cells irradiated with high-intensity pulsed electrons. *Radiat. Res.*, 1968, **34**: 320–325.
12. J.F. Fowler. Intervals between multiple fractions per day. *Acta Oncologica*, 1988, **27**: 181–183.
13. D.T. Goodhead. An assessment of the role of microdosimetry in radiobiology. *Radiat. Res.*, 1982, **91**: 45–76.
14. M.N. Gould, L.E. Cathers, K.H. Clifton, S. Howard, R.L. Jirtle, P.A. Mahler, R.T. Mulcahy, F. Thomas. The influence of *in situ* repair systems on survival of several irradiated parenchymal cell types. *Br. J. Cancer*, 1984, **49**: Suppl. 6, 191–195.
15. M.N. Gould, K.H. Clifton. The survival of mammary cells following irradiation *in vivo*: a directly generated single dose survival curve. *Radiat. Res.*, 1977, **72**: 343–352.
16. J. Gueulette, M. Beauduin, S. Vynckier, V. Grégoire, A. Wambersie. Étude microcinématographique de l'allongement du cycle cellulaire après irradiation par rayons X et par neutrons rapides. *C.R. séanc. Soc. Biol.*, 1985, **179**: 255–259.
17. E.J. Hall. Radiation dose-rate: a factor of importance in radiobiology and radiotherapy. *Br. J. Radiol.*, 1972, **45**: 81–97.
18. E.J. Hall. *Radiobiology for the radiologist* (3rd edn). J.B. Lippincott, Philadelphia, 1988.
19. R.H. Haynes, F. Eckardt, B.A. Kuntz. The DNA damage repair hypothesis in radiation biology: comparisons with classical theory. *Br. J. Cancer*, 1984, **49**; Suppl. VI: 81–90.
20. J.H. Hendry. Review: survival curves for normal tissue clonogens. *Int. J. Radiat. Biol.*, 1985, **47**: 3–16.
21. H.B. Hewitt, C.W. Wilson. A survival curve for mammalian cells irradiated *in vivo*. *Nature*, 1959, **183**: 1060–1061.
22. R.P. Hill, R.S. Bush. A lung colony assay to determine the radiosensitivity of the cells of a solid tumor. *Int. J. Radiat. Biol.*, 1969, **15**: 435–444.

23. S. Hornsey. Differences in survival of jejunal crypt cells after radiation delivered at different dose rates. *Br. J. Radiol.*, 1970, **43**: 802–806.
24. G. Iliakis, W. Pohlit. Quantitative aspects of repair of potentially lethal damage in mammalian cells. *Int. J. Radiat. Biol.*, 1979, **36**: 649–658.
25. R.L. Jirtle, G. Michalopoulos, J.R. McLain, J. Crowley. Transplantation system for determining the clonogenic survival of parenchymal hepatocytes exposed to ionizing radiation. *Cancer Res.*, 1981, **41**: 3512–3518.
26. M.C. Joiner. The dependence of radiation response on the dose per fraction, in: *The scientific basis of modern radiotherapy*, BIR report No. 19, pp. 20–26. British Institute of Radiology, London, 1989.
27. H.S. Kaplan, L.E. Moses. Biological complexity and radiosensitivity. *Science*, 1964, **145**: 21–25.
28. A. Kappos, W. Pohlit. A cybernetic model for radiation reactions in living cells. Sparsely ionizing radiations; stationary cells. *Int. J. Radiat. Biol.*, 1972, **22**: 51–65.
29. A.M. Kellerer, H.H. Rossi. The theory of dual radiation action. *Curr. Topics Radiat. Res.*, 1972, **8**: 85–158.
30. A.M. Kellerer, H.H. Rossi. A generalized formulation of dual radiation action. *Radiat. Res.*, 1978, **75**: 471–488.
31. A.M. Kellerer, P.L. Yuk-Ming, H.H. Rossi. Biophysical studies with spatially correlated ions — 4. *Radiat. Res.*, 1980, **83**: 511–528.
32. N.F. Kember. An *in vivo* cell survival system based on the recovery of rat growth cartilage from radiation injury. *Nature*, 1965, **207**: 501–503.
33. R. Latarjet, B. Ephrussi. Courbes de survie des levures haploides et diploides soumises aux rayons X. *C.R. Acad. Sci.*, Paris, 1949, **229**: 306–308.
34. J.B. Little. Factors influencing the repair of potentially lethal radiation damage in growth-inhibited human cells. *Radiat. Res.*, 1973, **56**: 320–333.
35. J.B. Little, G.M. Hahn, E. Frindel, M. Tubiana. Repair of potentially lethal radiation damage *in vitro* and *in vivo*. *Radiology*, 1973, **106**: 689–694.
36. N.J. McNally, J. de Ronde. Effect of repeated small doses of radiation on recovery from sub-lethal damage by Chinese hamster cells irradiated in the plateau phase of growth. *Int. J. Radiat. Biol.*, 1976, **29**: 221–234.
37. A. Michalowski. A critical appraisal of clonogenic survival assays in the evaluation of radiation damage to normal tissues. *Radiother. Oncol.*, 1984, **1**: 241–246.
38. J.S. Orr, C.S. Hope, S.E. Wakerley. A metabolic theory of survival curves. *Phys. Med. Biol.*, 1966, **11**: 103–108.
39. C.S. Parkins, J.F. Fowler. The linear quadratic fit to lung function after irradiation with X-rays at smaller doses per fraction than 2 Gy, *Br. J. Cancer*, 1986, **53**: Suppl. VI, 320–323.
40. T.T. Puck, P.I. Markus. Action of X-rays on mammalian cells. *J. Exptl. Med.*, 1956, **103**: 653–666.
41. M.R. Raju, S.G. Carpenter, J.J. Chmielewski, M.E. Schillaci, M.E. Wilder, J.P. Freyer, N.F. Johnson, P.L. Schor, R.J. Sebring. Radiobiology of ultrasoft X rays 1. Cultured hamster cells (v79). *Radiat. Res.*, 1987, **110**: 396–412.
42. H.H. Rossi. Radiation quality. *Radiat. Res.*, 1986, **107**: 1–10.
43. W.K. Sinclair. Cyclic X-ray responses in mammalian cells *in vitro*. *Radiat. Res.*, 1968, **33**: 620–643.
44. G.G. Steel, J.M. Deacon, G.M. Duchesne, A. Horwich, L.R. Kelland, J.H. Peacock. The dose-rate effect in human tumour cells. *Radiother. Oncol.*, 1987, **9**: 299–310.
45. M.R. Stienon-Smoes, M. Octave-Prignot, A. Baudoux, A. Wambersie. Tolérance de l'intestin de la souris à une irradiation par Co-60 à faible débit. Implications en radiothérapie. *C.R. séanc. Soc. Biol.* 1978, **172**: 774–778.
46. R.M. Sutherland, J.A. McCredie, W.R. Inch. Growth of multicell spheroids in tissue culture as a model of nodular carcinomas. *J. Natl. Cancer Inst.*, 1971, **46**: 113–120.
47. T. Terasima, L.J. Tolmach. X-ray sensitivity and DNA synthesis in synchronous populations of HeLa cells. *Science*, 1963, **140**: 490–492.
48. H.D. Thames. Effect-independent measures of tissue responses to fractionated irradiation. *Int. J. Radiat. Biol.*, 1984, **45**: 1–10.
49. J.E. Till, E.A. McCulloch. A direct measurement of the radiation sensitivity of normal mouse bone marrow cells. *Radiat. Res.*, 1961, **14**: 213–222.
50. I. Turesson, G. Notter. Accelerated versus conventional irradiation. The degree of incomplete repair in human skin with a 4-hour interval studied after post mastectomy irradiation. *Acta Oncologica*, 1988, **27**: 169–179.
51. E. van Rongen. Analysis of cell survival after multiple fractions and low dose-rate irradiation of two *in vitro* cultured rat tumor cell lines. *Radiat. Res.*, 1985, **104**: 28–46.

52. A. Wambersie, J. Dutreix. The initial slope of cell survival curves. Its applications in radiotherapy, in: *Proceedings of the fifth symposium on microdosimetry* (J. Booz, H. G. Ebert, B. G. R. Smith eds), Commission of the European Communities, Luxembourg, EUR 5452 d-e-f, pp. 679–713, 1976.
53. H. R. Withers. The dose-survival relationship for irradiation of epithelial cells of mouse skin. *Br. J. Radiol.*, 1967, **40**: 187–194.
54. H. R. Withers, M. M. Elkind. Microcolony survival assay for cells of mouse intestinal mucosa exposed to radiation. *Int. J. Radiat. Biol.*, 1970, **17**: 261–267.
55. H. R. Withers, N. Hunter, H. T. Barkley, B. O. Reid. Radiation survival and regeneration characteristics of spermatogenic stem cells of mouse testis. *Radiat. Res.*, 1974, **57**: 88–103.
56. H. R. Withers, K. A. Mason., H. D. Thames. Late radiation response of kidney assayed by tubule-cell survival. *Brit. J. Radiol.*, 1986, **59**: 587–595.
57. H. R. Withers, L. J. Peters. Biological aspects of radiation therapy, in *Textbook of radiotherapy* (3rd edn), (G. H. Fletcher, ed.), pp. 103–180. Lea and Febiger, Philadelphia, 1980.
58. E. M. Zeeman, J. S. Bedford. Dose rate effects in mammalian cells: V — Dose fractionation effects in non-cycling C3H 10 T1/2 cells. *Int. J. Rad. Oncol. Biol. Phys.*, 1984, **10**: 2089–2098.

Chapter 5.
Effects on normal tissues

The cells of which normal tissues are composed are not independent of one another; they form a complex structure in which, under normal conditions, there is a delicate equilibrium between birth and death. This occurs thanks to regulatory mechanisms which maintain the constancy of organization of the tissue and the number of cells in it. When tissue is damaged it is necessary to consider not only cell death itself but also the reaction provoked in the tissue by death of the cells. This necessitates an understanding of the organization and kinetics of the tissue. These two parameters can explain important differences in the timing and severity of reactions in two tissues which are composed of cells with the same radiosensitivity.

We will examine first the transition from cellular damage to early effects in tissues, showing with the aid of some examples how the expression of damage is conditioned by the structure and proliferative state of the tissue. We will then consider some serious late effects in which vascular damage often plays an important role.

5.1 From cellular effects to tissue damage

Cellular depletion

In Chapter 4 we studied the lethal effect of radiation on cells. *Reproductive death*, that is to say loss of proliferative capacity, is a probabilistic or random phenomenon. This explains why it is impossible to foretell among the population of apparently identical cells which will be killed and which will remain viable. After irradiation, each of the cells in a given tissue has a certain probability of being killed and this probability increases with the dose. At a given dose it varies with the tissue and with the type of cell in the tissue.

Given the large number of cells present in a tissue, at each dose a certain proportion of the cells will be killed. This proportion is never zero even for small doses. This may seem in contradiction with daily experience which shows that after small doses no effects are seen in the tissues, whereas lesions of increasing severity appear when the dose rises above a threshold level. The reason is that a macroscopic lesion appears only after death of a large enough proportion of the cells: the *threshold dose* corresponds to the proportion of cells killed, above which an effect becomes noticeable. For a given tissue it is about the same in every individual of a species and differs little from one mammalian species to another. The threshold dose, together with the delay before the lesion is observed, varies greatly from one tissue to another.

After doses of a few gray, reproductive cell death occurs at the time of one of the first cell divisions. Most of the non-viable cells can still divide a small number of times. The time at which the abortive mitosis takes place differs from one tissue to another and is related to the cell turnover rate of the tissue. For example, its duration is a matter of hours in intestinal epithelium and bone marrow, of days in skin and mucosa and of months in slowly proliferating tissues such as lung and kidney. In tissues where the cells divide only rarely, cellular damage remains latent for a long period of time and is revealed slowly. Damage in cells which are already partially differentiated and are destined to divide only a small number of times is of relatively little consequence for doses which are not too great. Many of them will still be able to pass through a few mitoses. On the other hand damage in stem cells has serious consequences: as they are programmed to perform a large number of divisions, they will be eliminated together with their descendants. Thus cells on the road to differentiation appear much less radiosensitive than stem cells. This explains the observations of Bergonié and Tribondeau in 1906 who noted that tissues appear to be more radiosensitive when their cells are less differentiated, have a greater proliferative capacity and divide more rapidly.

In each tissue, target cells can be identified which are usually the stem cells and whose number and radiosensitivity depends on the tissue. Changes in the number of cells present in the tissue depend therefore on several factors, notably the proportion of cells capable of division and their rate of proliferation. *In vitro*, cells remaining viable after irradiation multiply more slowly than unirradiated cells and this alteration in the kinetics of division increases with the dose. This difference is shown by a reduction in the mean size of the colonies. For example, colony size is reduced to a half after a dose of 2 Gy owing to the presence of small colonies formed by the descendants of cells which are viable but divide only slowly. The proportion of slowly proliferating but viable cells increases with dose, going, for example, in the experiments of Joshi (20), from 7 to 70% when the dose is increased from $0 \cdot 2$ to $3 \cdot 8$ Gy. *In vivo*, these phenomena are more complex due to stimulation caused by homeostatic mechanisms. Nevertheless both these effects occur: reduction in the number of viable cells and reduced response to a stimulus causing the viable cells to proliferate. Both factors are reduced when a given total dose is divided into a series of fractions.

This emphasizes that in addition to reproductive cell death, other phenomena play a role in the expression of tissue damage. Cells do not react to radiation as autonomous units; they are linked to adjacent cells by intercellular junctions, they receive and emit short-range and long-range microenvironmental signals such as growth factors and inhibitors of cell division. Thus the lesions in some cells in a given tissue can elicit abscopal effects in other tissues or organs. This interdependence of cells should never be overlooked; it contributes to the explanation of several untoward reactions initiated by radiation damage. Some early effects are not mediated through mitotic death but by injury to the cell membrane; e.g. acute erythema is associated with injury to blood vessels.

Before describing tissue damage we will remind the reader briefly of the kinetics of cell proliferation in tissue.

Kinetics of proliferation in tissue

A description of the cell cycle was given in Section 3.1. The proportion of labelled cells seen on an autoradiograph after a brief administration of [³H] thymidine is called the *labelling index* (LI). This index is equal to the proportion of cells in S phase. In a population where all the cells are in cycle, the labelling index is equal to the ratio T_s/T_c, that is the duration of S phase (T_s) divided by that of the cycle (T_c).

After mitosis a cell may enter a quiescent state in which it does not progress into a new cycle. This phase is called G_0; the cell can rejoin the cycle when stimulated to do so.

The *growth fraction* (GF) is equal to the ratio of the number of cells in proliferative cycle (N_p) to the total number of cells (N):

$$GF = N_p/N = N_p/(N_p + N_q)$$

where N_q is the number of cells in G_0. In a tissue under steady state conditions the numbers of cells being born and dying are equal. The *turnover rate* is equal to the proportion of cells born per unit time.

Delay in cell division

After irradiation the progress of the cells through the cell cycle may be delayed for periods up to a few tens of hours. In 1929 it was noted that after irradiation of a population of cells, the proportion in mitosis (mitotic index) is reduced; this

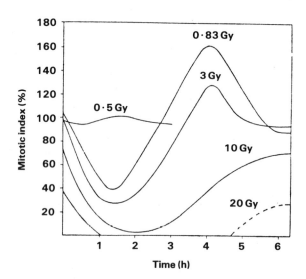

Figure 5.1. Changes in the number of mitoses (as a percentage of the mitotic index before irradiation) in chick fibroblasts after irradiation by radium γ-rays at a dose rate of 20 Gy h⁻¹.

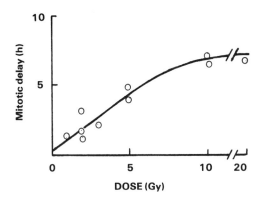

Figure 5.2. **Length of the premitotic delay as a function of dose — leukaemia cells L 51 784.** After [40].

phenomenon has been observed since then in all types of cell. In contrast with cell death which is an all or nothing effect, the duration of mitotic arrest is proportional to dose [42] (Figures 5.1 and 5.2).

The radiation-induced reduction in mitotic index results from a slowing down in the progression of cells through the cycle. Irradiation of synchronized cells (see Section 4.4), that is to say cells which are all in the same phase of the cycle, has shown that the length of this delay depends on the phase of the cycle at which the cells are irradiated. The longest delay is seen for cells irradiated in G_2; it is essentially due to a block before mitosis. The speed of progression from G_1 to S and from S to G_2 is reduced to a relatively small extent (Figure 5.3). The accumulation of cells in G_2 (pre-mitotic arrest) is connected either with a surveillance mechanism blocking the cells with radiation-induced lesions which prevents cell division, for example chromosomal lesions, or to a slowing down in the synthesis of proteins necessary for mitosis. *In vitro*, after irradiation at a high dose rate, mitotic delay is about 1–$3\,h\,Gy^{-1}$. *In vivo*, the duration of this delay depends on the power of the homeostatic mechanisms; this helps to explain the variation from one tissue to another. For example, it is 7–$10\,h\,Gy^{-1}$ for epidermis [16]. Some experimental results suggest that it is proportional to the duration of the cell cycle. In slowly renewing populations, the cells also accumulate at the G_1/S boundary. Accumulation of cells in G_2 is also seen during irradiation at low dose rate (Table 5.1).

After irradiation with doses of a few gray given at a high dose rate, the number of mitotic cells diminishes at first and later increases and can exceed

Table 5.1 **Percentage of cells in different phases of the cycle during continuous irradiation at $0 \cdot 5\,Gy\,h^{-1}$ (NCTC 2472 ascites cells, by cytophotometric analysis).**

	G_1	S	G_2
Controls	32	63	5
6h	25	65	10
12h	15	59	26
24h	17	45	38
40h	10	28	61

After [13].

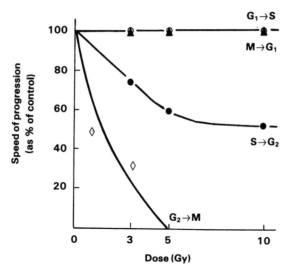

Figure 5.3. Effect of irradiation on the speed at which a cell passes from one phase in the cell cycle to the next. For Ehrlich ascites cells and at all doses, irradiation does not modify passage from G_1 to S or from M to G_1. Passage from S to G_2 is slowed down. For doses above 3–5 Gy, passage from G_2 to M is temporarily blocked. After [21].

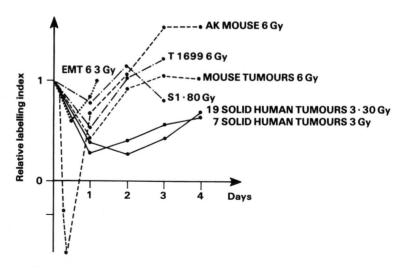

Figure 5.4. Changes in labelling index (i.e. in the percentage of cells in S phase) after irradiation of solid tumours, experimental and human. The 19 solid tumours which had received a dose of 3·3 Gy were reported by Malaise *et al*, [24] and the 7 others by Hendrickson [17].

the normal level when the cells blocked in G_2 enter mitosis together. In this situation the total number of mitoses is unchanged but their distribution in time is modified. This slowing down in the progression of cells through the cycle also causes variations in labelling index (Figure 5.4).

The cells whose premitotic block was longest have the greatest probability of dying. Most of the non-viable cells die at mitosis, which is the reason why the

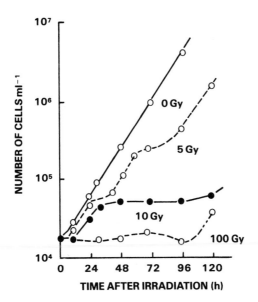

Figure 5.5. Delay in the growth induced by increasing doses of X-rays — leukaemia cells L 51 784.
After [40].

upsurge in mitoses is accompanied by the appearance of degenerating cells, particularly if the dose was large. The presence of non-viable cells destined to die explains the difference between changes in the labelling index and the proportion of viable cells in S phase. Moreover, in addition to cell death, mitotic delay contributes to the slowing down of the proliferation rate, particularly after small doses. Figure 5.5 shows the delay in the growth of a population of tumour cells induced by increasing doses of radiation.

Slow repair

This phenomenon plays a role in tissues with a low rate of proliferation [9]. Indeed in these tissues there may be delays of several weeks or months between irradiation and cell division. During this long period it seems that cellular lesions can be partially repaired, a phenomenon analogous to the repair of potentially lethal damage but whose speed is much slower. In certain tissues with low mitotic activity such as vascular endothelium, if proliferation is stimulated at different times after irradiation, the proportion of viable cells increases and the frequency of chromosome aberrations diminishes with increasing delay between irradiation and stimulation. The practical importance and the mechanism of this slow repair, which is never complete, remain controversial. Slow repair must be distinguished from regeneration due to cellular proliferation, which is sometimes difficult.

Repopulation

The cells in normal tissues are controlled by powerful homeostatic mechanisms.

The constancy in the number of each type of cell is a result of regulatory mechanisms such that the cells divide only to replace losses due to death by senescence. Cellular renewal is rapid when the lifespan of the differentiated cells is short.

A lesion involving a cellular deficit (trauma, toxicity, irradiation) triggers the proliferation of normal cells to compensate for the losses [31, 33]. For example, after a cut there is a loss of continuity in the skin. The gap is filled after a few days. Rapid multiplication of the cells at the edges of the wound enable the original morphology to be restored exactly. Similarly, after partial hepatec-tomy in the rat, the initial weight and form of the liver is restored in a few days. In this case the cells begin to multiply 12–15 h after the insult, due to a stimulus which acts on all the hepatic cells wherever they may be. For example, if some hepatic tissue has been grafted in a different anatomical site such as the spleen, the grafted cells also begin to proliferate. This shows that the stimulus has been transmitted by means of the blood stream. The stimulating factor has recently been isolated.

The regulation of proliferation in normal tissue is due to an equilibrium between growth factors and inhibitors [12, 36]. Stimulation can result from a reduction in the concentration of inhibitors, for example if the number of cells which secrete them is reduced, or from an increase in the secretion of growth factors. After irradiation both phenomena have been seen. The delay between irradiation and the homeostatic response varies from tissue to tissue. The response can be triggered by a deficit of cells in the proliferative compartment or later by an ensuing deficit in the non-proliferative functional compartment.

Scheme of tissue organization

Schematically, three categories of cells or tissue compartments can be distinguished. *Stem cells* are capable of dividing a very large number of times and give birth both to identical stem cells and to cells which will differentiate. The stem cells, which are capable of reproducing themselves, apparently escape from the link between cell division and differentiation which exists in other cells whereby a cell loses a little of its proliferative potential after each mitosis and finally differentiates into a functional non-dividing cell. During the course of a human life the stem cells seem to lose none of their proliferative capacity; however, experiments with successive transplantations show that the number of mitoses is limited. Normally almost all of them are in G_0 but they can enter rapidly into cycle after stimulation (see Figure 5.16). The term clonogenic cell is used to describe a cell capable of giving birth to a clone or colony composed of at least 100 cells. Stem cells and clonogenic cells are not synonymous terms since the definition of the latter is operational whereas that of the former is conceptual; in practice however the two terms are very close.

At the other extreme there are *differentiated* or *functional cells*: for example, circulating granulocytes and cells of the intestinal mucosal villi. These are usually incapable of division and die by senescence. All the cells of a given type have a similar lifespan but there are large variations between one cell type and another: it is 120 days for red cells and less than 1 day for granulocytes.

Maturating cells. Between these two compartments there is an intermediate compartment composed of cells in the process of maturation. In this compartment the partially differentiated cells which are descendants of the stem cells are multiplying while completing their differentiation. For example, in the bone marrow the erythroblasts and granuloblasts represent intermediate compartments. In some cases several successive cell types can be identified morphologically. When there is a large number of divisions in this compartment, each stem cell gives rise to a large number of differentiated cells. If, for example, there are four divisions during maturation, each stem cell entering the compartment will produce 16 differentiated cells. On the assumption that there is no cell death, the ratio between the number of cells entering and leaving a compartment is called the *amplification factor*.

The *transit time* of a cell in a compartment is the interval of time between its entry and exit (or that of its descendants) by death or differentiation. It can be measured by labelling with [^{3}H] thymidine. As irradiation mainly affects the stem cells without greatly modifying the lifespan of the differentiated cells, the lesions are expressed later when the transit time is longer.

The structure of many tissues corresponds to this model of hierarchical organization, e.g. haemopoietic bone marrow, intestinal epithelium, epidermis, epithelium of the bladder. However, others such as liver, thyroid and dermis have a different organization and are composed of cells which divide only rarely under normal conditions. After an insult such as partial hepatectomy or thyroidectomy, homeostatic mechanisms stimulate a large proportion of the cells to enter into cycle [41]. It is not certain whether there are any real stem cells in the tissue; in any case it is impossible to distinguish between stem cells and differentiated cells.

Models of effects in tissue

To interpret the effect of radiation on different tissues we must remember that the radiosensitivity of cells depends on their type and, within each type, on their degree of differentiation. Stem cells are the most radiosensitive; as a rule D_0 is about 1 Gy but for certain stem cells it can be as low as $0 \cdot 1$ Gy. The initial part of the survival curve also shows considerable variation. The sensitivity of maturing cells is lower and diminishes as differentiation becomes more complete. Fully differentiated cells which no longer divide are very radio-resistant. After irradiation the least differentiated compartments are therefore the most damaged, particularly as these contain the smallest numbers of cells. Cells which are differentiated but capable of proliferation when stimulated to do so, e.g. hepatocytes, have a lower radiosensitivity (D_0 of several gray), perhaps because they seldom divide.

When the same dose of radiation is given to tissues whose clonogenic cells have the same radiosensitivity, the appearance and repair of damage may have different time courses [41]. For example, the stem cells of the intestine and testis have similar radiosensitivities. However, in the first case the damage is expressed in a few days and repaired in 2 weeks whereas in the second the reduction in spermatogenesis may last for many months. These differences can be explained by the organization of the tissues and by the cellular homeostatic mechanisms. To interpret these reactions two types of tissue model have been proposed [41].

Hierarchical model

Hierarchical tissues (described above) are those in which there are at least two compartments, one of stem cells and one of cellular maturation. As we have seen, damage begins to be expressed after a delay proportional to the transit time and with a time course which is linked with the death of the functional cells by senescence and is therefore independent of dose. The later development of damage depends only on the lifespan of functional cells which is usually not altered by irradiation. This is confirmed experimentally, in agreement with the model (Figure 5.6). As the dose is increased, the stem cell compartment is progressively depleted; the time at which the depletion and the intensity of the reactions reaches its peak is later (Figure 5.7) and regeneration is slower.

However, in certain tissues regeneration of the stem cell compartment can be more rapid when the aplasia is deeper, i.e. after higher doses. Thus, in bone marrow aplasia develops earlier and regeneration is more rapid after higher doses (Figure 5.14). Absence of a simple relation between dose and the period of regeneration is therefore explained by the assumptions that after moderate doses the cells can divide a small number of times before dying [26] and that the stimulus for regeneration is more intense when the cellular depletion is greater [36]. Surviving maturing cells can contribute initially to a spurt in the production of new cells. However, proliferation of stem cells is required to initiate recovery of all the cell types in a lineage.

Flexible model

Flexible tissues are, as we have seen, those which apparently have no compartments and where there is no strict cellular hierarchy. After damage by surgery or chemical or physical agents, all the cells, including the functional cells, enter the mitotic cycle. In such a tissue, when a cell dies by senescence it is replaced by division of another cell. After irradiation, if mitoses do not give birth to viable cells, death of a cell by senescence leads to a series of divisions. The total number of cells falls progressively; when the critical level is reached it sets in motion a compensatory proliferation (Figure 5.8) and therefore the entry into mitosis of a large number of cells. As a result, most of the cells die by a phenomenon of avalanche, leading to rapid expression of the damage [25, 41].

In this case the time at which the damage becomes apparent is a function of the dose (Figure 5.8). If this is small the damage is expressed much later, as the cells divide infrequently and the lesions remain concealed for a long time due to the late expression of homeostatic mechanisms. For example, functional failure of the thyroid may be delayed for 10 or 15 years after irradiation. Moreover, in such a case the cells which are capable of only a few divisions may play an important role. By dividing even a small number of times they help to maintain the population of cells in the tissue at least for a certain time. This subclonogenic proliferation can result in pronounced curvature of the dose–response relationship for the tissue even if the dose–response curve of the clonogenic cells is exponential. Furthermore, there is no connection between the surviving fraction of clonogenic cells and the extent of the damage to tissue during an intermediate period which may be long [26].

These two models (hierarchical and flexible) are at extreme ends of a spectrum

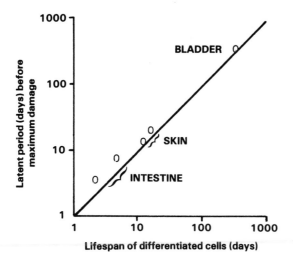

Figure 5.6. Length of the interval between irradiation and the appearance of maximum tissue damage as a function of the lifespan of the differentiated cells. After [25].

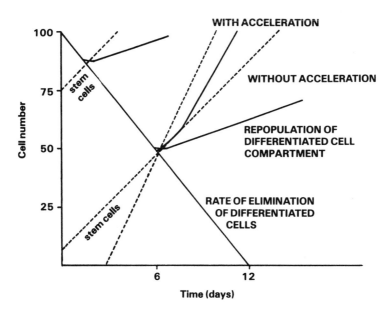

Figure 5.7. Depletion of differentiated cells in a hierarchical tissue. Almost all the stem cells have been killed by irradiation; as no more differentiated cells are formed, the number of cells diminishes steadily at a rate depending on the death of the cells by senescence, a rate which is the same whatever the dose. By contrast, regeneration can be accelerated to a smaller or greater extent by homeostatic mechanisms, depending upon the tissue. In the figure the time course of depletion corresponds to that of the basal cells of the epidermis (see [1]). The dashed lines correspond with various speeds of regeneration of the stem cell compartment.

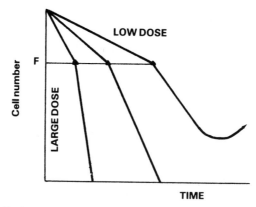

Figure 5.8. Post-irradiation changes in the number of cells in a flexible type tissue. After a large dose cellular homeostatic mechanisms come into action which, beyond the level F, lead to the entry into cell cycle of a large number of cells, resulting in the death of a large number of them — the avalanche phenomenon. After [25, 43].

of proliferative structures; many tissues are more realistically represented by hybrid models in which most cells are subclonogens capable of a small number of divisions while there may exist a minority population of stem cells. These hybrid tissues have two important features of a flexible type model: accelerating decline of population size with time (avalanche effect) and dependence of the shape of the dose–response curve on the properties of the subclonogenic cells. However, at variance with the flexible type, there is a theoretical possibility of radioprotection by post-irradiation stimulation of stem cell proliferation accompanied by an inhibition of proliferation of functional cells.

5.2 Late effects

After accidental irradiation received as a single dose, late effects are not usually of great importance, whereas the early toxicity dominates the clinical picture. On the other hand, in radiotherapy acute reactions are kept below a tolerable level and it is the late reactions which become the critical factor in limiting the dose that can be given. Severe late effects include fibrosis of deep tissue, osteoradionecrosis, intestinal obstruction, fistulae, oedema of the larynx, pulmonary and mediastinal fibrosis, paraplegia, etc. Some of these will be described later but we will discuss first their pathogenesis.

Pathogenesis of late effects

It is conventional to distinguish the early reactions, appearing during the first few days or weeks following irradiation, from the late effects which appear after a delay of several months or years. The early reactions are due to the death of a large number of cells and occur in tissues with a rapid cell turnover rate, whereas late reactions occur in tissues with slow cellular renewal. Although this contrast is correct it is oversimplified.

The timing of early reactions depends on the proliferation rate of the cells [25] which in certain tissues may be very slow. For example, because of the long lifespan of bladder epithelial cells the delay may extend to 3 months (Figure 5.6), but these lesions retain the pathogenesis of acute reactions. Sometimes, as for example in the lung, the early and late reactions merge without any symptom-free interval between them. The difference between the two types of lesion lies in their progression: acute damage is repaired rapidly and may be completely reversible, whereas late damage, even if it improves, is never completely repaired [29, 31]. In the first case, rapid multiplication of stem cells regenerates the tissue after rebuilding the various compartments. In the second case it is as though the stem cells had lost part of their proliferative capacity, either because of the damage which they have undergone [4], or because of the microenvironment in which they exist [28] and/or the lack of proliferative stimulating factors, or finally because the relevant stem cells have only a limited power of multiplication. Consequently the tissue undergoes progressive atrophy. Reduction in the proliferative capacity of haemopoeitic stem cells after repeated irradiation, changes caused by vascular damage, and development of damage in the thyroid illustrate these three mechanisms [18, 29, 32].

In addition to the prominent role of vascular damage, late reactions are in part due to a reduction in the number of stem cells [43]. For example, renal damage may be caused by loss of stem cells in each of the nephrons which constitute the renal parenchyma; if a nephron (containing about 3000 cells) no longer contains any stem cells capable of regenerating it, the nephron disappears and death of a large number of nephrons leads to renal atrophy. Biochemical changes can also be caused by loss of cells; e.g. if there is a reduced number of fibroblasts in the dermis the production of collagen molecules is slowed down, the molecules become 'aged' and cross-links are formed between them.

Moreover, if all late complications were of vascular origin, the dose–effect relationship would be the same in all tissues. This, however, is not the case and tolerance depends on the tissue, as shown in Table 5.2. For example, after irradiation of the hypophysis, hormonal disorders are mainly connected with the functions of the anterior lobe whereas vascular lesions would be the same in both lobes.

The latent period before the appearance of late effects in many tissues (contraction of the skin, development of paraplegia after irradiation of the spinal cord; Figure 5.9) becomes shorter as the dose is increased [41]. This suggests an avalanche type of phenomenon as we have seen previously in Section 5.1. After small doses the delay may be very long; however, the fragile equilibrium of the irradiated tissue which remains apparently normal can be broken by a second insult such as surgery or chemotherapy [29].

Whether the critical cells responsible for late effects are those of the vascular endothelium or are other cells, it has been shown from their radiobiological properties, both clinically and experimentally, that they are not the same as the cells responsible for acute effects, particularly with respect to their response to fractionation. For a given total dose, an increase in the dose per fraction increases late effects much more than early effects, as we will see in Chapter 8. The fact that fractionation has a similar effect on all late reactions suggests that the cells responsible have a powerful capacity for repair after small doses

Table 5.2 Tolerance of different tissues.

Organ	Type of damage	TD (Gy) 5/5	TD (Gy) 50/5	Total or partial organ irradiation (Field size or length)
Bone marrow	Aplasia, pancytopenia	2·5/30	4·5/40	Total/partial
Liver	Acute and chronic hepatitis	25/15	40/20	Partial/total
Stomach	Perforation, ulcer, haemorrhage	45	55	100 cm²
Intestine	Ulcer, perforation, haemorrhage	45/50	55/65	400 cm²/100 cm²
Brain	Infarction, necrosis	50	60	Whole
Spinal Cord	Infarction, necrosis	45	55	10 cm
Heart	Pericarditis and pancarditis	45/70	55/80	50%/25%
Lung	Acute and chronic pneumonitis	30/15	50/25	100 cm²/total
Kidney	Acute and chronic nephrosclerosis	15/20	20/25	Total/partial

TD: tolerance dose (5/5 and 50/5: 5% and 50% of severe complications at 5 years) The alternatives in the last column refer to the alternative values of dose and to total or partial organ irradiation. For example, 2·5 Gy to the whole bone marrow results in 5% severe complications and 4·5 Gy gives 50%. For partial irradiation the doses are 30 Gy and 40 Gy.
After [29].

(shallow slope of the initial part of the survival curve), perhaps because they seldom divide. Besides, it would be artificial to allocate different causes for late reactions as they are often associated, e.g. in skin fibrosis, atrophy and contraction result both from a reduction in the number of cells in the dermal connective tissue and a reduction in blood flow. Moreover, reduction in the number of clonogenic stem cells is important only if their reproduction becomes limited, otherwise only a few remaining viable cells would be enough to repopulate the tissue. This may be due to a reduction in the proliferative capacity of the cells or to an alteration in the stroma.

The concept of tolerance in radiotherapy

Owing to the variability of individual reactions and to statistical fluctuations (see Section 6.1) one can only speak of the probability of lesions. Any statement of the dose giving rise to a given complication in 5, 50 or 95% of irradiated subjects is subject to considerable statistical uncertainty. However, the collective experience of radiotherapists does make it possible to estimate the threshold of tolerance in radiotherapy (Table 5.2). The meaning of this term depends on whether the complication is very serious, e.g. paraplegia, or whether it can be endured without great loss of quality of life, e.g. muscular or articular damage. In the first case a probability of 5% is not acceptable whereas in the second a considerably greater probability can be allowed. In the same way, while one cannot risk inducing a neurological lesion in the spinal cord or the brain stem, it can be accepted in a silent region of the brain. In radiotherapy the concept of accepted risk must take account of the benefit to be expected from irradiation, together with the existence of other possible methods of treatment. For example, contraction and sclerosis of the thoracic wall caused by irradiation of breast cancer cannot be accepted if surgical removal is possible, whereas

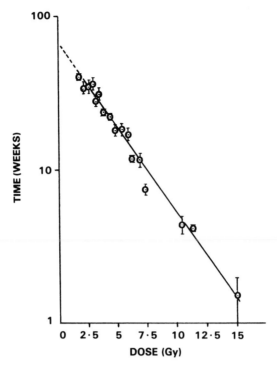

Figure 5.9. Variation with dose of the latent period between irradiation and induction of paraplegia in the rat.
After [14]

similar lesions seem legitimate in the treatment of osteosarcoma of the iliac bones or of a single bony metastasis.

Age also plays an important role. A given irradiation of the brain may cause an unacceptable intellectual deficit in a child but would have no appreciable mental effect in an adult.

Another reason for ambiguity in the notion of tolerance dose is the distinction between early and late complications. The two are not parallel and have different consequences. Irradiation of the kidney and bladder will illustrate this point. After a dose of 50–60 Gy, a very painful acute cystitis develops a few weeks later, but this can heal without serious sequelae; on the other hand a lower dose given to the whole of one kidney produces no early clinical reaction but initiates a progressive atrophy leading to functional loss of the kidney. In practice, late reactions are generally more important because they are irreversible and sometimes fatal. Early and late reactions have a different dependency on the fractionation scheme. The dose per fraction and the number of fractions must therefore be chosen to avoid serious late reactions.

In addition, chronic damage may result in death or remain latent depending on the environmental conditions. Thus rats whose kidneys have been irradiated survive much longer if they receive a diet containing little protein than if they are fed on a standard diet. In the same way patients who have been irradiated with very large fields seem to have normal haemopoiesis until the fragile equilibrium is broken by the administration of cytostatic drugs.

5.3 *Examples furnished by certain tissues*

As it is impossible to review every tissue we will take several examples, indicating for each the early and late effects, as well as the influence of fractionation. Chapter 8 will return to this point.

Radiotherapy and chemotherapy are often combined. Numerous articles and general reviews have shown how the addition of chemotherapy modifies the effects of radiation [5, 11, 28, 29, 38] and we will limit ourselves to some brief indications. The combined effect of the two modes of treatment may be additive or superadditive (synergistic). The first occurs if the drug and irradiation act by different mechanisms. Irradiation acts essentially by reduction in the number of stem cells and by its effect on connective tissue and the vascular system, whereas chemotherapy has little effect on the vasculature, its late effect being due essentially to the death of a large proportion of cells. For sequential administration of the two agents these additive mechanisms predominate. A synergistic effect may be seen when the two agents are administered simultaneously or close together in time. The quasi-synchronization produced by one of the two agents as well as the entry into cell cycle of stem cells and accelerated proliferation during the phase of repopulation can then lead to an increase in the sensitivity of certain normal tissues. Depending on the drug, the tissue and the chronology, the result of these combinations may be very different. In view of the variety of drugs and of mechanisms of action, it is difficult to foresee the immediate, and even more the late, effects of such combinations; great care is therefore always necessary.

Drugs or irradiation sensitize tissues to a later insult. Radiotherapy or chemotherapy given to patients who have already been treated may therefore reveal lesions which until then had been tolerated and occult. In other cases the latent lesions may only manifest themselves later during normal ageing of the tissue [28, 29].

Intestinal mucosa

Two techniques have been used to study the proliferation kinetics of the intestinal mucosa after irradiation or administration of cytotoxic agents: (1) counting the number of surviving crypts in a segment of the intestine, (2) injection of [3H] thymidine.

1. As a single viable clonogenic cell is able to repopulate a crypt, the technique of counting crypts makes it possible to measure the proportion of surviving clonogenic cells. As we have seen (Chapter 4), this method can only be used over a rather narrow range of doses, between 9 and 14 Gy. By using fractionated irradiation an approximate value of the ratio α/β can be obtained (Table 8.2).
2. After injection of [3H] thymidine it is possible to identify by autoradiography the cells in S phase and thus to define the region where the intestinal cells proliferate. After large doses of the radioactive label, the cells which have incorporated [3H] thymidine are killed (suicide effect) and in this way the proportion of clonogenic cells in S phase can be measured.

Normal intestine

There are no proliferating cells in the villi or the upper third of the crypt. On the other hand active proliferation (a high proportion of labelled cells after injection of [³H] thymidine) is seen in the central part of the crypt (Figure 5.10). Four hours after labelling, the labelled cells begin to differentiate. They then migrate towards the upper part of the crypt without further division, completing their maturation at the summit of the villus where they are desquamated. In the rat this journey takes about 3 days, but a little longer in old animals in which migration is slower. In germ-free animals the lifespan of differentiated cells is longer; consequently the villi are taller and the migration time longer (about 5 days). In man the cell transit time on the villus is 3–4 days.

The stem cells are located near the bottom of the crypt; they divide seldom and in the normal intestine administration of large doses of [³H] thymidine has little effect on their number. The number of stem cells is rather small, about 20 per crypt, out of a total of 250 cells of which 150 are in rapid proliferation [28]. Proliferation in the crypt follows a circadian rhythm leading to variations in radiosensitivity.

Early effects of acute irradiation

There is a large initial shoulder on the survival curve ($\alpha/\beta=12$ Gy). Between 9 and 14 Gy D_0 is about 1·2 Gy. However, certain stem cells situated near the bottom of the crypt seem to be much more radiosensitive [28]. Radiosensitivity is lower ($D_0=2$ Gy) a few days after a first irradiation, during cellular regeneration.

Immediately after a dose which sterilizes 99% of the clonogenic cells, the morphology of the intestine is apparently normal. In the central region of the crypts the cells continue to divide, differentiate and migrate in a quasi-normal fashion and their lifespan is not shortened. About 3–6 h later, pyknotic cells begin to appear near the base of the crypt where the stem cells are to be found. The number of mitoses then diminishes and 24 h after a dose of 6 Gy there are no cells in S phase, reflecting the arrest of cell multiplication. As a result the height of the villus is steadily reduced. After 24 h the percentage of crypt cells in proliferative cycle increases. It reaches a maximum much greater than the

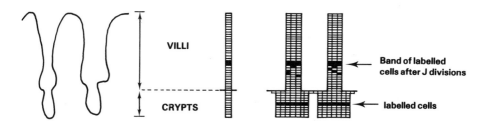

Figure 5.10. Diagram of an intestinal crypt. The cells multiply in the central part of the crypt, the only region in which there are cells in S phase which incorporate a DNA precursor. The cells then migrate along the villi and are shed into the intestinal lumen when they die.

normal value at about the fourth day, at the time when there is the smallest number of cells on the villus. Thereafter it slowly falls [28].

In germ-free rats the percentage of labelled cells reaches a minimum at the same time as in normal rats, but regeneration is slower and the maximum percentage of cells in proliferation is reached later. The decrease in the total number of cells is also slower, which is not surprising as their lifespan is longer. Proliferation in the crypt seems to depend on the number of differentiated cells in the upper part of the crypt and the villus, suggesting that these cells secrete an inhibitor of cellular proliferation.

After doses of a few gray, there are several foci of regeneration in each crypt; after doses of the order of 10 Gy there is on average only one focus of regeneration per regenerating crypt, suggesting that there is a single surviving clonogenic cell. With higher doses, a normal crypt density is restored by a process of longitudinal fission of surviving crypts.

During regeneration, acceleration of proliferation results from: (i) shortening of the cell cycle from 18 to 12 h; (ii) extension of the zone in which the cells proliferate towards the upper part of the crypt. This movement of the boundary between the zones where the cells divide and where they differentiate without dividing causes a considerable increase in cell production. It is observed at the moment when the reduction in height of the villus corresponds to a loss of about 50 cells (minimum quantity of inhibitor?). With higher doses the mucosa becomes ulcerated after 4 or 5 days, exposing the underlying tissue. The symptoms (diarrhoea, anorexia, infection) are a consequence of depletion of the cells lining the intestine.

Other cytotoxic agents have different effects on the intestinal mucosa, e.g. hyperthermia kills the differentiated cells, producing lesions which appear sooner and are repaired more rapidly.

Late effects [8, 30]

After fractionated irradiation, late effects may occur even if there have been no early reactions. In small animals, about 6 months after fractionated irradiation to a total dose of 50 Gy the number and cellularity of the capillaries are reduced; submucosal fibrosis develops progressively and by 12 months leads to a considerable reduction in the intestinal lumen.

In humans the late effects usually appear between 12 and 24 months after the end of radiotherapy but sometimes after several years. After localized irradiation the mobility of the intestinal loops reduces the dose received by each, except for the terminal portion of the ileum which is fixed; this is perhaps the reason why this is the part most frequently damaged [8]. The risk of intestinal damage is increased when there are intestinal adhesions due to surgery before irradiation (splenectomy and staging laparotomy). The intestinal wall of the damaged segments is thickened and indurated with oedema and fibrosis. Stenosis of the intestinal lumen is frequent, with short zones of concentric restriction and fibrous peritonitis. Superficial ulcerations are common. The mesentery is also thickened and indurated. The existence of endoarteritis and perforation in the necrotic zones suggests the role of vascular damage. Surgical intervention is dangerous as manipulation of the intestine may damage fragile blood vessels.

Clinically the patient presents with abdominal cramps, difficulty in digesting fat and alternation between diarrhoea and constipation; there are peritoneal masses consisting of intestinal loops adhering to one another. Complications, sometimes tell-tale (subacute or acute obstructions, perforations, fistulae) may require sugical intervention. Medical treatment of these enteropathies is important. During radiotherapy itself, a *residue-free diet* with frequent and small meals reduces the frequency of later complications. Once these become established, symptomatic care and antibiotics are useful. When large fields are used for irradiation of the abdominal cavity, and particularly if there has been previous surgery, these complications are seen with moderate doses (40–45 Gy). After doses of 50–60 Gy they occur with variable severity in one third of the patients. They are more frequent when the dose per fraction exceeds 2·5 Gy which appears to constitute a limit.

The combination within 1 year of irradiation to 60 Gy with chemotherapy (5-FU and Me-CCNU) increases the frequency of late complications (fistulae and perforations), as though the moderate cellular depletion produced by chemotherapy was not tolerated by an atrophic and poorly vascularized tissue [8, 29].

The colon and rectum are less radiosensitive. Damage may be seen after doses of 55 Gy; after 60–70 Gy, one third of the patients are affected. The size of the irradiated volume plays a critical role.

The skin

Reminder of anatomy

The skin is composed of two tissues, the epidermis and the dermis [28]. The epidermis is derived from a basal layer of actively proliferating small cells, the keratinoblasts. It also contains other cells: melanocytes which synthesize melanin and Langerhans cells which belong to the immunological system.

The basal layer is covered by three or four layers of non-dividing differentiated cells containing nuclei, which are wider and thinner (Figure 5.11). These cells are themselves covered by about 10 layers of keratinized cells which are very thin and do not contain nuclei. These cells are arranged roughly in columns. At the base of each column there is an *epidermal proliferative unit* composed of about 10 basal cells lying in a single plane. This layer is covered by a large cell which is incapable of division and is surmounted in turn by other cells arranged one on top of the other in a column reaching to the surface where the most superficial keratinized cells are desquamated. In the mouse each proliferative unit produces about one cell per day. This migrates towards the surface while differentiating and becoming flat, covering the whole proliferative unit and pushing up the cells above it. The cycle time of the basal cells in a proliferative unit in man is on the average about 200 h. This is a long time but some of the cells probably have shorter cycles. The total transit time, between the moment when the cell differentiates while leaving the basal layer and the time at which it is desquamated, is about 14 days (between 7 and 21 days depending on the body site), much longer than for cells of the intestinal mucosa.

The dermis is a dense connective tissue, generally 1–2 mm thick, within which there are scattered fibroblasts which produce most of the dermal

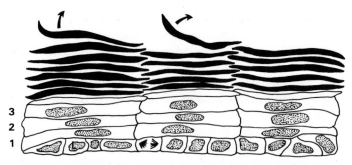

Figure 5.11. **Diagram of the epidermis of the mouse. In the basal layer there are proliferative units containing a stem cell at the centre. This cell divides and is surrounded by about 10 cells in the process of maturation but still capable of division. When a cell is fully differentiated (and becomes incapable of division) it passes into the layer above and extends laterally, a single cell covering the whole proliferative unit. It then migrates towards the surface, keratinizes, dies and is desquamated. In the basal layer there are also melanocytes and Langerhans cells.**
After [28].

proteins. It is a slowly proliferating tissue. The vascular elements of the dermis play a major role in the radiation response.

After irradiation the surviving clonogenic cells regenerate the tissue. Their number is reduced with increasing dose. The cell survival curve makes it possible to estimate by extrapolation the number of clonogenic cells in the unirradiated normal epidermis. Whereas there are about 20 000 basal cells per mm^2 of epidermis grouped in about 1500 proliferative units, the number of clonogenic cells is of the order of 1000–2000 per mm^2. This suggests that there is only one stem or clonogenic cell in each proliferative unit. The other cells in the unit must therefore be cells which are differentiating; moreover, by injection of [³H] thymidine one can distinguish among them several varieties of cells corresponding to different stages of maturation and with different cell cycle times. The most differentiated cells leave the unit to migrate towards the surface about 2 days after the last mitosis.

The number of hair follicles in the skin varies in different regions. In these follicles there are stem cells which are capable of participating in regenerating the epidermis.

Acute effects of a single dose: macroscopic reaction [8]

Several types of reaction can be distinguished.

EARLY ERYTHEMA
A few hours after doses greater than 5 Gy there is an early erythema similar to sunburn which is due to vasodilation, oedema and loss of plasma constituents from the capillaries. It lasts for a few days.

SECONDARY REACTIONS RELATED TO CELL DEATH [8]
These occur after doses of about 10 Gy and begin about 10 days after irradiation. This delay, together with the speed at which the lesions subsequently develop, is not influenced by the dose but varies with the species and the anatomical

region. The severity and to some extent the timing of the peak depends on the dose to the basal layer of the epidermis: dry desquamation after 10 Gy, moist desquamation after 15 Gy, etc. The time required for regeneration becomes longer as the dose is increased, probably because the number of surviving basal clonogenic cells becomes smaller. After very large doses, repair of the epidermis takes place mainly from the periphery.

COMBINATION OF RADIOTHERAPY WITH CHEMOTHERAPY
Administration of cytotoxic drugs during irradiation increases the effects and reduces the threshold. For example, a dose of 50 Gy in 5 weeks (telecobalt) produces only a dry desquamation, but if adriamycin is given simultaneously moist desquamation occurs, sometimes even leading to necrosis. If an interval of 1 week is allowed between giving the two agents this additivity disappears.

Radiobiological interpretation of the development of macroscopic lesions [8, 28]

As with the intestine, the method of colony assay makes it possible to measure in animals the number of surviving clonogenic cells, by counting the number of regenerating foci 10–14 days after irradiation. After doses greater than 8 Gy each focus develops from a single cell. The survival curve measured by this method has a value of $D_o=1\cdot3$ Gy. The parameters of the initial part of the curve can be determined by using fractionated irradiations; these suggest that there is a large shoulder with an initial slope of about $4\cdot5$ Gy. The ratio α/β is high, about 20 (see Table 8.2). After 2 Gy the proportion of surviving cells is about 50%, after 15 Gy there remain only about 1 clonogenic cell mm^{-2} and after 30 Gy there are about 10^{-4}–10^{-5} cells mm^{-2}. D_o is increased when the dose rate is reduced. The severity of the effects and the survival of clonogens is markedly dependent on the area of skin irradiated between 1 and 400 cm^2.

Even after high doses there are no pyknotic cells above the basal layer. In the basal layer the number of degenerating cells is small and shows little dependence on dose between 5 and 35 Gy. The number reaches a maximum at 3 or 4 days, but even with doses sterilizing all the clonogenic cells and leading to ulceration it does not exceed 10%, i.e. the approximate proportion of stem cells in this layer. Denudation is therefore not due to cell death but to cessation of cell production. This is different from what is seen after irradiation with UV; the number of degenerating cells is then very high as the differentiated cells are damaged, leading to the earlier appearance of damage.

Labelling with [³H] thymidine confirms that the maturing cells can still synthesize DNA, divide and migrate after doses which kill almost all the clonogenic cells. The progressive depopulation of the basal layer is therefore due to the differentiation and migration of the cells which are programmed to differentiate and whose fate is not altered, while their production is reduced or interrupted by the death of the stem cells. The time course of the damage is therefore independent of dose as it corresponds to the time needed for death by senescence of the cells of the differentiated layers and the maturing cells in the proliferative units. Moreover, both denudation of the epidermis due to desquamation of the keratinized cells and depletion of the basal layer by maturation and migration have the same time-scale of about 20 days after irradiation. Various factors can accelerate denudation, e.g. infection and poor attachment of the cell layers situated above the basal layer when the latter is depleted, leading to rapid loss of cells from the upper layers when the density of cells in the basal layer becomes very small.

Regeneration begins about 1 week after irradiation, when small islands of cells in rapid proliferation can be seen with labelling index greatly above normal.

The cutaneous reaction is only seen if the dose exceeds a *threshold*, as a small depletion of the basal layer does not lead to any detectable macroscopic reaction, but doses below the threshold, even below 1 Gy, do reduce the number of stem cells in the basal layer. This residual damage reduces the tolerance to later irradiation. Thus the doses needed to produce skin reactions are reduced by about 10%. Several months after irradiation, administration of actinomycin D may lead to the appearance of localized erythema in the irradiated areas (recall). In the same way certain drugs given after irradiation may cause subcutaneous fibrosis.

Late effects

After radiotherapy, as after accidental or occupational irradiation, delayed reactions occur predominantly in the dermis [8]. These are more serious than the early reactions because they are irreversible. The skin becomes thin and fragile; small injuries may lead to ulceration which heals poorly. Telangiectasis is also seen, demonstrating damage to the vasculature. If the irradiation was very superficial the damage is limited to the dermis and the epidermis. With X- and γ-rays of high energy the dose to the skin is reduced (Section 1.3) and the early reactions are slight, enabling higher doses to be delivered at a depth; fibrosis of the subcutaneous tissues is then observed.

There is a lack of parallelism between the early reactions (dry or moist desquamation) and the late damage, particularly when the fractionation is varied (the ratio α/β is about 3 for the late effects, very different from that measured for the acute effects, Figures 8.4 and 8.5). In contrast with what is seen with early skin reactions, late damage develops earlier when the dose is increased. The mechanisms of induction are therefore not the same and the origin of the late damage is to be found in the dermis.

The pathogenesis of this effect which appears between 6 months and 2 years after irradiation remains controversial [18]. Vascular damage plays an important role. Experimentally, the existence and severity of the late damage had been correlated with the reduction of blood flow measured 3 months after irradiation. This is due to vascular lesions in the dermis (partial or total obliteration of arterioles by endothelial cells). Ultimately the blood flow becomes normal again despite dermal atrophy and contraction of the irradiated skin. It is possible that reduction in blood flow leads to death of cells in the dermis. However, the reduction in fibroblasts is probably due to a direct effect: several decades after irradiation, chromosome aberrations can still be found in the fibroblasts. The rapid growth of tumour fragments implanted in subcutaneous tissue suggests that the cells in the irradiated vessels are capable of rapid proliferation.

Whatever may be the cause, the reduction in the number of dermal fibroblasts leads to a slowing down in the renewal rate of collagen molecules and to their incomplete resorption. As a result cross-links are formed between and within the collagen molecules, leading to a loss of elasticity in the skin.

Effects on mucosa

The cellular organization of the mucosa, for example the oropharyngeal mucosa, is very similar to that of the skin. There is a basal layer where the cells multiply. The cells then leave this zone to migrate towards the surface while differentiating. However, the lifespan of the differentiated cells is much shorter than in the epidermis, which is the reason for the more rapid appearance of reactions. Several degrees of severity have been distinguished: erythema with oedema and dilatation of the capillaries, ulceration by plaques or simple mucositis, confluent mucositis with pseudo-membranes and finally extensive ulceration requiring hospitalization. Regeneration sets in quickly and is completed more rapidly than in the skin; in the course of fractionated irradiation, regeneration can be seen in spite of continued irradiation. Several successive waves of mucosal reaction can be observed. A submucosal fibrosis sets in during the weeks and months following irradiation. The shape of the cell survival curve is similar to that seen for the epidermis but varies markedly from one region to another.

As with skin, concomitant administration of cytotoxic drugs aggravates the damage and sometimes reduces considerably the threshold of tolerance. For example, in a clinical trial organized by the European Organisation for Research in the Treatment of Cancer (EORTC), administration of bleomycin during radiotherapy made it necessary to interrupt the treatment of a high proportion of the patients [5]. Also, if the treatments are given sequentially instead of simultaneously, the additivity of the effects is greatly reduced and the immediate tolerance increased.

Epithelium of the bladder

The epithelium of the bladder consists of a basal layer formed of small diploid cells, followed by three or four layers of rather larger transitional cells and at the surface by a layer of very large polyploid cells with a thick membrane capable of resisting the irritation caused by urine. The rate of cell renewal is very low and the lifespan of the superficial cells very long, of the order of several months or more [31].

After damage by trauma or a chemical agent, the cells of the basal layer are quickly triggered into proliferation. On the other hand *after irradiation*, accelerated proliferation of the basal cells begins about 4 months later. This long delay is probably due to the long life span of the differentiated cells (200 days). It is only after the death by senescence of the differentiated cells that mitosis of the basal cells reveals latent cellular damage. The increase in the labelling index coincides with the onset of functional difficulties. Frequency of urination increases in parallel with bladder damage, loss of surface cells and epithelial hyperplasia. In spite of hyperplasia of the basal layer, the large polyploid cells at the surface are not formed, as though differentiation is not proceeding normally. The absence of these protective cells explains the irritation by urine of the deeper cellular layers, leading to stimulation of cellular proliferation for a period of several months [28, 31].

The damage is expressed more rapidly with higher doses. The ratio $\alpha/\beta=7$ Gy; prolongation of treatment does not modify the reactions because of the absence of repopulation. The late effects are related to fibrosis and reduction in the capacity of the bladder. Combination of radiotherapy with chemotherapy accelerates the appearance of bladder damage but does not accelerate the appearance of late effects; this shows that there is no direct relationship between denudation of the bladder wall and late effects.

Haemopoietic tissues

In healthy adult man the liver and spleen have no haemopoietic activity and the haemopoietic tissues are located only in the bone marrow which can be regarded as a diffuse single organ with structural organization. This can be seen by histological examination and can be investigated by functional studies.

Reminder on haemopoiesis and the effects of irradiation

Figure 5.15 indicates the series of compartments which can be distinguished in the bone marrow, showing the degree of differentiation from the pluri-potential stem cells to the functional end cells which can circulate in the blood and no longer divide. The distribution of the different types of blood cell depends on the distance from the bony wall and on the dimensions of the cavities in which haemopoiesis takes place. This emphasizes the role of the stromal cells and intercellular interactions.

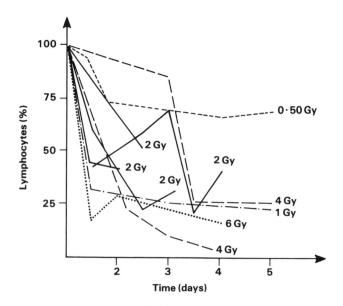

Figure 5.12. Changes in the number of lymphocytes (expressed as a percentage of the number before irradiation) in 10 patients given total body irradiation in preparation for an organ graft.
After [37].

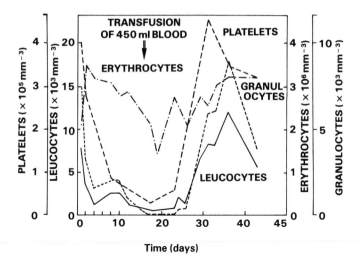

Figure 5.13. Changes in the number of blood cells in a patient given total body irradiation of 4·3 Gy in preparation for a kidney graft.
After [37]

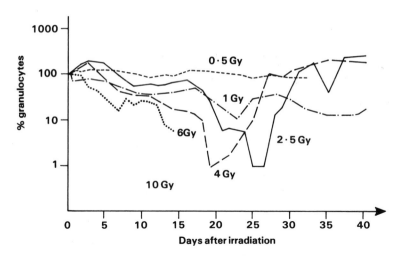

Figure 5.14. Changes in the number of granulocytes after total body irradiation with different doses in preparation for organ grafting.
After [37].

Pluripotential stem cells and progenitors

In the mouse the four lines of blood cells originate from the same multi-potential stem cells. When bone marrow cells from a normal mouse are injected intravenously into a mouse which has been irradiated with a dose big enough to cause bone marrow aplasia (10 Gy), they restore haemopoiesis, particularly in the spleen. In this organ cell colonies are formed in which all the cells have a single common ancestor, demonstrated by the presence of the same chromosome marker in all the cells of a given colony. Some of these colonies contain erythro-

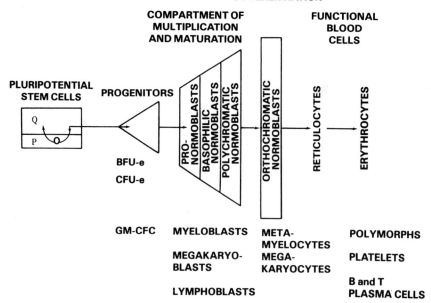

Figure 5.15. Diagram of the different cellular compartments of the bone marrow. The four haemopoietic lines originate from the same pluripotential stem cells. These differentiate into specific progenitors for each of the lines. As an example the diagram represents the erythropoietic line. The cells multiply and differentiate progressively in the progenitor compartment, followed by the compartments containing pronormoblasts and normoblasts which contain haemoglobin. The orthochromatic normoblasts differentiate but do not divide and give birth to reticulocytes and then erythrocytes.

cytes, myelocytes, megakaryocytes and sometimes even lymphocytes, showing that these cell lines develop from a single stem cell. The stem cells constitute about 0·2% of the bone marrow cells and have two characteristic properties: (i) a capacity for *indefinite self-reproduction*, or at least the ability to divide several hundred times as shown by transplantation experiments; and (ii) *pluripotentiality*, i.e. the capacity to differentiate towards any of the four lines.

This population of cells is probably not homogeneous and some of the stem cells have a lower capacity for repopulation. Similarly the stem cells do not all respond in the same way to a stimulus. These variations are at least partly related to the cellular microenvironment. After irradiation, the ability of surviving stem cells to renew themselves and differentiate depends upon the survival of an appropriate microenvironment in the stroma.

Between the pluripotential stem cells (or CFU-S, *colony forming units in spleen*) and the first cells which are recognizable morphologically, there are intermediate cells which are not identifiable morphologically and which are the committed stem cells or progenitors. These cells give rise only to a single cell line but have a large capacity to reproduce themselves, although the number of divisions which they can make without differentiating is limited.

The transit time between the pluripotential stem cell in the bone marrow and the haematocyte is about 4 days in the mouse and a week in man. During this time the cells are multiplying in the compartment of proliferation and maturation; they then differentiate without division in the compartment of differentiation (Figure 5.15).

The proliferative state of the stem cells can be studied by the *suicide method* [12, 13, 39]. The cells are incubated with large quantities of [³H] thymidine; the cells in S phase incorporate a considerable amount and are killed by the radioactivity. For example, if injection of 10^{-5} bone marrow cells results in the formation of 20 spleen colonies but only 10 colonies if they are first incubated in the presence of [³H] thymidine, it shows that 10 stem cells out of 20 were in the DNA synthetic phase.

In normal marrow more than 90% of the CFU-S are in resting phase [39]; on the other hand the progenitors are dividing rapidly and their proliferation is not accelerated during regeneration of the tissue. When regeneration is needed to maintain a constant rate of haemopoesis, for example after loss of cells from the more differentiated compartments, some of the CFU-S differentiate into progenitors while others enter the proliferative state. If a drug which kills the

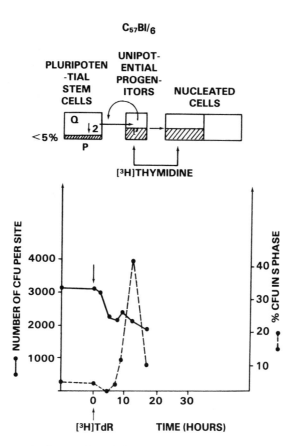

Figure 5.16. Changes in the number of pluripotential stem cells (CFU-S) and the percentage of cells in S phase after administration of [³H] thymidine. As most of the stem cells are quiescent, the [³H] thymidine only irradiates and kills the more differentiated cells which are rapidly multiplying. This causes differentiation of the stem cells, reducing the number of cells in the stem cell compartment and causing these cells suddenly to enter cycle about 10 h after administration of [³H] thymidine. After [39].

cells in S phase is given, e.g. hydroxyurea or [³H] thymidine, the quiescent CFU-S are not damaged but about half the cells in the compartment of proliferation and differentiation are killed. About 10 h after administration of the drug a large proportion of the CFU-S enter S phase (Figure 5.16).

In the same way, after partial irradiation, i.e. with part of the marrow shielded, two indirect effects are seen in the shielded marrow [7]: first a reduction in the number of CFU-S due to differentiation which increases with increasing dose to the irradiated parts; this then triggers proliferation of the remaining CFU-S (Figure 5.17). These two effects increase the number of cells in the proliferative compartment; they are caused by humoral factors whose presence can be detected in the plasma [12].

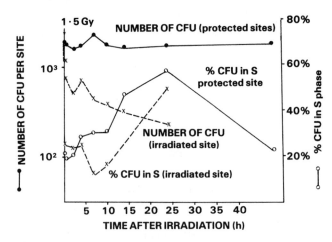

Figure 5.17. Effect of partial irradiation of the bone marrow to a dose of 1·5 Gy on the irradiated and shielded marrow. At this dose, the number of stem cells in the shielded marrow remains almost constant but, because of the liberation of a stimulating factor by the irradiated tissue, the percentage of stem cells in S phase in the shielded marrow increases rapidly 15–20 h after irradiation. It also increases, but later, in the irradiated marrow, probably because the irradiated cells react more slowly to stimulation.

The erythrocyte line

Several precursors of the erythrocyte line can be identified from their morphology. Beginning with the least mature, they are pronormoblasts, basophilic normoblasts, polychromatic normoblasts, orthochromatic normoblasts and reticulocytes. All these cells contain haemoglobin and incorporate radioactive iron which can therefore be used to label the whole line. After differentiation, the labelled cells are transformed into reticulocytes which pass into the blood and become red blood cells (Figure 5.15). As the labelled pronormoblasts differentiate into reticulocytes, they are replaced by unlabelled pronormoblasts arising from differentiation of the progenitors† of the erythrocyte series as these do not contain haemoglobin. In this way the transit time between pronormoblasts and red cells can be measured; it is 8 days. The number

---

†The least mature of these are called BFU-E and the more differentiated CFU-E.

of cell cycles and their duration in each of the sub-compartments can be assessed by means of experiments with [³H] thymidine. The acidophils (orthochromatic normoblasts) are the only cells of the erythrocyte line which do not synthesize DNA; maturation from acidophil to reticulocyte therefore takes place without cell division.

Knowing the length of the transit time, the percentage of cells in division and the duration of the cell cycle, one can calculate the number of cells leaving the proliferative compartment for every progenitor cell entering it. This is called the *amplification factor*. For example, if all the cells are proliferating, the transit time is 5 days and the cell cycle is 24 h, for every cell entering the compartment 32 cells must leave. The amplification factor is then 32. Normally there are between five and eight divisions in the human marrow. However, all the cells are not in cycle and the cycle time is of variable duration. Also some of the cells may die in the course of proliferation. The amplification factor may therefore be considerably lower but can increase when needed. This variation in amplification plays an important role in the regulation of cell production.

All the cells of the bone marrow are radiosensitive but the youngest cells, the least mature, are the ones for which loss of part of their proliferative capacity is the most critical.

After total body irradiation to a moderate dose, the number of red cells and reticulocytes in the blood at first remains normal thanks to maturation of pronormoblasts into reticulocytes. The production of reticulocytes is reduced about 1 week after irradiation (Figure 5.13). Twelve to fifteen days after irradiation to several gray, the production of red cells stops and starts again later, at the same time as the other blood cells. The number of reticulocytes is a better indication of erythropoiesis than changes in the number of red cells because of the long lifespan of the red cells and the possibility of haemorrhage or haemolysis.

Granulocyte line

Because of the short lifespan of the circulating granulocytes, their number faithfully reflects granulopoiesis. Their progenitors, GM-CFC, can be counted by culturing *in vitro*. The ratio between the number of granulocyte progenitors and the number of metamyelocytes makes it possible to measure the amplification factor. A large amplification indicates an increased number of divisions in the compartment of maturation; this is seen during regeneration of the bone marrow.

Changes in the proportions of blood cells after total-body irradiation

The effects of total body irradiation on blood cells have been known for a long time. A dose of 0·3 Gy leads to a reduction in the number of blood lymphocytes both in animals and man, lymphocytes being among the most radiosensitive cells in the body (Figure 5.12).

After larger doses the number of blood cells is altered and this constitutes the first warning sign. Lymphopenia is followed by granulopenia, then thrombopenia and finally anaemia. These changes are similar in all subjects who have received the same dose. For example, after total-body irradiation to

4–6 Gy (Figure 5.13), there is a temporary and variable increase in the number of granulocytes during the first few days (due to mobilization of the reserve pool) followed by a rapid fall by the end of the first week. The number then remains steady for a few days and may even increase due to recovering haemopoiesis from precursor cell populations, before falling again to a minimum value below 200 granulocytes per mm^3 18–20 days after irradiation. After a week of aplasia, regeneration is rapid and takes place simultaneously in all the cell lines (platelets, reticulocytes, granulocytes) [37].

When the dose is higher (Figure 5.14) the minimum number of cells is reached earlier and the period of aplasia may be longer, increasing the danger of haemorrhage and infection (see Chapter 12). For lower doses of the order of 1 Gy the depression in the number of granulocytes is less marked but its duration is longer and regeneration less rapid [37]. With whole body doses above 6 Gy, the critical level of granulocytes (300 μl^{-1}) is reached in 7–9 days. The bone marrow cellularity is reduced by 30% one day after 3–4 Gy and by 80% after 8 Gy. It reaches a minimum value 3–4 days after 5 Gy or above and regeneration can be detected in the marrow at day 6 by the presence of colonies of undifferentiated cells. After doses up to 8 Gy, regeneration begins earlier than after lower doses. After many small doses (chronic irradiation) there are changes in blood count which will be discussed in Chapter 12.

The reduction in the number of blood cells is a relatively sensitive biological criterion. The haemopoietic stem cells are particularly radiosensitive. The extrapolation number of the survival curves is close to 1 (between 1·2 and 1·5) with a very small shoulder (which explains the small protective effect of fractionation) and a very high ratio α/β of 20 Gy; the value of D_0 is low, about 0·9 Gy. Some experimental and clinical findings suggest that the D_0 of some stem cells may be even lower [28]. The radiosensitivity of the progenitors (GM-CFC, etc.) is a little lower and their survival curves have small shoulders with extrapolation numbers about 4. Fractionation does not influence the proportion of survivors. The slope of the curve of CFU-S survival versus dose is practically identical at high and low dose rates. This indicates that there is no significant repair of sublethal damage.

The damage becomes manifest very quickly because of the rapid cell turnover. However, the number of circulating blood cells gives no indication of the severity of damage to haemopoietic tissues and in particular to stem cells. Peripheral blood counts can sometimes be maintained despite severe damage inflicted on progenitors because a compensatory increase in production of circulating cells can originate from maturing cells; e.g. cells in the early erythroid-committed stages can increase their production by extra divisions during maturation. Conversely, relatively low acute doses of radiation can temporarily suppress production of blood cells.

Interpretation of changes in the production of erythrocytes and granulocytes

As discussed above, the survival of stem cells determines the subsequent performance of the bone marrow. During the first few hours following *total body irradiation* there is a sudden decrease in the number of pluripotential stem cells and progenitor cells. This is due partly to the lethal effect of the irradiation and partly to differentiation which takes place in response to depletion of the more differentiated compartments [36]. However, when the number of stem cells is reduced below a critical level their differentiation becomes blocked; this results in depletion of cells in the compartment of proliferation and maturation, followed by an arrest in the production of functional end cells about 10 days after irradiation when there are no more cells in the last stage of maturation (erythroblasts, acidophils or metamyelocytes). Production of functional cells then remains almost zero until partial regeneration of the stem cell compartment, due to their rapid proliferation, once more allows differentiation and rapid repopulation of the cell line. Regeneration is then truly explosive (Figures 5.13 and 5.14). Administration of haemopoietic growth factors (CSF) can markedly shorten the duration of aplasia and accelerate blood-cell regeneration.

After *repeated (fractionated) irradiations* there is a reduction in the pool of stem cells and progenitors. However, the small production of progenitors is compensated by an increase in the amplification factor. This occurs due to a prolongation of the transit time with a larger number of mitoses within this compartment (up to five or six additional mitoses), particularly in the least differentiated cells. Moreover, this mechanism compensates for the mortality of cells in this compartment. During protracted continuous irradiation, the initial shape of the stem-cell survival curve is identical to that found with single doses. However, when the dose rate is low there is an abrupt change of slope when the stem cell survival becomes very small. The CFU-S population may remain constant (at $0.7\,\mathrm{Gy\ day^{-1}}$) or even increase (at $0.5\,\mathrm{Gy\ day^{-1}}$) despite the irradiation because the stem cells are cycling at their maximum rate. Therefore, as a result of both the increase in proliferation rate of CFU-S and an increased number of mitoses in the maturation compartment, mice can have almost normal numbers of circulating blood cells while receiving more than $30\,\mathrm{Gy}$ at low dose rate to the whole body.

Partial body irradiation

In the irradiated volume the effects of partial body irradiation are analogous to those of total body irradiation. In the unirradiated marrow the stem cells enter the mitotic cycle a few hours after irradiation (Figure 5.17) and a compensatory hyperplasia occurs which ensures that the total production of blood cells is not reduced [7, 27, 34]. In addition there is an extension of haemopoiesis into marrow volumes such as those in the long bones which are not normally haemopoietic in the adult human, together with extramedullary haemopoiesis in the spleen and liver [27, 29]. With fractionated irradiation the pool of stem cells in the unirradiated volumes falls progressively owing to acceleration of differentiation. Also total production may be reduced in spite of increased proliferation; this persists after irradiation until normal activity is resumed in the irradiated volume. With doses greater than $30\,\mathrm{Gy}$, haemopoiesis never returns to normal in the irradiated volume and the hyperplasia and extension of the active bone marrow in unirradiated volumes persists indefinitely [27].

Repopulation in the irradiated volume is greater when this is more extended. In man the activity of the irradiated volumes remains low after irradiation of 20% of the marrow; on the other hand if 50 or 60% of the marrow is irradiated it partially regenerates even after relatively high doses, probably because of the intense stimulation to which it is exposed [27].

Sequelae and late effects

There is always a reduction in the number of stem cells after irradiation of the bone marrow. This returns very slowly to normal, which is why patients remain more sensitive to a new insult for several months or years after total body irradiation or cytotoxic treatment [29, 37], a long time after the blood count has returned to normal. Regeneration of the stem cell compartment is slower when the total dose has been greater.

When haemopoiesis starts again in the irradiated volumes there is a considerable mortality of progenitor cells (ineffective haemopoiesis). Late failure can be seen both in animals and man after periods of variable duration during which the blood count is normal [6]. Several interpretations have been put forward for these late effects [28, 29]: (i) destruction of the 'niches', that is to say, tissue structures where the stromal cells play an important role and in which the stem cells find a favourable microenvironment for self-renewal; (ii) changes in vascularization; and (iii) residual damage in the stem cells which reduces their repopulating ability [4]. None of these explanations is sufficient by itself.

Combination with cytotoxic agents

Some of the drugs used in chemotherapy act essentially on cells in cycle. Others can also kill cells out of cycle in G_0. The cycle-specific drugs have little effect on the stem cells since over 90% of them are in G_0 unless the marrow is regenerating, e.g. after irradiation [29]. This explains why these drugs have additional toxicity when they are administered shortly after radiotherapy.

Whatever the time interval, the marrow of a patient who has been irradiated over a large volume has increased sensitivity to drugs, partly as we have seen because the marrow is hyperactive, and also because of the reduction in the pool of stem cells. This is not seen after localized irradiation. Some drugs, in particular busulphan, reduce the proliferative capacity of the surviving stem cells and thereby considerably diminish tolerance to irradiation of extended volumes [4]. On the other hand, small doses of drugs given before total body irradiation reduce the radiation effect, probably because they trigger the stem cells into proliferation [3].

The immunocompetent tissues, the lympho-immune system

The immunological system is composed of two types of cell: macrophages and lymphocytes. The *macrophages* are derived from the same progenitors as the granulocytes, the GM-CFC. These give birth to monocytes which are transformed into macrophages. This line is relatively radioresistant but the macrophages do not all have the same radiosensitivity nor the same functions.

The *lymphoid cells*, in particular the lymphocytes, are derived from the same pluripotential stem cells (CFU-S) as the other haemopoietic lines. Two cell lines can be distinguished:

1. *The B line* (bursa of Fabricius) which gives rise to B lymphocytes and plasmocytes. These cells are responsible for humoral immunological responses (secretion of immunoglobulins). The lifespan of these lymphocytes is about 7 weeks and that of plasmocytes from 2–3 days.
2. *The T line.* These cells pass through the thymus where they accomplish part of their maturation and then become T lymphocytes. Several types can be distinguished, some responsible for cellular immunity (cytotoxic reactions), others for regulation of the immune system, notably by secreting lymphokines. The lifespan of the T lymphocytes is about 5 months. Differentiation of the B and T lymphoid cells can be followed by means of specific membrane antigens and the corresponding monoclonal antibodies.

There are other cell lines (lymphocytes which are neither T nor B) such as the *killer cells* (K) responsible for antibody-dependent cytotoxic reactions, and the *natural killer cells* (NK) which have no specific recognizable function.

The immunological reactions of the B and T cells result from complex cellular interactions which involve *helper T cells* or suppressors. As the radiosensitivity and chemosensitivity of these various types of cell and their precursors are different, irradiation or administration of a cytotoxic drug modifies immune responses by perturbing the interactions and balance between the various types of cell [19, 28].

Effects of radiation on the various types of lymphoid cell

Total body irradiation leads to a rapid fall in the number of circulating B and T lymphocytes (Figure 5.12). The number of lymphocytes returns to normal only after several weeks, this delay becoming longer as the dose is increased [37].

The lymphoid tissues (nodes, spleen, etc.) are very radiosensitive and are depleted of cells by small doses of radiation. After partial body irradiation their regeneration is accelerated by migration of cells from non-irradiated volumes which thereby become partially depleted themselves (Table 5.3). After total body irradiation regeneration is due essentially to proliferation and differentiation of the bone marrow stem cells. However, surviving lymphocytes may also be able to multiply. Although lymphocytes are among the most radiosensitive cells (a dose of $0 \cdot 2$–$0 \cdot 3$ Gy is enough to kill a large proportion of them in interphase, i.e. by rapid lysis), some of them are relatively radioresistant. In general B cells are more radiosensitive than T cells and subpopulations of T cells have varying radiosensitivity. Also irradiation produces complex perturbations in the equilibrium between the different subpopulations of T cells; in particular the helpers (T_4) are more radiosensitive than the suppressors (T_8); in addition the suppressors regenerate more quickly. The ratio T_4/T_8 is reduced for several months or years after total body irradiation or radiotherapy with large fields [19]. The activity of natural killer cells is restored earlier.

The radiosensitivity of lymphocytes, measured by assaying the proportion capable of giving rise to a colony, is close to that found for haemopoietic stem cells ($D_0 = 0 \cdot 8$–1 Gy, $n = 1$–$1 \cdot 2$), probably because the population of clonogenic lymphocytes studied in this way is less radiosensitive than most of the lymphocytes. In general the radiosensitivity of lymphocytes which have been stimulated to proliferate by an antigen or mitogen is lower than that of resting lymphocytes.

Table 5.3 Changes in spleen weight after total or partial body irradiation of rats to a dose of 10 Gy. Whether the spleen is irradiated or not, the greater the proportion of the animal irradiated the more marked its splenic aplasia. This suggests rapid renewal of splenic cells, the weight of the organ indicating the degree of lymphoid aplasia.

	Time interval (days)	Body weight (g)	Weight of the irradiated region (g)	Spleen weight (as % of controls)
	2	197±9	197	63
	5	185±8	185	33
	2	226±8	115	49
	5	238±16	115	39
Protected spleen	2	257	56	64
	5	269	58	67
	2	185	0·6	82
	5	180	0·6	94
Irradiated spleen	2	251±12	110	55
	5	253±8	110	41
	2	237	145	57
	5	240	155	39

The shaded zone corresponds to the irradiated region.
After [35].

The thymus is remarkably radiosensitive but is rapidly repopulated after irradiation, perhaps because the cells multiply quickly; however, there is a subpopulation of relatively radioresistant cells in the thymus. The spleen is also very radiosensitive; the regeneration of T cells in the spleen precedes that of B cells [8, 28]. Nodal lymphoid tissues are also very radiosensitive. Doses above 30 Gy cause destruction of the stroma, vascular lesions, atrophy and fibrosis [8].

Effect of irradiation on immune function

The effect of irradiation on immune function is complex. It depends on the number of surviving cells and their capacity to migrate and become lodged in the microenvironment which they need for normal functioning (homing). It depends also on the irradiated volume and on the time-course of the irradiation with respect to the antigenic stimulus.

Total body irradiation to a large dose (3·5–4·5 Gy) inhibits the immune response against a new antigen. Advantage is taken of this inhibitory effect when preparing a patient for an organ graft (kidney or bone marrow). The effect of total body irradiation is much smaller on the response to an antigen to which the organism is already sensitized (for example, a new skin graft in a subject who has already received a graft from the same donor). Similarly, irradiation is less effective when it is given after challenge with a new antigen and may even increase the immune response. This lack of effectiveness is due to several factors: (i) there is a large number of cells sensitized against this antigen; (ii) lymphocytes in proliferation are much less radiosensitive than resting lymphocytes; (iii) the functional memory of the lymphocytes is radioresistant.

The graft-versus-host reaction (GVH), after bone marrow transplantation, is relatively radioresistant, perhaps because the T cells which were damaged by irradiation produce a factor which is able to stimulate them.

Partial body irradiation such as that occurring in radiotherapy has only a limited effect on the immune response. Nevertheless it leads to a reduction in the number of B and T cells due to irradiation of the circulating blood and of the lymph nodes which are situated in the irradiated volume [19]. If the irradiated volume is sufficiently large the depression of T lymphocytes lasts longer than that of B lymphocytes [28]. This seems to be due not to an absence of regenerative capacity of the T cells but to the relative radioresistance of suppressor T cells which inhibit the return to normal of the number of helper T lymphocytes [19] (reduction in the ratio T_4/T_8). This prolonged T cell lymphopenia does not reduce resistance to infection. The only illness whose frequency seems to be increased in irradiated subjects is *herpes zoster*; also this is more frequent after combined radiotherapy plus chemotherapy than after radiotherapy alone. Its effect on metastatic dissemination is controversial.

Total lymphoid irradiation

Total lymphoid irradiation to 30–40 Gy such as that given for the treatment of lymphomas leads to a long-lasting immune paralysis by T cell lymphopenia. It can be used for preparing a subject for an organ transplant and also for the treatment of autoimmune diseases, particularly chronic progressive polyarthritis [22, 28]. The autoimmune diseases are due, at least in part, to malfunction of homeostasis of the immune system, the reaction of a subject against his own cells being normally controlled or suppressed by a subpopulation of suppressor T cells [19]. The effects of total lymphoid irradiation on autoimmune diseases may be very different depending on the dose delivered.

The liver

The liver is an organ with very slow cell renewal. The mean lifespan of a hepatocyte is about 1 year and therefore the rate of normal cell proliferation is very slow. Also, the stem cells in the hepatic parenchyma have not been identified, and under the intense stimulation caused by partial hepatectomy all the hepatic cells enter the proliferative phase (see Section 5.1). If partial hepatectomy is performed at different times after irradiation a very slow intracellular repair, is demonstrated by an increasing percentage of surviving cells during the weeks and months following irradiation.

After irradiation, some malfunction can be seen such as lack of uptake of radioactive colloids, but this does not appear to have any functional consequences. Even a relatively large dose is apparently well tolerated for the first few months after irradiation. However, hepatic function then deteriorates progressively. Fatal hepatitis may develop after 3–6 months when the dose received by the whole liver exceeds 35 Gy in 4 weeks. The functional consequence of partial irradiation of the liver is limited thanks to compensatory hypertrophy of the unirradiated regions.

The parameters of the survival curve of hepatocytes seem to be: $n=2$, $D_0=2\cdot5$ Gy (Figure 5.18).

The long latent period before the damage becomes manifest is due to the fact that the irradiated hepatic cells retain normal functional activity but are no longer able to divide [8, 28]. Their disappearance therefore leads to progressive aplasia, particularly as this depopulation causes other cells to enter the cell cycle and leads to an acceleration of cell death by the avalanche phenomenon (Figure 5.8).

In animals partial hepatectomy after irradiation produces the same avalanche phenomenon. Acute liver failure has been seen in children whose liver has been irradiated for nephroblastoma and who have undergone partial hepatectomy shortly afterwards for removal of a hepatic metastasis [10]. On the other hand, partial hepatectomy followed a few weeks later by radiotherapy seems to be better tolerated.

The damage inflicted by actinomycin D enhances that of irradiation. Other antimitotic agents such as busulphan, cytosine arabinoside and 6-thioguanine are also capable of damaging the liver [29]. The pathogenesis of the radiation effect is damage to the centro-lobular veins with reduction in their calibre and

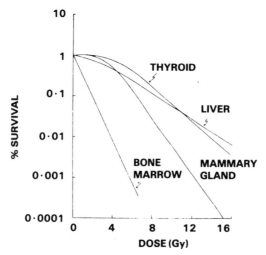

Figure 5.18. Survival curves of four types of cell maintained *in situ* after irradiation. The parameters of the curves are as follows: mammary cells $D_0=1\cdot3$ Gy, $n=17$; liver cells $D_0=2\cdot5$ Gy, $n=2$; thyroid cells $D_0=2$ Gy, $n=10$; bone marrow cells $D_0=0\cdot8$ Gy, $n=1$. After [14].

finally occlusion. It leads to retrograde congestion, haemorrhagic foci and centro-lobular atrophy. Certain drugs (nitrosoureas) cause similar lesions while others increase the damage produced by radiation [8, 28, 29].

The radiosensitivity of the liver varies considerably between species. In the rat, injection of radioactive colloids may cause cirrhosis in the same way as a combination of irradiation with a low protein diet.

Thyroid

The proliferation kinetics of thyroid cells are even slower than those of liver cells. Under normal conditions only a very small percentage of the cells are dividing (mitotic index $0 \cdot 03\%$, labelling index $0 \cdot 1\%$) but a large proportion of the cells enter the proliferative phase after partial thyroidectomy. The labelling index then reaches 5%, suggesting (taking account of the relative length of S phase) that about a quarter of the cells are proliferating [28].

The proportion of clonogenic cells seems to be of the order of 5%. The cells in the process of maturation seem to be capable of two to four divisions while the differentiated cells, which represent about 75% of the total, seem incapable of division.

Initially, the functional capacity of the thyroid is remarkably resistant to radiation because cells which have lost their proliferative capacity may persist and function for long periods. Hence for the thyroid, as for the liver, tolerance in the short term is apparently excellent, even after large doses. However, as the damaged cells are eliminated from the population, the thyroid stimulating hormone (TSH) titre increases and further mitoses are stimulated, giving rise to an accelerated round of mitoses and cell loss. If cell survival is sufficiently low this may provoke atrophy accompanied by functional failure occurring several years later, even 10 or 20 years after irradiation. About 2–4% of hyperthyroid patients treated with radioiodine become hypothyroid every year depending on the dose.

An irradiated thyroid synthesizes hormones normally in spite of the damage inflicted, but stimulation by TSH does not increase its capacity for iodine uptake as it is already functioning at the limit of its capability. Normal thyroid tissue becomes hyperplastic under the influence of prolonged oversecretion of TSH, whether this is caused by administration of an antithyroid drug or by partial thyroidectomy. After irradiation, this hyperplastic capacity is reduced due to a reduction in the number of cells capable of proliferation and perhaps to a reduction in the number of divisions of which each cell is capable. This reduction in hyperplasia becomes greater as the dose is increased; a dose of 7–8 Gy (at high dose rate) reduces to half the weight gain caused by administration of a goitrogen. On the assumption that this effect is due to a reduction in the number of cells capable of division, it is possible to determine the parameters of the cell survival curve *in vivo*: they are $n=2$, $D_0=4 \cdot 5$–$5 \cdot 5$ Gy [28]. These values are close to those obtained by cloning *in vitro*. They are different from those obtained by transplantation techniques where the number of surviving cells is evaluated by counting the number of thyroid nodules seen in the fatty pads ($n=4$, $D_0=2$ Gy). But if the potentially lethal lesions are allowed to be fully repaired the extrapolation number rises to 10 [15], showing the effectiveness of *in situ* repair (Figure 5.18). However, the significance of these different tests is not the same, as the cells which only divide two or four times make a contribution to the increase in weight but not to a transplantation assay nor to an assay of clonogenic cells *in vitro*. Furthermore, the inhibition of goitrogen-induced thyroid growth does not allow evaluation of surviving fractions below $0 \cdot 1$ so that the data correspond to cell survival in the shoulder region. There is a discrepancy between the limited ability of thyroid regeneration *in situ* and the results of culture *in vitro* or cell transplantation experiments which show a practically unlimited capacity for division of surviving clonogenic cells. The impairment of clonogenic cell proliferation *in situ* may be due to stromal damage or to alterations of cell–cell interactions.

The method of goitrogen growth inhibition makes it possible to compare the effects of external irradiation using X-rays, with those of endogenous irradiation at low dose rate given by ^{131}I (half-life 8 days); in the latter case D_0 is 55 Gy, indicating a great reduction in effect. This is due to the low dose rate, as irradiation with radioiodine of short half life (^{132}I, half-life 2 h) has an effectiveness similar to that of external irradiation.

The testis

Reminder of its anatomy and physiology

The seminiferous tubules are composed of two types of cell.

Sertoli Cells These cells play a role in the microenvironment, enabling the germinal cells to proliferate and differentiate and allowing hormonal regulation of spermatogenesis. They secrete a hormone, inhibin, which controls secretion of FSH by the hypophysis.

Germinal Cells The hierarchy of these cells is strictly defined and the chronology of spermatogenesis is well understood. The undifferentiated stem cells have been identified; they divide seldom and their cycle time is long. They are the undifferentiated type A spermatogonia which give rise to intermediate spermatogonia A_1, A_2, $A_3 \ldots$, then type B. From this point the kinetics of differentiation are precisely fixed and are not altered by irradiation or cytotoxic agents. The yield or amplification factor in the compartment of spermatogonia type A is lower than would be expected from the number of cell divisions, indicating considerable cell mortality. This is not seen for the intermediate or type B spermatogonia. There is a very strict synchronization between division and differentiation. When spermatogonia type B divide they give birth to spermatocytes which are the cells in which meiosis occurs. After meiosis each spermatocyte gives rise to four spermatids; in practice the number is lower, evidence of a new wave of cell death. Also a considerable number of spermatids die at various stages of maturation. All these losses explain why the production of spermatozoa is much lower than would be expected on the basis of the number of mitoses. The complete transit time from the stem cell in the seminiferous tubules to the spermatozoa is 74 days in man.

Interstitial or *Leydig cells* are also found in the testis. They secrete testosterone and their function is regulated by pituitary gonadotrophins, prolactin and luteinizing hormone (LH). The level of prolactin may stimulate or inhibit spermatogenesis. Testosterone and the protein secreted by the Sertoli cells control spermatogenesis.

Effects of irradiation

Spermatogenesis is affected by quite low doses [2, 8]. In man a dose of 0.08 Gy leads to a temporary reduction in the number of spermatozoa and 0.2 Gy causes a considerable depression which lasts for several months. A dose of 0.5 Gy reduces the number of spermatozoa to less than 2%. Azoospermia lasting for 1–2 years occurs after a dose of 2 Gy; after 6 Gy there is usually permanent azoospermia although regeneration has been seen after delays as long as 10 or 14 years. On the other hand, even with larger doses of the order of several tens of gray there is little effect on the Leydig cells in the adult. Irradiation of the testis therefore leads to sterility but has no effect on secondary sex characteristics or libido.

Increasing dose produces a greater reduction in sperm production than it does in stem cell survival because it also affects the rate of formation of differentiating cells and the yield of sperm per spermatogonium. However, late effects are mostly correlated with killing of stem cells. The parameters of the stem cell survival curve are approximately $D_0 = 3$ Gy, $n = 4$. The stem cells seem, however, to be more radiosensitive in man than in other mammals. They are less sensitive to ionizing radiation and cytotoxic drugs than the differentiating spermatogonia. They are the basis of regeneration and repopulation of the seminiferous tubules; when their number is only slightly reduced, regeneration is rapid. On the other hand, if few stem cells remain they multiply without differentiation until there is partial reconstitution of the compartment. This explains why the duration of azoospermia becomes longer as the dose is increased. The extreme radiosensitivity of spermatogenesis is explained by the radiosensitivity of the differentiating spermatogonia first noted by Regaud in 1906. The death of a single spermatogonium type A leads to death of the whole line in the syncytium due to cytoplasmic bridges which link the cells of a compartment. Spermatogonia of types A and B disappear completely after a dose of 1–1.5 Gy. The intermediate and type B spermatogonia seem to be the most sensitive. Spermatocytes which have received doses above 2 Gy are incapable of maturation. After meiosis, the cells (spermatids, spermatozoa) are radioresistant in terms of survival but are more susceptible to the induction of mutations than the less differentiated cells; their time course of differentiation is little modified by irradiation. The maturation of post-meiotic cells is the reason why in man the number of spermatozoa and consequently fertility is unchanged for the first 6 weeks after irradiation. However, if conception occurs the probability of genetic abnormality is about double that seen after conception at a later time.

Between the 6th and 9th weeks, the rapid fall in the number of spermatozoa reflects the disappearance of the spermatogonia. After the 10th week, the descendants of the cells which were already engaged in the cycle of proliferation and maturation have left the seminiferous tubules and the spermatozoa now come from the surviving stem cells whose proliferation has been stimulated by the depopulation of the spermatogonial compartment. This is the reason why it is advisable to wait for at least 3 months after irradiation before procreation in order to diminish the risk of genetic abnormalities.

Regeneration of the spermatogonial epithelium is much slower in man than in other mammals. It becomes longer as the dose is increased. After a dose of 2 Gy, nuclei of spermatogonia reappear only after several months. Incomplete regeneration might be due to residual damage in the surviving stem cells or to homeostatic mechanisms limiting the proliferation of stem cells after depletion of their number; the latter explanation is a likely possibility. This would explain why the recovered level of sperm production is dependent on the initial number of surviving stem cells and independent of how these cells were killed. Recovery of fertility corresponds to the time at which the number of spermatozoa exceeds 10% of the normal value. Concomitantly with histological changes, there are increases in serum gonadotrophins (follicle stimulating hormone (FSH) and LH) after doses greater than 0·2 Gy. Testosterone levels are unchanged. Before puberty, doses of 3–10 Gy (for treatment of a tumour) lead to an increase in the level of FSH after puberty.

In animals, chronic irradiation at a very low dose rate (1 cGy day^{-1}) is enough to perturb spermatogenesis. Fractionated irradiation is equally effective as a single dose.

The Sertoli cells divide seldom, but nevertheless the progressive reduction in their number may play a role in the alteration of spermatogenesis after high doses.

A number of cytotoxic drugs have an important effect on spermatogenesis, e.g. the alkylating agents present in MOPP, a combination of drugs used for the treatment of Hodgkin's disease, lead to complete sterility in almost all patients. These drugs act in the same way as radiation, by killing the stem cells.

The ovary

The effects of radiation on the ovary are different from those in the testis because, after the foetal stage, the oocytes no longer divide. They are all present at birth and their number diminishes steadily with age: about 2 million at birth, 100 000 at puberty of which about 400 ovulate, 8000 at 40 years and of course zero at the menopause. The loss of oocytes is irreversible [2, 8].

Oocytes are extremely radiosensitive as D_0 is of the order of 0·12 Gy, the lowest value of all mammalian cells [2]; like lymphocytes they die in interphase. However, the radiosensitivity of oocytes varies with the stage of maturation and the early oocytes are relatively radioresistant. Both the mature follicles and those in the process of maturation are damaged equally; sterilization is therefore immediate. The effects of fractionation and dose rate vary with the species.

Oocytes are remarkably insensitive to mutation induction. For doses too low to sterilize all the follicles, the genetic consequences of irradiation are much less than after irradiation of the testis (see Chapter 12).

Hormonal secretion is associated with follicular maturation; absence of primordial follicles capable of development therefore leads to arrest of the secretion of hormone at the end of a few weeks after disappearance of the mature follicles. Irradiation of the ovary therefore results in castration. The dose which causes this varies with age from 12–15 Gy, depending on fractionation, in a woman of 20, to 5–7 Gy at 45 years of age. A dose of a few gray results in temporary sterility and a transitory hormonal disequilibrium; women who have suffered a long period of amenorrhoea after a dose of 3–4 Gy may later become pregnant. In girls irradiated for cancer, a high level of gonadotrophins (FSH and LH) is seen when the ovary has received 20–30 Gy in a month, demonstrating irreversible damage to the ovary. Several cytotoxic drugs may lead to temporary amenorrhoea or even castration.

The nervous system

Neurological complications affect the spinal cord, the brain and the peripheral nerves [8, 28]. The neurons do not divide but the vascular endothelium, the Schwann cells and the glial cells must be considered. The latter divide to become astrocytes (protective shielding of neurones) and oligodendrocytes which are involved in the formation of the myelin sheath. Loss of oligodendrocytes leads to segmental demyelinization, leaving a bare unprotected axon. Remyelinization may occur by proliferation of glial cells since these cells retain their ability to revert to proliferation. Normally their turnover rate is very slow but their growth fraction may increase 2–3 months after irradiation. A subgroup of astrocytes (β-astrocytes) may be glial progenitors mainly committed to the oligodendrocyte cell lineage. Schwann cells are involved in myelinization and regeneration of spinal nerve roots and peripheral nerves.

Early myelopathy

Early reversible myelopathies may appear a few weeks after the end of irradiation with doses of 50–60 Gy. They are characterized by 'diffuse demyelinization'. In man, after irradiation of the spinal cord they become manifest through paraesthesia and peripheral sensations of electric shock (tingling) provoked by hyperflection of the neck (Lhermitte's sign). After irradiation of the brain they lead to mild or pronounced somnolence. Remyelinization can be observed after about 2 months.

Late effects

After a latent period of about 4–6 months, distinct areas of necrosis develop in the white matter. This probably arises from two causes. The rapid progression from focal demyelinization into areas devoid of glial nuclei, followed by tissue necrosis, suggests the role of loss of oligodendrocytes in the central nervous system (CNS) and of Schwann cells in peripheral nerves. Below a critical level of cell survival, necrosis develops very quickly (2 weeks), probably by reason of an avalanche phenomenon. However, the occurrence of vascular damage (haemorrhage) suggests a precipitous role of these vascular lesions in the expression of predominantly glial cell damage. Capillary obstructions, reduced blood flow in individual arterioles, can cause areas of local ischaemic necrosis. After very long time intervals, several years, a different type of vascular damage is observed: telangiectasia, haemorrhagic infarcts and hyaline degeneration of the vessels. These vascular disorders result in later damage which affects the white matter as much as the grey matter and develops after lower doses.

Paraplegias

Paraplegias are rare but extremely serious as they are irreversible. They appear from 6 months to 4 years after irradiation and may develop suddenly or progressively, causing a Brown–Sequart syndrome or a flaccid paraplegia (see Chapter 8). In practice paraplegias are most often due to overdosage at the junction of two fields, particularly in the treatment of lymphomas and cancers of the lung. In terms of pathology, there is atrophy of the spinal cord visible on myelography or magnetic resonance imaging (MRI), demyelinization and necrosis. The threshold dose is 44 Gy in 4 weeks, but the incidence remains relatively low after 50 Gy in 5 weeks given in five sessions per week. Above that level a small increase in dose (3–5 Gy) greatly increases the risk. Animal experiments have emphasized the importance of the length of the segment of irradiated cord and the dose per fraction [28]. The latent period becomes shorter as the dose is increased (Figure 5.9). The sparing conferred by fractionation shows that the spinal cord has a large capacity to repair sublethal injury. The ratio α/β ranges from $1\cdot5$–$2\cdot5$ Gy. For vascular damage α/β is $2\cdot8$ Gy. The differences are small but imply the existence of different target cells.

Small variations in the intervals between fractions have little effect. The sparing conferred by fractionation is due mostly to intracellular repair but there is also some long-term repair of residual injury. In rats an increasing number of functional cells (oligodendrocytes ?) after 2–3 months is reflected by an increase in the tolerance dose for white matter necrosis. Despite these phenomena, in the clinic it must be recognized that the residual damage after irradiation is repaired to only a small extent and remains significant even after long periods of time.

Damage to the brain

Damage to the brain occurs 1–3 years after irradiation [30]. For a dose of 50 Gy in 5 weeks to the whole brain, significant damage occurs in about 5% of the patients. Tolerance is greater for localized irradiation and the risk is acceptable for a dose of 55 Gy in $5\cdot5$ weeks to the posterior fossa; 65–70 Gy can be given to a small field. The acceptability of the risk depends on the gravity of the disease; e.g. for an astrocytoma grade III or IV, 50 Gy to the whole cranium plus a boost of 15–20 Gy are considered acceptable.

In children, the dose limit for prophylactic irradiation of the brain in acute leukaemia seems to be 30 Gy in 3 weeks; with higher doses intellectual development is impaired. Combination with chemotherapy, in particular methotrexate, reduces tolerance and late damage has been seen after doses of 30 Gy in 3 weeks. Damage to the choroid plexus caused by irradiation allows methotrexate to penetrate into the brain, thereby increasing its toxicity. When this drug is administered intrathecally, the dangers of complications due to the combined treatment are increased. Many other drugs have an effect on the brain but the target cells are generally different from those damaged by radiation and there is no evidence of an enhanced toxicity of these drugs after irradiation.

The lung

For a long time it was thought wrongly that the lungs were relatively radio-resistant. In fact, when the dose exceeds 40 Gy of fractionated irradiation, about 10% of patients have pulmonary symptoms of variable severity [8, 29, 30].

In the mouse, after irradiation of the thorax, the mean lethal dose (LD 50) is about 12 Gy. Two waves of damage have been identified. Radiation pneumonitis occurs between 3 and 6 months after irradiation and is characterized by interstitial oedema and oedema in the air spaces. Animals surviving this first phase exhibit a second wave of damage after the 9th month. This later wave of injury is not a secondary consequence of the pneumonitis phase; it has been suggested that it is a result of lung fibrosis but this interpretation remains controversial.

The alveolar collapse, with atelectasis and the passage of blood transudates into the alveolar lumen which characterizes pneumonitis, may be due to loss of production of alveolar surfactant and to damage to the alveolo-capillary interface. Therefore the two most likely target cells are the endothelial cells and type 2 alveolar cells (granular pneumocytes). Type 2 cells are associated with production of surfactant which is the surface-active material responsible for preventing collapse of the alveoli. Type 2 cells are a proliferating population and are the progenitors of type 1 cells (membranous pneumocytes) which do not divide. The turnover time of type 2 cells is about 1–2 months. During the first few days after irradiation these cells release surfactant; they then swell and finally are detached from the basement membrane. In man the presence of surfactant in alveolar lavage liquid during the first few days after irradiation should therefore be of prognostic value and should correlate with the severity of the damage.

After irradiation of experimental animals, the expression of injury occurs sooner after higher doses. However, the survival time is dose-dependent only over a small dose range. In man, early acute pneumonopathy appears 2–4 months after irradiation. The only symptom is often the discovery of an opacity on an X-ray of the chest, but it may also be accompanied by functional signs: cough, dyspnoea, and respiratory difficulties. In anatomical terms the damage arises from pneumonia with oedema, swelling of the alveolar cells, congestion and often secondary infections. These lesions may be reversible.

Nevertheless, progressive pulmonary fibrosis develops in most of these patients. Fibrosis may appear in patients who had previously been asymptomatic; it then begins towards the end of the first year after irradiation. In addition to radiological signs, there is progressive alteration in respiratory function: reduction in respiratory capacity, fall in lung compliance and vascular perfusion and increase of arterial hypoxia. These difficulties may increase in severity for 1–2 years before stabilizing. They are generally irreversible. In their most serious form they convert the patient into a cripple or lead to death. Their frequency and severity depends on three factors: the volume of lung irradiated, the dose and the fractionation. Fractionation plays a critical role as the lung is particularly radiosensitive when the dose per fraction exceeds 2 Gy. Animal experiments suggest that reduction to 0·5 Gy per fraction markedly increases tolerance. Results for the end point of fibrosis are consistent with a linear–quadratic relation with $\alpha/\beta = 3$ Gy.

Single doses of radiation in man (irradiation of the trunk for bone metastases or total-body irradiation before marrow grafting) may lead to pneumonopathy with doses above 6 Gy. In some series its frequency reaches 10% for 8 Gy and 50% for 10 Gy. The steepness of the dose–response curve could be interpreted by a D_0 value for the target cells of about 0·6 Gy. Progression leading to death in 4–6 months occurs in a significant proportion of the patients. For this type of irradiation the lung is the critical organ which limits the dose. The pathogenesis of these pneumonopathies is complex. Viral infection (cytomegalovirus) plays an important role, probably enhanced by immunosuppression. This explains the precautions taken to reduce the dose to the lung during total-body irradiation for acute leukaemia before marrow grafting. In man, as in the mouse, a small variation in dose can have a considerable effect on the frequency of pneumonopathy.

With fractionated irradiation of both lungs, as used for treatment of subclinical pulmonary metastases from osteosarcoma, the maximum tolerated dose is of the order of 22–24 Gy, when given at 2 Gy per fraction and 5 fractions per week. A small increase in dose (20%) increases the frequency of pneumonopathy from 5 to 50%. With localized irradiation, the damage depends on the size of the field; if this is not too large, doses of 45–50 Gy are usually tolerated on condition that the dose per fraction does not exceed 2·5 Gy. During the acute phase, treatment includes administration of corticosteroids at moderate doses. Above all it is necessary to avoid secondary infection.

Pulmonary damage may also occur after treatment with several chemotherapeutic agents, notably bleomycin, cyclophosphamide and mustine. Combination of radiotherapy with these drugs reduces lung tolerance as has been shown by animal experiments, even though the mechanisms of action are different.

The heart

Irradiation of the heart and mediastinum produces damage to the pericardium and myocardium [8, 18, 29].

Serofibrinous pericarditis usually runs a benign course but may be transformed into constrictive pericarditis requiring pericardectomy. It generally appears about a year after irradiation but may develop later. It may be associated with myocarditis. This usually gives no clinical symptoms but may lead to fatal heart failure. Systematic electrocardiograms have shown that these problems are less rare than had been thought. Coronary damage due to irradiation is exceptional.

In terms of pathology, the pericardium is thickened due to dense and diffuse fibrosis. In the myocardium there is an alteration in the capillary network with damage to endothelial cells, thickening of the walls, thrombosis and appearance of microscopic areas of fibrosis. In animals, muscular atrophy and arrhythmia are seen after 6 months with a substantial reduction in cardiac output. This damage is strongly influenced by fractionation ($\alpha/\beta = 3$ Gy).

The frequency of these complications depends on the dose and the volume of heart irradiated. When a large proportion of the heart (more than 50%) receives 45 Gy in 4 weeks the incidence is about 5%, but it reaches 40% for doses greater than 60 Gy. Protection of part of the heart considerably reduces the incidence. Animal experiments have demonstrated the role of arteriolar and capillary lesions in the production of fibrosis and myocardial damage, whereas they have shed no light on the origin of pericarditis.

Combination with chemotherapy by adriamycin increases the severity of these complications; the toxic effects are additive although adriamycin acts on the myocytes of the cardiac muscle which radiation does not damage directly. In addition adriamycin may reveal latent radiation damage even many years after radiotherapy.

The kidney

Irradiation of both kidneys [8, 28, 29] with moderate doses (30 Gy in 5 weeks) results in nephropathy with arterial hypertension and anaemia after latent periods of 1–5 years. The tolerance dose is about 23 Gy in 5 weeks. Irradiation of a single kidney is relatively well tolerated and causes, if needed, compensating hypertrophy of the opposite kidney. Irradiation of the superior pole of the left kidney during splenic radiotherapy with a dose of 40 Gy causes atrophy of the irradiated region but seldom has any functional consequence [23]. In animals, unilateral nephrectomy of the opposite kidney accelerates development of the damage.

Histologically there is sclerosis and atrophy of the glomeruli and tubules but physiological and histological studies have not permitted the identification of a single target cell, nor any consensus about the pathogenesis. In experimental animals, radiation may cause direct vascular injuries and progressive thrombosis of the glomerular capillaries. Tubular cell injury is related to dose. Damage to the tubules may result from sterilization of all the cells in a tubule, about 1000 cells. A surviving fraction of 10^{-4} would then be enough to lead to the disappearance of more than 90% of the tubules. Reduction of kidney function by primary damage to the tubules or glomeruli could cause chronic renal vasodilation with resulting elevation of glomerular pressure and flow. In man, hypertension is probably a consequence rather than a cause of the nephropathy. Drugs, in particular cisplatin, act only on the tubules, so here again the mechanism of action is different, but nevertheless the combination with radiation reduces total tolerance. Kidney damage shows a dose–effect relation of the linear–quadratic type with a ratio $\alpha/\beta = 3$ Gy.

In children, lower doses (10–15 Gy) slow down or stop growth of the kidney. In the young rat, unilateral nephrectomy normally leads to hypertrophy of the remaining kidney, but this is inhibited temporarily after a dose of 7·5 Gy and permanently after 10 Gy.

Blood vessels and the vascular system

The action of radiation on blood vessels is particularly important because, as we have seen, late reactions are to a large extent probably due to disturbance of the vasculature [8, 18]. Arterial damage is seen after doses of 50–70 Gy, but capillaries are damaged from 40 Gy.

The structure of blood vessels is complex. The internal surface is covered by a monolayer of endothelial cells. These rest on connective tissue whose thickness varies with the type of vessel. In arteries and arterioles there are smooth muscles and networks of collagen fibres which are capable of changing the lumen of the vessel and thereby controlling the blood flow.

The radiosensitivity of the endothelial cells has been measured, both *in vitro* and *in vivo*, by evaluating proliferative capacity after stimulation. The value of D_0 for the clonogenic cells is about 2 Gy whether measured *in vivo* or *in vitro*. The tissue appears much more radioresistant ($D_0=c.$ 10 Gy) when the cells which perform only a few divisions are included in the study. Survival of the endothelial cells, or the regenerative capacity of the blood vessels, is increased when the level of cellular proliferation is low at the time of irradiation. Fractionation considerably reduces the damage, as in all tissues with a low rate of cellular renewal ($\alpha/\beta=2$ Gy).

The proliferation rate of endothelial cells is low; about 1% of the cells are in S phase. The labelling index increases 3 weeks after irradiation, at a time when the layer of endothelial cells still seems to be normal; it then remains high while the number of endothelial cells rapidly diminishes, as they die at the moment when they try to divide. Reduction in endothelial cell number is significant at 2–3 months after irradiation, reaching a minimum at 6 months. The severity of the diminution is dose-dependent. The loss of cells results in an abnormal proliferation of viable cells. Regions of constriction appear due to this proliferation (resembling a string of sausages) (Figure 5.19). As a result there are vascular occlusions and a loss of capillary vessels leading to a reduction in the density of the vascular network. Denudation of the internal surface of the vessels leads to formation of thromboses and capillary necrosis.

In the smooth muscle of the vessel walls, cell proliferation is very slight (of the order of 0·1%) which is the reason why the number of these cells only diminishes about a year after irradiation. This loss of muscular fibres plays an important role in the genesis of late damage which appears from 9 months to a few years after irradiation. The walls of the vessels become thicker and contain fewer cells. The muscle cells are replaced by collagen fibres. The calibre of the

BEFORE IRRADIATION

VIABLE CELL

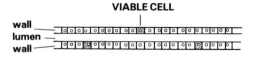

6 MONTHS AFTER IRRADIATION

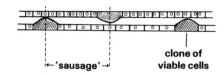

Figure 5.19. Formation of stenoses and telangiectasia after irradiation of blood vessels. After irradiation, most of the cells in the vessel wall are sterilized. Stimulation of the viable cells to proliferate leads to the formation of clones which reduce the lumen of the vessels, creating this appearance of 'a string of sausages'. After [18].

vessels diminishes and the walls lose their elasticity. Telangiectasis of the capillaries is also seen. Blood flow diminishes during the first few weeks as the endothelial damage develops, becomes normal again and then diminishes once more. The consequence of this vascular damage varies from tissue to tissue.

Unlike radiation, chemotherapeutic agents have little effect on the vascular network.

Bones and cartilages

Growth cartilage is particularly radiosensitive. Irradiation even at a dose of 10 Gy slows or temporarily stops growth owing to death of chondroblasts in the proliferative zone and to disorganization in the structure [8, 28]. A dose of 10–20 Gy causes some delay in growth and above 20 Gy the deficit in growth is irreversible. If the vertebrae are irradiated the result is a diminution in their height together with scoliosis.

Disturbances of growth are more serious when the dose is higher and the child younger. The sequelae are particularly serious in children of less than 2 years; until puberty they lead to a significant deficit in stature. This is the reason why the dose in Hodgkin's disease in children is limited to 20 Gy.

In experimental animals, a single dose of 6–12 Gy leads to a temporary arrest of growth; this continues later at a normal rate, even with a reduced number of chondroblasts, but the delay is not made up. 30 Gy leads to a permanent arrest in growth and ossification in addition to disturbances of vascularization.

In the adult, osteonecrosis of the lower maxilla is a serious complication in cancers of the buccal cavity. The incidence is about 6% for doses of 40–50 Gy and reaches 20% for 60–70 Gy. The dimensions of the irradiated area, the state of dentition and buccal hygiene have an important influence on the incidence of this complication, its severity and development. Secondary infections are particularly serious. In more than half the cases conservative treatment is possible.

Spontaneous fractures of the femoral neck are seen with doses greater than 65 Gy but affect less than 1% of the patients treated for cancer of the uterine cervix. In patients treated for cancer of the breast, fractures of the ribs and clavicle are frequent but not serious.

References

1. S. E. Al-Barwari, C. S. Potten. A cell kinetic model to explain the time of appearance of skin reaction after x-rays or ultraviolet light irradiation. *Cell Tissue Kinet.*, 1979, **12**: 281–289.
2. M. Bianchi. Cytotoxic insult to germinal tissue, in: *Cytotoxic insult to tissue* (C. S. Potten, J. H. Hendry, eds), pp. 258–328. Churchill Livingstone, Edinburgh, 1983.
3. N. Blackett, M. Aguado. The enhancement of haemopoietic stem cell recovery in irradiated mice by prior treatment with cyclophosphamide. *Cell Tissue Kinet.*, 1979, **12**: 291–298.
4. L. E. Botnik, E. C. M. Hannon, S. Hellman. Late effects of cytotoxic agents on the normal tissue of mice. *Front. Radiat. Ther. Oncol.*, 1979, **13**: 36–47.
5. Y. Cachin, A. Jortay, H. Sancho, F. Eschwege, H. Madelain, A. Desaulty, P. Gerard. Preliminary results of a randomized EORTC study comparing radiotherapy and concomitant Bleomycin to radiotherapy alone in epidermoïd carcinomas of the oropharynx. *Eur. J. Cancer*, 1977, **13**: 1389–1395.
6. H. Croizat, E. Frindel, M. Tubiana. Long term radiation effects on the bone marrow stem cells of C3H mice. *Int. J. Radiat. Biol.*, 1979, **36**: 91–99.

7. H. Croizat, E. Frindel, M. Tubiana. The effect of partial body irradiation on haemopoietic stem cell migration. *Cell Tissue Kinet.*, 1980, **13**: 309–317.
8. L. F. Fajardo. *Pathology of radiation injury.* Masson Inc., New York, 1982.
9. S. B. Field, S. Hornsey, Y. Kutsutani. Effects of fractionated irradiation on mouse lung and a phenomenon of "slow repair". *Br. J. Radiol.*, 1976, **49**: 700–709.
10. R. M. Filler, M. Tefft, G. F. Vawter, C. Maddock, A. Mitus. Hepatic lobectomy in childhood: effects of X-ray and chemotherapy. *J. Pediat. Surg.*, 1969, **4**: 31–41.
11. G. H. Fletcher, C. Nervi, H. R. Withers (eds). *Biological bases and clinical implications of tumour radioresistance.* Masson Inc., New York, 1983.
12. E. Frindel, H. Croizat, F. Vassort. Stimulating factors liberated by treated bone marrow: *in vitro* effect on CFU kinetics. *Exp. Hematol.*, 1976, **4**: 56–61.
13. E. Frindel, C. Hahn, D. Robaglia, M. Tubiana. Responses of bone marrow and tumour cells to acute and protracted irradiation. *Cancer Res.*, 1972, **32**: 2096–2103.
14. J. P. Geraci, P. D. Thrower, K. L. Jackson, G. M. Christensen, R. G. Parker, M. S. Fox. The relative biological effects of fast neutrons for spinal cord injury. *Radiat. Res.*, 1974, **59**: 496–503.
15. M. N. Gould, L. E. Cathers, K. H. Clifton, S. Howard, R. L. Jirtle, P. A. Mahler, R. T. Mulcahy, F. Thomas. The influence of *in situ* repair systems on survival of several irradiated parenchymal cell types. *Br. J. Cancer*, 1984, **49**, Suppl. VI: 191–195.
16. M. A. H. Hegazy, J. F. Fowler. Cell population kinetics and desquamation: skin reactions in plucked and unplucked mouse skin. II Irradiated skin. *Cell Tissue Kinet.*, 1973, **6**: 587–602.
17. F. R. Hendrickson, C. G. Hibbs, Radiation effects on cell cycle dynamics. *Radiology*, 1964, **83**: 131–139.
18. J. W. Hopewell, D. Campling, W. Calvo, H.S. Reinhold, J. H. Wilkinson, T. K. Yeung. Vascular irradiation damage: its cellular basis and likely consequences, *Br. J. Cancer*, 1986, **53**, Suppl. VII: 181–191.
19. G. Job, M. Preundschuh, M. Bauer, J. Zum Winkel, W. Hunstein. The influence of radiation therapy on T-lymphocyte subpopulations defined by monoclonal antibodies. *Int. J. Radiat. Oncol. Biol. Phys.*, 1984, **10**, 2077–2081.
20. G. P. Joshi, W. J. Nelson, S. H. Revell, C. Shaw. Discrimination of slow growth from non-survival among small colonies of diploid syrian hamster cells after chromosome damage induced by a range of X-ray doses. *Int. J. Radiat. Biol.*, 1982, **42**: 283–296.
21. J. H. Kim. T. C. Evans. Effects of x-irradiation on the mitotic cycle of *Ehrlich ascites* tumour cells. *Radiat. Res.*, 1964, **21**, 129–143.
22. B. L. Kotzin, G. S. Kansas, E. G. Engleman, R. T. Hoppe, H. S. Kaplan, S. Strober. Changes in T-cell subsets in patients with rheumatoid arthritis treated with total lymphoid irradiation. *Clin. Immunol. Immunopathol.*, 1983, **27**: 250–260.
23. J. P. Le Bourgeois, M. Meignan, C. Parmentier, M. Tubiana. Renal consequences of irradiation of the spleen in lymphoma patients. *Br. J. Radiol.*, 1979, **52**: 56–60.
24. E. P. Malaise, N. Chavaudra, F. Pene, J. M. Richard, M. Tubiana. Cell proliferation kinetics and growth rate of irradiated human tumour cells. Ed. D. F. Nygaard, H. I. Adler, W. K. Sinclair. Academic Press 1975. Congress Radiat. Res., pp. 850–858.
25. A. Michalowski. Effects of radiation on normal tissues: hypothetical mechanisms and limitations of *in situ* assays of clonogenicity. *Radiat. Environ. Biophys.*, 1981, **19**: 157–172.
26. A. Michalowski. A critical appraisal of clonogenic survival assays in the evaluation of radiation damage to normal tissues. *Radiotherapy Oncol.*, 1984, **1**: 241–246.
27. C. Parmentier, N. Moradet, M. Tubiana. Late effects on human bone marrow after extended field radiotherapy. *Int. J. Radiat. Oncol. Biol. Phys.*, 1983, **9**: 1303–1311.
28. C. S. Potten, J. H. Hendry, (Eds). *Cytotoxic insult to tissue. Effects on cell lineages.* Churchill Livingstone, Edinburgh, 1983.
29. P. Rubin. Late effects of chemotherapy and radiation therapy. A new hypothesis. *Int. J. Radiat. Oncol. Biol. Phys.*, 1984, **10**: 5–34.
30. P. Rubin, G. W. Casarett. *Clinical radiation pathology.*, W. B. Saunders, Philadelphia, 1968.
31. F. A. Stewart. Mechanism of bladder damage and repair after treatment with radiation and cytostatic drugs. *Br. J. Cancer*, 1986, **53**, Suppl. VII: 280–291.
32. K. R. Trott. Chronic damage after radiation therapy, challenge to radiation biology. *Int. J. Radiat. Oncol. Biol. Phys.*, 1984, **10**: 907–913.
33. M. Tubiana. Cell kinetics and radiation oncology. *Int. J. Radiat. Oncol. Biol. Phys.*, 1982, **8**: 1471–1489.
34. M. Tubiana, C. I Bernard, C. Lalanne. Modification de l'érythropoïèse après radiothérapie pelvienne. *Acta Radiologica*, 1959, **52**: 321–335.
35. M. Tubiana, M. Boiron, C. Paoletti, A. Dutreix, R. Gerard-Marchant. Lésions spléniques provoquées chez le rat par irradiation segmentaire ou globale de l'organisme ou par irradiation sélective de la rate. *J. Radiol. Electrol.*, 1956, **39**, 45–48.
36. M. Tubiana, E. Frindel. Regulation of pluripotent stem cell proliferation and differentiation: the role of long range humoral factors, *J. Cell Physiol.*, 1982, Suppl. 1: 13–21.

37. M. Tubiana, C. M. Lalanne. Evolution hématologique des malades soumis à une irradiation totale pour transplantation d'organes. *Ann. Radiol.*, 1963, **6**: 561–580.
38. J. M. Vaeth (Ed.). Combined effects of chemotherapy and radiotherapy on normal tissue tolerance, in: *Frontiers of radiation therapy and oncology*, vol. 13. New York, S. Karger, 1979.
39. F. Vassort, M. Wintherholer, E. Frindel, M. Tubiana. Kinetic parameters of bone marrow stem cells using *in vivo* suicide. *Blood*, 1973, **41**: 789–796.
40. I. Watanabe, S. Okada. Study of mechanisms of radiation-induced reproductive death of mammalian cells in culture: Estimation of stage at cell death and biological description of processes leading to cell death. *Radiat. Res.*, 1966, **27**: 290–306.
41. T. E. Wheldon, A. S. Michalowski. Alternative models for the proliferative structure of normal tissues and their response to irradiation. *Br. J. Cancer, 1986,* **53**, Suppl. VII: 382–385.
42. G. F. Whitmore, J. E. Till, S. Gulyas. Radiation induced mitotic delay in L-cells. *Radiat. Res.*, 1967, *30*: 155–171.
43. M. V. Williams. The cellular basis of renal injury by radiation. *Br. J. Cancer*, 1986, **53**, Suppl. VII: 257–264.

Bibliography

K. F. Clifton, Thyroid and mammary radiobiology: radiogenic damage to glandular tissues, *Br. J. Cancer*, 1986, **53**, Suppl. VII: 237–250.

J. Denekamp. Cell kinetics and radiation biology. *Int. J. Radiat. Biol.*, 1986, **49**: 357–380.

M. C. Joiner, J. Denekamp. The effect of small radiation doses on mouse skin. *Br. J. Cancer*, 1986, **53**, Suppl. VII: 63–66.

M. L. Meistrich. Relationship between spermatogonial stem cell survival and testis function after cytotoxic therapy. *Br. J. Cancer*, 1986, **53**, Suppl. VII: 89–101.

C. S. Parkins, J. F. Fowler. The linear quadratic fit to lung function after irradiation with X-rays at smaller doses per fraction than 2 Gy. *Br. J. Cancer*, 1986, **53**, Suppl. VII: 320–323.

R. Schofield. Assessment of cytotoxic injury to bone marrow. *Br. J. Cancer*, 1986, **53**, Suppl. VII: 115–125.

E. L. Travis and S. L. Tucker. Relationship between functional assays of radiation response in the lung and target cell depletion. *Br. J. Cancer*, 1986, **53**, Suppl. VII: 304–319.

I. Turesson, G. Notter. Dose–response and dose latency relationships for human skin after various fractionation schedules. *Br. J. Cancer*, 1986, **53**, Suppl. VII: 67–72.

UNSCEAR. Sources, effects and risks of ionizing radiation. A report to the general assembly. New York, United Nations 1988.

A. J. Van der Kogel. Radiation induced damage in the central nervous system: an interpretation of target cell responses. *Br. J. Cancer*, 1986, **53**, Suppl. VII: 207–217.

Chapter 6.
The effects of radiation on tumours.
The biological bases of radiotherapy

Radiotherapy was born in 1896, the year following the discovery of X-rays. It remained ineffective until systematic researches were made at the Institut Curie (Paris) from 1919 to 1930, under the direction of Regaud. With the aid of his collaborators, notably Coutard, he showed that it was possible to obtain a differential effect between two tissues by adjusting the fractionation. One of his studies was made on the testis of the ram: whereas a single dose of radiation large enough to stop spermatogenesis also caused severe cutaneous reactions, this could be avoided by giving the radiation in a number of fractions [48]. Regaud and Coutard showed that a differential effect is also obtained for a tumour and the normal tissues surrounding it: fractionation improves the therapeutic ratio, i.e. the effect on the tumour compared with that on the normal tissues. In this way they emphasized that in radiotherapy one cannot consider the effect on the tumour in isolation but that one must also study the effects on critical normal tissues. As the response of tumours is variable between one tumour and another, the tolerance of normal tissues represents the essential reference level.

Since this time the importance of fractionation for increasing the tolerance of normal tissues has been established. During a period of 60 years, attempts to find more effective schemes of fractionation have, until recently, ended in failure because the scientific basis of fractionation was poorly understood (see Chapter 8).

It must be noted that use of experimental tumours in animals has been of only limited value. Transplanted animal tumours are different from spontaneous human tumours: their growth rate is greater and they often provoke strong immunological reactions as they are composed of cells foreign to the organism. Their reactions to treatment may therefore be misleading; over-confidence in the results obtained has been at the origin of a number of disappointments in the history of experimental cancer therapy.

After 1930 the progress of radiotherapy was at first due to developments in dosimetry and technology: more penetrating X-rays and better collimated beams. As long as the technical conditions were unsatisfactory, it was hoped that by improving them it would be possible to control all tumours without irreversible damage to normal tissues. When it became possible to irradiate tumours in a satisfactory way, it became clear that because of the variability in response of normal tissues and tumours it was impossible to cure 100% or even 80% of the tumours with zero probability of serious complications in normal tissues. In other words, when the dose is increased in order to increase the percentage of sterilized tumours, there is an increasing risk of irreversible complications in the tissues close to the tumour (Figure 6.1). The severity and frequency of complications can be reduced by means of good technique and care of the patients under treatment, but with doses effective against the tumour the risk is never zero (Figure 6.1).

From this arose the concept of *optimal dose* and the *philosophy of accepted risk*. For example, in the case of bladder cancer it is possible to quantify this

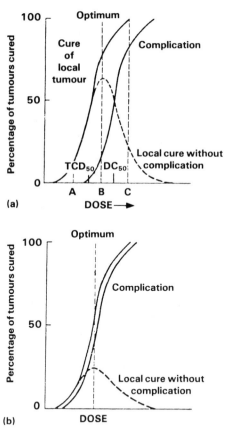

Figure 6.1. Theoretical dose–effect relationships for the percentage of local control of one particular type of tumour and the appearance of complications in the irradiated normal tissues.
(a) Tumour of average radiosensitivity;
(b) to a more radioresistant tumour than (a), cure without complication is possible only for a small proportion of tumours. At A, cure without complication; B, the optimal dose; C, cure of all the tumours but with a high proportion of complications. TCD$_{50}$, dose to cure 50% of the tumours. DC$_{50}$=dose resulting in a complication in 50% of the patients.

concept. The dose causing 50% of complications (DC 50) is greater than that required for local control of 50% of the tumours (TCD 50), but the difference is relatively small; thus the TCD 50 results in complications in 30% of the patients. For a complication frequency of 10% the percentage of cures is 25% [41].

A quantitative approach to this problem requires an understanding of various parameters of each type of cancer, in particular the DC 50 and TCD 50. According to Moore *et al.* [41], the DC 50 (mean value for fractionated treatment, 68 Gy) is greater than the mean TCD 50 value (62 Gy) for a large variety of cancers but the difference between the two varies with the type of cancer.

Animal experiments show that for normal tissues, when the dose per fraction is increased the slope of the curve becomes greater, i.e. a small increase in dose causes a considerable increase in the frequency of complications but produces a smaller increase in tumour control [41]. There is therefore a greater margin of safety with small doses per fraction, a point which we will return to in Chapter 8.

6.1 Theoretical considerations on the local control of tumours

Dose–effect relationship

The relationship between the probability of local cure and the dose has some common features for all types of tumour. The cure probability is minimal below a certain dose which represents a practical threshold; it increases progressively with dose and may reach a value close to 100% for some tumours, but is often restricted to a smaller value on account of the limit imposed on the dose by the tolerance of normal tissues. The threshold dose, and the maximum value clinically achievable, depend on the pathology, extent and location of the tumour. The steepness of the curve relating the variation of tumour control probability with dose (Figure 6.1) depends on the range of radiosensitivity among the tumours of a particular type.

Analysis of the dose–effect relationship is based on simple statistical considerations. The only important tumour cells are those which are able to multiply indefinitely. These *clonogenic cells* are the equivalent of the stem cells in normal tissues. In experimental solid tumours the proportion of clonogenic cells varies between 0·1% and 100%; it can be measured by determining the number of cells which must be injected into an animal of the same strain to produce a 50% tumour take (TD 50) (see Section 4.2). As we will see below, in human tumours it probably varies between 0·01% and 1%.

It is generally assumed that a tumour is controlled only if all the clonogenic cells have suffered reproductive death and are incapable of further multiplication. For example, we will consider a tumour of 100 g, containing 10^{11} cells of which 1% are clonogenic. It contains therefore 10^9 clonogenic cells. We have already seen (Section 4.5) that the cell survival curve for fractionated irradiation is exponential. Let us assume that the surviving fraction after each dose of 2 Gy amounts to 50%, corresponding to an effective D_0 of 2·9 Gy. After 30 fractions, or a total dose of 60 Gy, the proportion of surviving cells will be 10^{-9} and there will remain on average one surviving cell per tumour. This reasoning assumes a cell population with an uniform cell sensitivity which does not significantly change during the course of treatment.

If there are 100 similar tumours each of which receive 60 Gy there will be a total of 100 surviving cells; after 62 Gy there will be 50. In both cases there will be some tumours without any surviving cells and which are therefore cured and others in which there will remain one or more surviving cells able to give rise to a recurrence. The number of cured tumours can be estimated from statistical theory. For a mean number n of surviving cells per tumour the proportion of tumours in which there are no survivors is equal to e^{-n} according to the Poisson distribution. Thus if $n=1$, there will be 37% of tumours with no surviving cells (37% with 1 cell, 18% with 2 cells and 8% with 3 or more). The percentage of cured tumours is therefore 37%. If there is an average of $0 \cdot 5$ surviving cells per tumour the percentage of cured tumours is about 60%. It is 50% (the TCD 50) for a mean survival of $0 \cdot 69$ cells per tumour. It is 10% for an average of $2 \cdot 3$ cells per tumour and 90% for $0 \cdot 1$ cells per tumour (10 surviving cells per 100 tumours).

This calculation shows that the dose must be increased by 3 D_o, in this example about 5×2 Gy, to increase the cure rate from 10 to 90% (Figure 6.2). The probability P of controlling a tumour, or the *control percentage* for a series of identical tumours, depends on three parameters, namely :(i) the initial number of clonogenic cells n_o; (ii) the total dose $D=N \times 2$ Gy; (iii) the proportion s of surviving cells after each session of irradiation. s depends upon the radiosensitivity of the clonogenic tumour cells and their proliferation rate between the end of one session and the beginning of the next. The role of the three

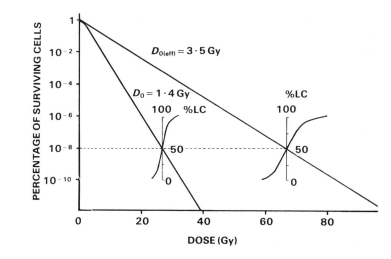

Figure 6.2. Cell survival curves for tumour cells and the probability of local cure as a function of dose. The lower curve shows the survival of tumour cells irradiated with a single dose ($D_o=1 \cdot 4$ Gy, extrapolation number $n=2$) and the upper curve represents the survival of tumour cells after fractionated irradiation ($D_{o(eff)}=3 \cdot 5$ Gy). In both cases it is assumed that all the cells have the same radiosensitivity and that the dose to cure 50% of the tumours is equal to that giving a cell survival of 10^{-8}. With slightly greater or lower doses, the percentage of local tumour cures (LC) is increased or reduced in accordance with the probability of at least one viable cell remaining in the tumour (see text). As the value of D_o is larger for fractionated irradiation, the difference between the doses curing 0% and 100% of the tumours is also greater.
After [19].

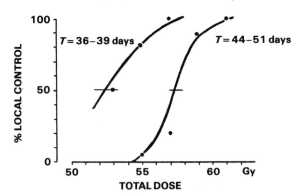

Figure 6.3. **Example of relationship between dose and the probability of cure of a human tumour. Results obtained with cancers of the larynx, stages 3 and 4, depending on whether the fractionated treatment is given over 36–39 days or 44–51 days. These curves emphasize the importance of both dose and total time which governs repopulation of the tumour.**
After [33].

parameters D, n_o and s is illustrated in Figure 6.3 which shows the rapid variation of P as a function of total dose. The steepness of the curves depends only on s. For example, if $s=0\cdot5$, P increases from 20 to 80% when the dose is increased by approximately 3×2 Gy.

Relationships between dose and probability of local control have been observed in several clinical studies [16, 41, 77] (Figure 6.4). However, the steepness of the dose–effect curves varies widely among different groups of tumours. In the review of Moore *et al.* [41] the mean dose increment corresponding to 34% increase in probability of local control was equal to 20% of the TCD 50 but varied from 10 to 30%. Williams *et al.* [77] analyzed 26 series of patients in whom local control values of 40% and 60% were reported. In about half of the studies the dose increment was less than 12% which is only slightly greater than the theoretical value for uniform radiosensitivity in all tumour cell populations. However, in several series the required dose increment was markedly higher, e.g. it was equal to 20% in the prospective study of Morrison [42] on bladder tumours.

A likely interpretation is that the tumour series anlayzed consist of subsets of tumours of different radiosensitivities [16]. For instance, if a series comprises four subsets with TCD 50 of 40, 50, 60 and 70 Gy, in proportions of 25% each, at 45 Gy almost all the tumours of the first subset are cured but practically no tumours of the second subset: thus, the cure rate of the series amounts to 25%. At 55 Gly, all tumours of the second subset are cured and the cure rate is 50%. The increase of cure rate from 20 to 80% spans the range 42 to 68 Gy. When the response curve is steep, a sensible conclusion is that the series consists of tumours of uniform radiocurability and the only problem is assessment of the optimal dose, taking into account the normal tissue tolerance. When the control probability increases slowly with dose, the dose required to obtain a large proportion of controls is much higher than necessary for most of the tumours in the series. Identification of the radioresistant tumours would permit a significant reduction of the dose for many patients. This should encourage

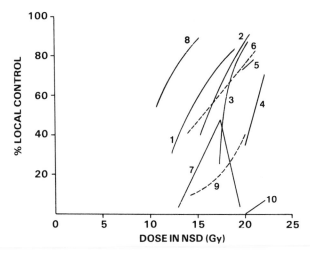

Figure 6.4. **Relation between dose and the probability of local control in various types of human tumour.**
Curves 1 to 5: tumours of the head and neck;
curve 6: cancer of the bladder;
curve 7: relation between dose and survival for T_3 tumours of the uterine cervix (the maximum is due to the fact that after doses which are too great the patients die of complications; the shape of the curve illustrates the existence of an optimal dose);
curve 8: probability of local cure of subclinical disease;
curves 9 and 10: tolerance of two normal tissues. To enable comparisons to be made between treatments given with different regimes of fractionation, the dose is expressed in NSD by means of the Ellis formula.
After [68].

study of the significance of the initial response to treatment as well as anlaysis of the pathological and clinical features correlated with the response, and the development of predictive radiobiological tests.

Similar statistical considerations make it possible to estimate the consequences of non-uniform irradiation. For example, if a dose of 60 Gy leaves on average only one surviving cell in a tumour (cure rate 37%), an underdosage to 50 Gy in one tenth of the tumour increases the number of surviving cells to four and the cure rate becomes only 2%. Inversely an overdosage of 70 Gy produces only a very small increase in cure probability to 40% but considerably increases the risk of complications.

Statistical considerations also explain why there is no sudden change for normal tissues from zero effect (complete tolerance) to 100% effect (serious complications in all patients), but a gradual increase in the severity and frequency of the damage over a certain range of dose (Figure 6.1). However, for normal tissues, variations in radiosensivity from one subject to another seem to be smaller than for tumours (Figure 6.2).

Relation between tumour volume and probability of cure

Clinical experience has shown that large tumours are more difficult to cure than small ones. For this reason bigger doses are used for the treatment of large tumours.

This can be explained in part by the cell survival curve. A tumour of 1 g is the smallest which is clinically detectable and a tumour of 100 g (diameter 5·5 cm) is already very large. To obtain the same absolute number of surviving tumour cells, the surviving fraction for the larger tumour must be reduced by a factor of 100, requiring an additional dose of about 7×2 Gy. This is about the same as the difference between the doses given by radiotherapists on purely clinical grounds (Table 6.1). Empirically it has been found that when the tumour volume is increased by a factor of 10 the dose must be increased by about 10 Gy. However, clinical observation [19] shows that certain large tumours react badly to radiotherapy in spite of increased dosage; this suggests that besides the total number of cells there must be other factors involved such as hypoxia, better repair of potentially lethal damage due to a large proportion of quiescent cells or tumour heterogeneity with the presence of cell lines of increased radioresistance (Figure 6.5). The slope of the dose–effect relationship is shallower for large tumours than for small ones, suggesting a greater variability of response from one tumour to another.

When there is no clinically detectable tumour the dose required to sterilize suspected subclinical metastases is much lower but must be given to large volumes, e.g. the afferent lymph nodes [19]. The diameter of these occult metastases is less than 5 mm; they therefore contain less than 10^8 cells, about 1000

Table 6.1. Relation between the diameter of the tumour and the dose required for local control of almost all the tumours of the upper aerodigestive tract.

	Subclinical tumour	Diameter (cm)			
		<2	2–4	4–6	>6‡
DOSE†	50 Gy 5 weeks	60 Gy 6 weeks	70 Gy 7 weeks	75 Gy 7·5 weeks	75 to 80 Gy 8 weeks

†In all treatments the dose was given in 5 fractions per week.
‡Non-infiltrating tumours more than 6 cm diameter.
After [19].

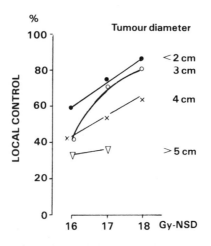

Figure 6.5. Relationship between dose and probability of local control for tumours of the larynx of different sizes. The dose is expressed in NSD.
After [25].

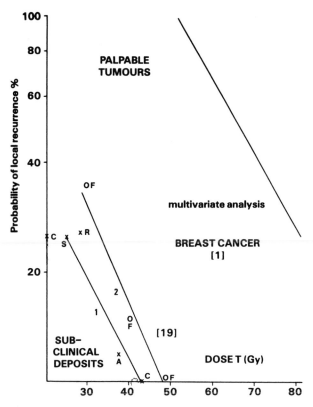

Figure 6.6. Comparison between the dose-effect relations for control of palpable tumours and subclinical deposits (breast cancer). After [1].

times less than the tumour of 100 g taken in the previous example. Assuming that the proportion of clonogenic cells is the same, it is adequate to give a dose equal to two thirds of the dose needed for the 100 g tumour, 40–50 Gy for the example given above, as a cell survival of 10^{-6} is needed instead of 10^{-9}. However, a larger dose may be needed if there is a large number of occult metastases. In addition, two other factors contribute to an explanation of why relatively modest doses are adequate. (i) Tumours with dimensions less than 1 mm³ are well oxygenated. (ii) Their radiosensitivity is greater because of the absence of quiescent cells [55].

Clinical findings confirm these theoretical results. This is an important matter, as Fletcher has emphasized [19], since 50 Gy is a dose which is well tolerated even when given to a large volume. For example, in the conservative treatment of cancer of the breast, when all macroscopic disease has been removed surgically, this dose seems adequate for the residual subclinical deposits (Table 6.1, Figure 6.6).

In the same way these considerations justify the reducing field technique. At the beginning, irradiation is given to a large volume encompassing not only the palpable tumour but also neighbouring tissues and lymph nodes which are likely to be affected. The field size is then progressively reduced in order to avoid acute reactions caused by high doses given to a large volume. Finally, irradiation is given to a small field centred on the tumour itself even if meanwhile it has completely disappeared. The justification of this technique is that higher doses must be given to the tumour itself even if it has shrunk and is no longer palpable: a residual tumour of less than 5 mm in diameter is no longer detectable but may nevertheless contain about 10^8 cells.

Relation between tumour regression and the number of surviving cells

This question is particularly important when radiotherapy is combined with chemotherapy. By how much can one reduce the radiation dose if chemotherapy has previously caused partial or total regression of the tumour? Partial regression is defined as a reduction to 50% of the tumour volume. If this corresponds to death of about 50 % of the clonogenic cells, it would allow only a small reduction in dose. In the previous example of a 100 g tumour, if this is reduced to 50 g it would still be necessary to give 58 Gy insted of 60 Gy. Quasi-total regression corresponds to a residual tumour of the order of 10^8–10^9 cells (that is to say 10^6–10^7 clonogenic cells, assuming these to be 1% of the total). If there is complete clinical disappearance of the tumour (tumour diameter between 0 and 5 mm) there may still be as many as 10^8 cells; in this last case it would still be prudent to deliver 45–50 Gy [68].

The preceding argument was based on the hypothesis that the cells were of uniform sensitivity in the whole tumour, independent of its volume and whether it is growing rapidly or slowly. It is obvious that this is not the case and that the radiosensitivity of tumour cells is influenced by several factors, particularly their proliferation kinetics.

6.2 Proliferation kinetics of human tumours: response to irradiation

The growth of a tumour can be considered from a macroscopic point of view, i.e. from its rate of growth, or histologically from the proliferation kinetics of the tumour cells.

Rate of growth of human tumours

Measurement of the growth of human tumours began only about 20 years ago [67]. From successive radiographs of pulmonary metastases, Collins *et al.* [9] have shown that tumour volume usually grows according to an exponential law during the period of observation, i.e. between a mass of a few grams and a few hundred grams. During this period the rate of growth remains constant and can be characterized by the *doubling time*, the time interval during which the tumour volume increases by a factor of 2. Since then many hundreds of patients have been studied both for primary tumours (e.g. breast cancer by means of mammograms, colorectal cancer on radiographs of the digestive tract) as well as for metastases, mainly pulmonary. In the great majority of cases growth was found to be exponential [8, 58].

Table 6.2. Characteristics of different types of tumour (after 8, 35).

Histological type	Doubling time (days)	Labelling index (%)	Growth fraction (%)	Cell loss (%)	Rate of cell renewal per day %	Radiosensitivity (mean dose for tumour sterilization) (Gy)	Chemosensitivity
Embryonal tumours	27 (22–33)	30 (22–41)	90	94	42	25–30	++
Lymphomas	29 (23–37)	29 (22–38)	90	94	51	35–40	++
Mesenchymal sarcomas	41 (35–50)	3·8 (2·5–5·9)	11	68	5·5	85	−
Squamous carcinomas	58 (48–70)	8·3 (6·4–10·9)	25	90	10	60–70	+
Adenocarcinomas	83 (72–96)	2·1 (1·7–2·7)	6	71	1	60–80	±

Numbers in brackets are 95% confidence limits.
After [35].

Table 6.2 shows the doubling times (T_D) of several types of human tumour. T_D has an average value of 2–3 months but there are some tumours of very rapid growth with a T_D of about a week and others of very slow growth where T_D may reach a year [8, 58].

There is a relationship between T_D and histological type. Thus lymphomas and embryonic tumours (testicular tumours, nephroblastoma) usually have small T_D values. On the other hand adenocarcinomas have very large T_D values. The differences between the groups are statistically significant but within each there are large variations [8]. In general terms, poorly differentiated tumours have a faster growth rate than well differentiated tumours (Section 11.2). An important fact is that each tumour has a characteristic growth rate which remains almost constant during its growth and is also the same or perhaps a little faster for a local recurrence. Moreover the value of T_D for the metastases seems to be correlated with that of the primary tumour, though in general it is rather shorter. This suggests that the rate of growth is connected with characteristics of the genome of the tumour cells.

Many studies have been made on experimental tumours. All the transplanted tumours arising from a given cell line have the same growth curve, emphasizing the connection between the biological characteristics of the cell and the shape of the growth curve [58].

For all animals tumours which have been followed over a period of 25–30 T_D (from a few cells to 10^9 cells), the growth rate is not constant but becomes steadily slower. This variation can be represented by mathematical functions of which the one most frequently used is that of Gompertz†: T_D is initially very short, of the order of 2–3 days, and becomes steadily longer, tending towards infinity when the tumour has reached its maximum size and is no longer growing [58]. This may seem in contradiction with what is observed in humans. In reality, in humans it is only possible to measure a relatively small portion of the growth curve, corresponding to a few doubling times. With such a small segment of the curve it is not possible to analyze the whole shape of the growth curve. It is therefore likely that, also in humans, growth of the tumour since its inception becomes steadily slower. However, this is not certain and there are also arguments in favour of a steady exponential growth with constant T_D.

Proliferation kinetics of tumour cells

The production of new cells in a tissue or a tumour is a function of two parameters:

the length of the cell cycle;
the percentage of cells engaged in the cell cycle, called the growth fraction.

Length of the cell cycle

As we have seen in Section 4.4, the length of the cell cycle can be measured by several methods. The most exact is that of labelled mitoses which requires an injection of [³H] thymidine. About 50 human tumours have been studied in this

---

†In the Gompertz function the doubling time increases exponentially with time.

way by various groups. The mean length of the cell cycle in human tumours is from 2 to 4 days, close to that of normal cells. Despite a very large variability from one cell to another in the same tumour, the mean length of the cycle shows little variation from one tumour to another [58].

Growth fraction

On the other hand the growth fraction varies widely. Its direct measurement is difficult and has been done in only a few human tumours [58, 67]. However, as the length of the cell cycle (T_C) and the ratio of the length of S phase to the total cycle time (T_S/T_C) are relatively constant, the *labelling index*, that is to say the percentage of cells in S phase, gives an approximate value of the growth fraction. It has been measured in several hundred human tumours and varies between 0·1% and nearly 40%. As the length of S phase is about one third of the total cycle time, the growth fraction varies between about 0·3% and 100%. These figures show the existence in tumours of a variable and often very high proportion of quiescent cells, i.e. cells not engaged in a cell cycle (Table 6.3).

Table 6.3. The different cellular compartments in a tumour

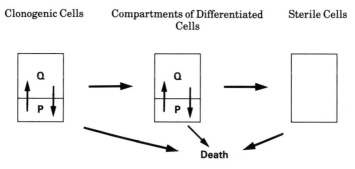

P: proliferating cells
Q: quiescent cells

   These *quiescent cells* are of several types and at the present time there is no reliable technique whereby they can be distinguished. (i) As in normal tissues, a tumour may contain differentiated cells which are incapable of division. (ii) There are also cells which are capable of division but are out of cycle, particularly in the regions of the tumour which are poorly vascularized, close to the necrotic zones and for this reason deficient in oxygen and other nutriments. (iii) Finally, it is possible that there are, as in normal tissues, cells truly in G_0, that is to say capable of division but waiting for a signal before entering into cell cycle. However, the existence of these G_0 tumour cells is plausible only in well-differentiated tumours.

Cell production and potential doubling time

Knowing the length of the cycle and the growth fraction, or T_c and LI, it is easy to calculate the rate of production of cells per unit time. When this production of cells is compared with the increase in tumour volume per unit time obtained by measuring the rate of growth, it is clear that the increase in the number of cells present in the tumour is much lower than the rate of cell production.

Cell loss

This shows that there must be loss of cells. This can be estimated by the difference between the actual measured doubling time of the tumour and the potential doubling time, i.e. what would be found if all the cells in cycle gave rise after mitosis to two viable cells which remained in the tumour [58].

These losses are of several types: (i) degeneration of the cells situated in poorly vascularized regions, close to the necrotic zones; (ii) mitotic death if mitosis is abnormal or if the daughter cells are not viable; (iii) death by senescence of the cells which have differentiated and become incapable of division, analogous to what is observed in normal tissues; (iv) migration out of the tumour of cells which pass into the blood stream or the lymph.

Whatever the cause, cell loss represents a very important percentage of cell production and may reach 90%. This figure indicates, for example, that the number of tumour cells, instead of increasing by one after each mitosis (two daughter cells for one mother cell) increases only on the average by $0 \cdot 1$, in other words 9 cells out of 20 are eliminated before the next division (10 mother cells produce only 11 daughter cells instead of 20). Cell loss is generally greater in rapidly proliferating tumours; many of the cells are proliferating and the daily percentage of losses is high. Cell renewal is therefore very important.

Thus, differences in growth rate of tumours are due essentially to two factors; the growth fraction and cell loss. Table 6.2 gives values of these parameters for several broad histological groups of human tumours; it indicates the very great radiosensitivity (and chemosensitivity) of rapidly proliferating tumours. We will discuss the possible causes later (see Section 6.3: *Differences in proliferation kinetics*).

Clonogenic cells

Until now we have been considering studies made on the whole population of tumour cells. However, most are incapable of multiplying or are already differentiated and are able to make only a small number of divisions. In terms of therapy it is only the clonogenic cells which count. Their kinetics are much less well understood as they cannot be distinguished when the labelling index is measured by means of autoradiography or cytofluorimetry. In experimental tumours the growth fraction of these cells has been measured by the 'suicide effect', i.e. by administration of cytotoxic agents which act only on cells in S phase [49]. The results suggest that there is also a large proportion of quiescent cells among the clonogenic cells; however, the growth fraction is usually greater in the clonogenic compartment than in the whole population and their proliferation is more rapid. However, this is far from always true (Figure 6.11).

One should also remember that in chronic myeloid leukaemia the stem cells responsible for the leukaemia may be pluripotential cells, very different from the leukaemic cells, as they are also capable of giving rise to a progeny of erythroblasts or megakaryocytes which are perfectly normal although carrying

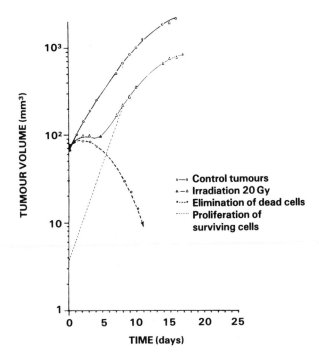

Figure 6.7. Changes in tumour size after irradiation. Upper curve: unirradiated controls. Middle curve: tumours given 20 Gy under anoxic conditions (tumour NCTC 2472). Lower curve: tumours given 70 Gy, showing the elimination of killed cells. Straight line (dotted): proliferation of surviving cells. The proportion of surviving cells after 20 Gy was estimated from the value of D_o measured *in vivo* and was used to estimate the initial tumour volume corresponding to the surviving cells.

the characteristic chromosome aberration of the leukaemia (Philadelphia chromosome). Therefore only a fraction of the descendants have neoplastic characteristics. This example illustrates the difficulties encountered in a human study of clonogenic tumour cells which constitute a very small proportion of the total, of the order of $0 \cdot 1\%$, and may be much less differentiated than the cells constituting almost the whole volume of the tumour in a spontaneous cancer.

Changes in tumour size after irradiation

The changes in the number of tumour cells after irradiation are a function of three parameters (Figure 6.7). (i) The proportion of non-viable clonogenic cells, the cells which have lost their capacity for indefinite multiplication. This is the parameter which is measured when establishing a cell survival curve. (ii) The rate of elimination of the non-viable cells; few pyknotic cells are seen in irradiated tumours although cell loss is important as shown by the technique of cell labelling [58]. The non-viable cells are eliminated either at the first attempt at mitosis or, as is often the case with moderate doses, after two or three cell divisions. The quiescent cells may therefore remain in the tumour for a long time with unchanged morphology. The delay before the non-viable tumour cells

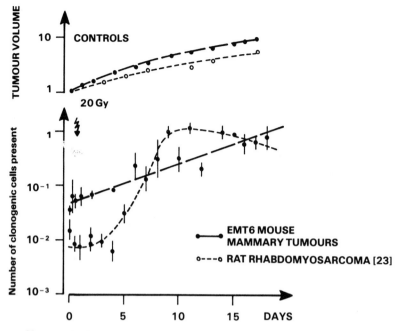

Figure 6.8. Changes in the number of clonogenic cells after irradiation of two experimental tumours. In the rhabdomyosarcoma studied by Hermens and Barendsen [23], by the eighth day there is a rapid increase in the number of clonogenic cells due to their rapid proliferation. In the EMT6 tumour (studied by Guichard *et al.* [22]) the number of clonogenic cells increases more slowly. This illustrates the variations which are found from one tumour to another.

are eliminated may be quite long (several weeks or months), particularly in those tumours in which the cells are dividing infrequently (small growth fraction) and remain for long periods of time without going into mitosis. (iii) The rate of proliferation of the surviving viable cells. After a pre-mitotic block lasting from one to a few days (Figure 5.4), the viable cells start to divide again (Figure 6.7). Moreover, in most tumours as in normal tissues there is *recruitment* of cells, that is to say entry into cycle of cells which had been in a quiescent state. Even when the proportion of surviving cells is small, if their doubling time is short they can quickly give birth to a large number of offspring (Figure 6.8). The tumour begins to grow again when the rate of production of cells is greater than the rate of elimination of non-viable cells (Figure 6.7). We will return to the problem of tumour repopulation later in this section.

The volume of the tumour is also influenced by the other constituents: (a) interstitial liquids: oedema may cause the tumour volume to increase even if the number of cells is constant or falling; (b) non-malignant cells: in some tumours the proportion of non-tumour cells (lymphocytes, macrophages, etc.) amounts to 30% or more of the cells present. In some experimental tumours a considerable increase in the number of these cells is seen after irradiation [5], which may mask the reduction in the number of tumour cells, or even lead to an increase in tumour size [5, 28] (Figure 6.9).

These facts explain why the variation in size of human tumours, the only parameter that can be measured in the clinic, gives unreliable information on

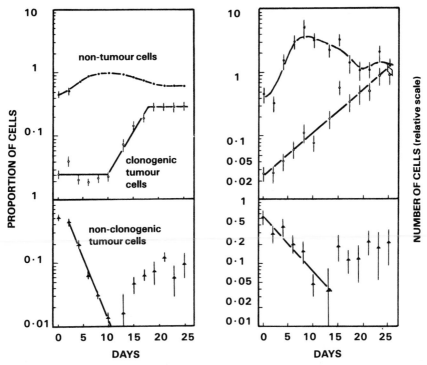

Figure 6.9. Comparison of changes in populations of cells present in a tumour after an irradiation of 15 Gy on day zero. The proportions of cells present are shown in the left-hand panel and the absolute numbers in the right panel. In the left-hand panel it appears that proliferation of clonogenic cells only begins on about the 10th day but in the right-hand panel it is clear that the absolute number of clonogenic cells is increasing steadily from day 1. •, number of non-tumour cells (essentially lymphocytes and macrophages), ○, clonogenic tumour cells; △, non-clonogenic tumour cells. Rhabdomysarcoma of the rat R_1H.
After [5].

what is the most important point, namely changes in the number of viable clonogenic cells. In tumours whose cells are proliferating rapidly, the non-viable cells are quickly eliminated. In tumours whose cells proliferate slowly, elimination of the non-viable cells is also slow. In any case the correlation between tumour regression during and after radiotherapy and tumour curability is not sufficiently reliable to be used in the clinic. Several studies have shown that changes in tumour size during treatment do not enable a reliable prognosis to be given of either tumour control or regrowth after partial or total regression. For example, in the work of Barkley and Fletcher [4] on patients with tumours of the oropharynx (T_2–T_3) with residual tumour at the end of radiotherapy, there were 50% of recurrences, while patients without residual tumour suffered 20% of recurrences. Sobel *et al.* [57] have shown that it is necessary to wait 2 or 3 months after the end of irradiation before persistence of the tumour has true prognostic value and can be correlated with local recurrence in 90% of the cases. In the study of Dawes [10] on 500 tumours of the head and neck, more than 20% of the tumours which were persisting one month after the end of irradiation never regrew and it was necessary to wait 3 months before this percentage fell below 15%.

Similar observations have been made on cancer of the uterine cervix [15] the proportion of long-term local control is better when the tumour has regressed at the end of treatment (69% when there is no tumour at the end of treatment compared with 30% when there is residual tumour).

Thus these studies show: (a) There is no strict correlation between radiocurability and speed of regression. The speed of regression depends essentially on the rate of cellular proliferation. In tumours with a slow rate of proliferation, e.g. medullary carcinoma of the thyroid or chondrosarcoma, there is very little regression during treatment but nevertheless a high proportion of these tumours are cured. Factors other than the death of clonogenic cells influence the speed of regression; thus in the study of Fletcher *et al.* [20] the speed of regression was greater in patients treated with a combination of radio-therapy and fluoro-uracil (FU) whereas the local cure rate was the same with or without FU. (b) Within a group of tumours of a given type, the probability of local cure is greater for tumours which have completely regressed at the end of treatment, but a considerable proportion of tumours which are undetectable will recur and a considerable proportion of persistent tumours will in fact be controlled. This last percentage falls slowly and it is necessary to wait 2 or 3 months after the end of treatment to obtain a satisfactory prediction of final remission. (c) It would be an error to reduce the intended dose because the tumour shrinks rapidly. A tumour which has become occult may still contain several million viable clonogenic cells despite its disappearance on clinical examination. The dose required to obtain complete clinical remission is only one third of the dose needed to sterilize all the tumour cells.

The number of neoplastic cells which are degenerating or morphologically normal can be estimated from histological measurements on tumour fragments removed during or after radiotherapy. This gives more information than a simple measurement of tumour size, but this type of examination is not completely trustworthy as only a very small number of viable clonogenic cells is needed to cause a recurrence.

Tumour repopulation and partial-synchronization

Repopulation

In experimental tumours, Malaise and Tubiana [37] and Hermens and Barendsen [23] have shown that after irradiation the birth rate of malignant cells was increased. This acceleration is due essentially to quiescent cells returning into cycle, a phenomenon called *recruitment*. This usually occurs 10–20 h after irradiation and seems to be triggered by humoral mechanisms; it is often but not always accompanied by a shortening of the cell cycle. Sub-sequently the growth fraction steadily falls and returns to its initial value. This recruitment and acceleration of proliferation is also seen after administration of cytotoxic drugs or partial surgical resection of the tumour. In some animal tumours it limits the effectiveness of fractionated irradiation [3]. In human tumours its importance is very variable.

Data concerning repopulation in human tumours have been obtained with three different techniques.

1. *Tumour doubling time before and after irradiation.* After a period of regression the tumour begins to grow again at the time when cell production, due to multiplication of the descendants of cells which remained viable, exceeds the elimination of non-viable cells (Figure 6.7). For experimental tumours as in humans the doubling time of the tumour is at first shortened and later becomes similar to what it was before irradiation (Figure 6.10). In 26 lung metastases of human tumours the ratio of the doubling times after and before irradiation varied from 0·1 to 0·5 [34].

2. *The time course of the percentage of tumour cells in S phase* (N_s). Following irradiation, N_s has been measured in a large number of experimental tumours and patients by *in vitro* incubation with [³H]thymidine or by flow cytometry, with or without administration of BrdU. An increase in N_s was observed in the majority of the patients but not in all. However, the drawback of this method is that it cannot distinguish the viable cells from those which are doomed to die or the clonogenic cells from the non-clonogenic. Rockwell *et al.* [49] have followed the time course of N_s of viable clonogenic cells and compared it with that of the other cells (Figure 6.11). Although the trends are similar, the information given by the N_s of the whole cell population can be misleading. Hence cell cycle parameters cannot give a reliable estimate of the extent of repopulation.

3. *Influence of protraction on TCD.* Clinically detectable growth of a tumour during treatment signals a rapid proliferation of cells, but lack of growth or even rapid tumour regression does not exclude an increased proliferation rate of surviving clonogenic cells (Figure 6.7). Late in treatment the absolute number of surviving clonogenic cells is so small that their rapid repopulation cannot have any detectable impact on the rate of change of the total tumour mass. The

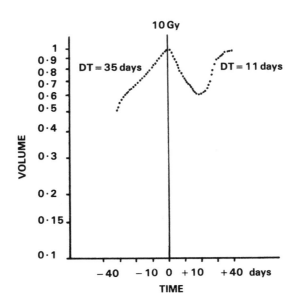

Figure 6.10. Changes in the mean size of 13 pulmonary metastases in 9 patients after a dose of 10 Gy. Three phases can be seen: regression of tumour volume, rapid growth (phase of intense repopulation), then return to the normal rate of growth (from the 40th day).
After [34].

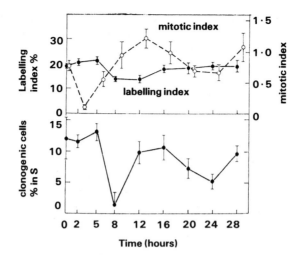

Figure 6.11. Changes of various parameters after a single dose of 3 Gy of X rays. Upper panel: mitotic index and labelling index. Lower: the proportion of clonogenic cells in S phase measured by the suicide technique with [³H]thymidine. The difference betweeen the curves, particularly between the labelling index and the proportion of clonogenic cells in S phase, shows that the labelling index of non-clonogenic cells and particularly of non-viable cells masks the changes in the proliferative state of the only cells which are important in therapeutic terms. EMT6 mouse tumour. After [49].

best way of detecting accelerated repopulation during treatment is therefore to determine the increase in the dose required for a given rate of tumour control with lengthening of the overall treatment time. Trott and Kummermehr [63], Fowler [21] and Withers *et al.* [78] have recently reviewed available clinical data; these retrospective analyses suggest the existence of rapid tumour repopulation in some tumour types, in particular in squamous cell carcinoma of the head and neck. In these tumours, accelerated repopulation becomes detectable after a lag period of approximately 4 weeks of radiotherapy. A dose increment of $0 \cdot 6$ Gy day^{-1} is then required to compensate for this repopulation. Such a dose increment is compatible with a 4-day average clonogenic doubling time; however, these mean values include a wide range of repopulation rates as well as times of onset of accelerated growth.

In split-course radiotherapy the schedule has a pre-planned rest interval of 1–3 weeks. Analysis of these studies has provided data on proliferation rates of malignant cells during the rest period. For head and neck tumours the data are consistent with repopulation corresponding to more than $0 \cdot 5$ Gy day^{-1} [27, 44, 46]. However, in pelvic malignancies (cervix, prostate, bladder) the local control rate was similar in the split-course and continuous treatment regimes when the total dose was the same [47]. This emphasizes the differences in repopulation rates between various types of cancer.

CLINICAL IMPLICATIONS OF REPOPULATION ON OPTIMUM OVERALL DURATION OF TREATMENT

Repopulation in the tumour may be a cause of failure of radiotherapy. Rapid multiplication of cells between fractions may in part compensate for the cell death produced by each fraction. If, for example, each fraction kills 50% of the tumour cells and if the survivors multiply by a factor of 2 during the 24 h separating the fractions, the total number of cells would remain constant whatever the total dose. Studies made on certain experimental tumours, particularly those by Barendsen and Broerse (Figure 6.13), show that this can be the situation in tumours which are capable of rapid repopulation, if the dose per fraction is too small or the interval between fractions is too long [3].

The importance of repopulation during treatment is evident in certain human tumours. In Burkitt's lymphoma, it has been found [43] that tumours which do not regress with irradiation given at one fraction per day may be controlled without increasing the total dose if the interval between treatments is shortened, for example by giving three treatments per day. The same observation has been made with certain inflammatory cancers of the breast. As we have seen, it is probable that repopulation plays an important role in many other types of tumour [53, 64]. However, optimization of total treatment time must take into account repopulation not only in the tumour but also in normal tissues [78].

Differences in the rate of repopulation between normal tissues and tumours, together with differences in the initial shape of the survival curve, are factors which explain how it is possible to sterilize a tumour without causing excessive damage to the surrounding normal tissues. Repopulation determines the choice of the total treatment time. Homeostatic mechanisms which maintain a constant number of cells in a tissue function much more effectively in normal tissues than in tumours. Moreover the very existence of a tumour, an autonomous proliferation of cells which have escaped at least in part from regulatory mechanisms, proves that these are deficient. Loss of a certain proportion of cells in normal tissues, particularly in epithelia, stimulates compensating mechanisms, i.e. an acceleration in cell proliferation which is much more marked than in tumours. In most acutely responding normal tissues repopulation probably begins about 2 weeks after the start of radiotherapy. In bone marrow the time interval between irradiation or administration of cytotoxic drugs and recruitment of stem cells is only 12 h.

This repopulation can generally balance the cytotoxicity of 10 Gy given in five fractions per week, so that during the latter part of a 6–7 week treatment the severity of the reaction remains stable or even decreases, whereas at this period approximately 4 Gy week^{-1} usually suffices to balance tumour clonogenic repopulation in most squamous cell carcinomas. Thus, despite the onset of tumour repopulation after 3–5 weeks, extension of treatment duration still increases the beneficial differential effect between normal epithelial tissues and the tumour. However, this beneficial effect does not exist for slowly proliferating late-responding normal tissues in which repopulation is negligible. Thus for these tissues the therapeutic differential declines when tumour clonogenic repopulation accelerates. The treatment duration should therefore aim at avoiding unacceptable acute normal tissue toxicity but it should also be as short as possible after the onset of tumour repopulation in order to protect the slowly proliferating tissues. Among the late responding tissues, blood vessels are particularly significant as vascular damage plays an important role in late effects.

In conclusion, the optimal overall duration of treatment depends on the tolerances of the early responding and late responding normal tissues and the magnitude and time of onset of tumour repopulation. The choice of dose per fraction is conditioned by the risk of late effects but the treatment strategy should consider simultaneously total dose, dose per fraction and treatment duration, in view of the interplay between these three parameters.

It would therefore be useful to identify the tumours in which repopulation is likely to contribute to radioresistance. Unfortunately, at present we have no satisfactory method for doing this with the exception of histological classification.

Partial-synchronization

The distribution of tumour cells in the different phases of the cell cycle is modified by irradiation for various reasons.

1. As we have seen, radiosensitivity varies in the course of the cell cycle. This is reflected by variations in the proportions of surviving cells.
2. Mitotic delay also varies with the phase of the cycle; the delay is longer for cells closer to mitosis at the time of irradiation, particularly during G_2. This leads to a build up of cells in G_2 (see Chapter 5).

These two phenomena, together with cell recruitment, lead to partial-synchronization, that is a preferential distribution of cells in certain phases of the cycle. After the end of the pre-mitotic block, when the cells start to progress again through the cell cycle, they are not equally distributed in the various phases and as a result there is a cyclic variation in radiosensitivity. This has been demonstrated in tissue culture and in experimental tumours *in vivo*. As far as radiotherapy is concerned, it must be noted that it is only the redistribution of viable clonogenic cells which is of importance, and this can only be studied by complex methods such as the 'suicide effect' [49] (Figure 6.11).

Attempts have been made to exploit this partial-synchronization by administering an agent with selective effectiveness against a particular phase of the cycle (for example, S phase), at the time when most of the tumour cells are passing through this phase. This method has given interesting results with certain experimental tumours but has not led to improvement in therapeutic results in the clinic. This is probably due to several reasons: (i) The length of the cell cycle in a human tumour is very variable from one cell to another. It is therefore difficult to obtain any synchronization and when it does exist it is very transitory. (ii) The growth fraction is usually small in human tumours and only a small proportion of the tumour cells is affected by this phenomenon. (iii) It is difficult to find the right moment to administer the drug as partial-synchronization also occurs in normal tissues. It is therefore not possible to increase the tumour effect without simultaneously increasing the effect on certain normal tissues [67].

On the other hand recruitment and repopulation are more open to therapeutic exploitation. Regeneration in normal tissues responsible for acute reactions (skin, mucosa, bone marrow) takes place earlier and is often more intense than that in the tumour; it therefore comes to an end before that in the tumour. The normal cells return to their usual rate of proliferation at a time when the malignant cells are still in a state of accelerated proliferation. At this time an agent acting on the cells in S phase will preferentially damage the tumour. Also differences between the speed of regeneration of bone marrow and that of tumours constitute the basis for the choice of the interval of time between two cycles of chemotherapy [70].

6.3 Factors affecting the radiosensitivity of human tumours

Clinical experience accumulated over more than half a century shows that there is great variation in the radiosensitivity of human tumours, both within any one type of histology but even more so between one histological type and another. Scales of radiosensitivity have been suggested [18]. They are generally but not universally agreed. Whatever may be their validity, it is clear that certain tumours, e.g. cancers of the colon, have very low radiosensitivity and have little chance of being controlled by radiotherapy, whereas others such as lymphomas and seminomas are very radiosensitive and are controlled by relatively low doses.

These differences in radiosensitivity are due to several factors. It had been considered for some time that the principal factor was variation in the proportion of anoxic tumour cells or differences in the rate of reoxygenation of tumours between fractionated treatments by radiotherapy. This hypothesis is discussed in Chapter 7 and we will not deal with it here. In any case the oxygen effect is not sufficient to explain all the differences seen in the clinic; other explanations must also be envisaged.

Differences in proliferation kinetics

Breur [6] showed with human pulmonary metastases that there was a correlation between growth rate and response to irradiation. This has been confirmed by other authors and it can be accepted that metastases with rapid growth regress not only more rapidly but also to a greater extent than those with a slow growth rate. The same has been found for experimental tumours. However, it is difficult to assess to what extent this is due to differences of renewal rate or of cell survival.

When comparing tumours of different histological types, it is clear that tumours with a high percentage of proliferating cells and a high rate of cell loss are those which are the most radiosensitive and the most radio-curable (Table 6.2). However, as the three factors (histological type, growth fraction and cell loss) are correlated, it is difficult to be sure which is the most important. Nevertheless certain remarks can be made.

1. During fractionated radiotherapy, the radiosensitivity of rapidly growing tumours is increased by the rapid regression of the tumour volume which improves blood perfusion and assists reoxygenation [13].
2. The distribution of cells in the different phases of the cycle is influenced by the rate of proliferation. As radiosensitivity varies during the cycle this affects tumour radiosensitivity (Chapter 4).
3. Repair of potentially lethal damage is more important in tumours with a

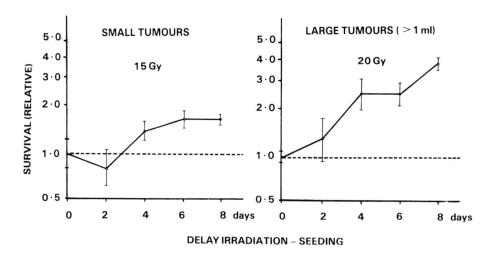

Figure 6.12. **Repair of potentially lethal damage in the NCTC tumour (fibrosarcoma of the mouse):**
left, in a small tumour (a few millimetres in diameter);
right, in a larger tumour (volume greater than 1 cm³). The repair of potentially lethal damage in the large tumour is greater and leads to a greater increase in the surviving fraction of cells.
After [30].

large number of quiescent cells than in those where a large proportion of the cells is proliferating rapidly. This has been shown with experimental tumours. With these the growth fraction falls as the tumour volume increases; the repair of potentially lethal damage is greater in large tumours than in small ones (Figure 6.12).

4. Quiescent cells seem to be more radioresistant than cells in cycle. Thus it has been shown that cell survival curves for very small tumours (a few milli-metres in diameter) have a steeper slope (smaller D_o) than for the same tumours when they have reached a volume of 1 cm³, at the same level of oxygenation (in one experiment the D_o of tumour cells increased from 0·89 to 1·1 Gy when the tumour volume increased from 0·5 to 500 mm³) [55]. The proportion of quiescent cells is smaller in the small tumours [55, 67]. In addition the quiescent cells are often located in regions which are poorly vascularized and therefore anoxic and poorly nourished which may be another factor leading to radioresistance.

It can be seen that there is a variety of possible causes for the radioresistance of slowly growing tumours but it is not yet posssible to estimate their relative importance.

Variation in the proportion of clonogenic cells

The proportion of clonogenic cells in human tumours is not well known. The methods of cloning *in vitro* and implantation in immunodeprived mice suggest that this proportion is of the order of 0·1%, but it is possible that it varies considerably with the type of tumour; e.g., it may be much greater in some melanomas.

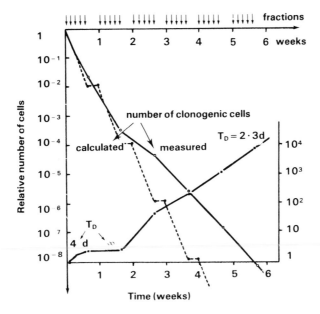

Figure 6.13. Repopulation in an experimental tumour treated by fractionated irradiation similar to that used in radiotherapy. The difference between the reduction in the number of clonogenic cells calculated from the survival curve (on the assumption that each fraction has the same effect) and the measured number of clonogenic cells present in the tumour makes it possible to follow the rate of proliferation of the cells and to measure their doubling time. Dotted line: calculated number of clonogenic cells. Continuous line: measured number of clonogenic cells.
Experimental data of Barendsen and Broerse [3]; calculation by Tubiana [66].

It has also been estimated from the effects of single doses of radiation on skin tumours [26, 65]. The dose to cure 50% of the tumours when given as a single irradiation is 22 Gy for tumours of 3–4 cm in diameter and 18·2 Gy for tumours less than 1 cm in diameter. The dose to give 50% skin necrosis is only a little greater (24·5 Gy). These data, together with other data obtained from fractionated irradiation, suggest that the clonogenic cells have a D_0 of 0·8–1·3 Gy with an extrapolation number between 5 and 10, or a ratio $\alpha/\beta = 13$ Gy. The calculation then shows that the proportion of clonogenic cells cannot be greater than 0·1% [65]. This percentage is compatible with that estimated indirectly by other authors [69].

Intrinsic cellular radiosensitivity

It is difficult to estimate the parameters of cell survival curves for clonogenic tumour cells from the relation between dose and the proportion of tumours cured by a fractionated irradiation, because of uncertainties in repair, reoxygenation and repopulation between fractions [41]. In animals, where some of these factors can be controlled, it seems that the ratio α/β is greater in experimental tumours than in most of the critical normal tissues, suggesting the value of small doses per fraction.

In man, measurements *in vitro* of the radiosensitivity of some 50 cell lines obtained from tumours of various histological types has provided useful information. In general the ratio α/β seems to be lower (Table 6.4) than that found in experimental tumours [77] (although it is similar to the values determined from clinical isoeffect curves, Chapter 8 — $\alpha/\beta = 10$ Gy for epitheliomas and $2 \cdot 5$ Gy for melanomas).

The first cell survival curves were relatively imprecise, particularly in their initial part (at doses less than 3 Gy) which is the most important in radiotherapy. More accurate measurements have shown that after doses of 2–3 Gy, considerable differences in cell survival are seen depending on the tumour lines studied [18]. These differences are amplified during fractionated irradiation and can explain large differences in cure rates. If the surviving fraction is $0 \cdot 5$ after a dose of 2 Gy, after 30 fractions survival is 10^{-9}; if the surviving fraction is $0 \cdot 6$ it becomes 2×10^{-7}, indicating that cure is not possible; if it is $0 \cdot 4$ the surviving fraction is 10^{-12}, corresponding to easy cure even for very large tumours. After doses of 2 Gy given to human or experimental tumours, the differences in survival from one line to another are even greater. In the study of Barendsen [2] the D_0 of the initial slope varies between $2 \cdot 8$ and 12 Gy, a huge range, whereas D_0 at high doses varies only from $1 \cdot 1$ to $2 \cdot 2$ Gy. Weininger [76] in a study *in vitro* of three human melonoma cell lines found surviving fractions between $0 \cdot 39$ and $0 \cdot 52$ after 2 Gy. The critical analysis of data from the literature made by Fertil and Malaise [18] has firmly established this role of variations in the intrinsic radiosensitivity of human tumour cells and has shown a statistically significant correlation between survival after 2 Gy *in vitro* of cell lines from tumours of different histologies and the dose necessary to control the tumours *in vivo*. After 2 Gy the surviving fraction varied from $0 \cdot 18$ (for a Burkitt's lymphoma) to $0 \cdot 90$ (for a melanoma). Table 6.4 (after [36]) brings together some values for cells from human tumours. Deacon *et al.* [12] have reported a value of $0 \cdot 11$ ($D_0 = 0 \cdot 9$ Gy) for neuroblastoma cells. When these cells are irradiated in the form of spheroids implanted into nude mice, the surviving fraction increases to $0 \cdot 26$ ($D_0 = 1 \cdot 5$ Gy) due to repair of potentially lethal damage and cell–cell contact phenomena, but it is still very small. Hypoxia seems to play no part in these variations. Variations in survival at 2 Gy among human tumours are mainly due to difference in the steepness of the initial slope of the cell survival curve (the α component in the linear-quadratic model). The β component makes little contribution to cell killing at 2 Gy and moreover it is similar in radiosensitive and radioresistant tumours [60].

Table 6.4. Radiosensitivity *in vitro* of human tumour cells of various histological types.

	Survival after 2 Gy	α Gy^{-1}	α/β Gy	$D_{0\,\text{eff}}$ for 2 Gy	Survival after 30 fractions of 2 Gy§
Glioblastomas (5)†	$0 \cdot 58$ (34%)‡	$0 \cdot 241$	$8 \cdot 3$	$3 \cdot 67$	$8 \cdot 0 \times 10^{-8}$
Melanomas (19)	$0 \cdot 51$ (28%)	$0 \cdot 255$	$4 \cdot 8$	$2 \cdot 97$	$1 \cdot 7 \times 10^{-9}$
Squamous carcinomas (6)	$0 \cdot 49$ (18%)	$0 \cdot 273$	$6 \cdot 1$	$2 \cdot 80$	$5 \cdot 1 \times 10^{-10}$
Adenocarcinomas (6)	$0 \cdot 48$ (37%)	$0 \cdot 311$	$5 \cdot 7$	$2 \cdot 72$	$2 \cdot 7 \times 10^{-10}$
Lymphomas (6)	$0 \cdot 34$ (27%)	$0 \cdot 451$	$8 \cdot 8$	$1 \cdot 85$	$8 \cdot 8 \times 10^{-15}$
Small-cell lung cancer (6)	$0 \cdot 22$ (42%)	$0 \cdot 650$	$8 \cdot 0$	$1 \cdot 32$	$1 \cdot 9 \times 10^{-20}$

†In parentheses, number of tumours studied.
‡In parentheses, variance.
§Assuming a constant proportion of survivors after each dose fraction and no repopulation.
After [36].

Deacon *et al.* [11] distinguished five groups of cell lines. The most radiosensitive are those of Burkitt's lymphoma and neuroblastoma, then small cell cancer of the lung and medulloblastoma, in the third group cancer of the breast and uterine cervix, in the fourth cancers of the colon, rectum and pancreas, and the fifth, the most radioresistant, melanoma, osteosarcoma and glioblastoma. However, within each histological category there is a large degree of variability. Thus differences in cellular radiosensitivity play an important role in radiotherapy, explaining both the differences in the results of treating tumours of different histology and different tumours of a given histology. It has been shown that in the course of tumour growth more resistant cell lines ('variants') may appear. Radioresistance as well as drug resistance has been observed in cell lines established from patients refractory to drugs [32]. Ensley *et al.* [17] reported that most of the tumours that initially failed to respond to chemotherapy (CT) subsequently did not respond to radiotherapy (RT). Also there is some evidence that cells from recurrences after radiotherapy may be more radioresistant than the cells in the original tumour. Hence the development of radioresistance due to prolonged administration of drugs or radiation is a possibility that should not be overlooked. Acquired radioresistance in human tumours might be more frequent than previously assumed.

Repair of potentially lethal damage (PLD)

As discussed above, a large capacity for repair of potentially lethal damage is another cause of radioresistance (Chapter 4). Repair has been found to be important in cell lines derived from clinically radioresistant tumours, cell survival being multiplied on average by a factor of 4, whereas repair of PLD was smaller in cells from radiocurable tumours [75].

Repair of PLD has been seen *in vivo* in experimental tumours (Figure 6.12), particularly in large tumours [30]; this type of repair is small but not zero after doses per fraction of about 2 Gy, particularly in slowly growing tumours in which a large proportion of the cells is quiescent, as is the case in many human tumours. Thus repair of PLD is one factor explaining both the radioresistance of certain categories of tumour such as melanoma, glioblastoma and osteosarcoma, and also differences in radiosensitivity among tumours of a given histological type.

In general this type of repair seems to be more important in the cells of normal tissues than in tumour cells, one of the reasons for the effectiveness of fractionated radiotherapy. The difference can be attributed to a greater proportion of quiescent clonogenic cells in normal tissues. The mechanisms whereby intercellular contact inhibits proliferation are much more powerful in normal tissues than in tumours.

Repair of sublethal damage

The rate of repair of sublethal damage also varies from one cell line to another (it seems to be slower in radioresistant cells). This may explain differences in survival after irradiation at low dose rate for cells with similar radiosensitivity when irradiated at high dose rate (1 Gy min^{-1}). The role of intercellular contact is also important for this type of repair, as has been shown by the differences in survival when cells are irradiated as a single cell suspension or in the form of spheroids (Chapter 4). The importance of these contacts can be quantified by measurement of electrical resistance and Guichard *et al.* [22] have demonstrated their role in human tumours implanted in nude mice. It is possible that the absence of intercellular junctions may explain the exceptional radiosensitivity of certain normal cells lines, for example haemopoietic stem cells and malignant haematogenous cells (leukaemias and lymphomas).

Predictive assays

Several assays capable of predicting the response of a tumour to radiotherapy have been proposed during the past few years. None have yet been proved to have clinical value, but continued study is well worthwhile.

1. *The labelling index (LI)* is correlated with the probability of distant metastasis [70] but also with the local aggressivity of the tumour and its resistance to treatment, perhaps because the least differentiated tumours have the highest labelling index. Some data suggest that a high LI is also correlated with the incidence of local recurrence, in particular when the percentage of S phase cells increases during radiotherapy, demonstrating a high rate of repopulation. The LI is on average higher in aneuploid tumours. Aneuploidy seems to be connected with genetic instability of the tumour, i.e. with a capacity to give rise to 'variant' cell lines some of which are resistant to various therapeutic agents. Ploidy can be evaluated by measuring the DNA content of the cells either by flow cytofluorimetry or histochemically on histological sections. The two variables (LI and aneuploidy) have limited predictive value and are not adequate to define an optimal choice of treatment.

2. The importance of measuring the *initial slope* of the oxic cell survival curve (or the survival at 2 Gy) was brought out by the work of Fertil and Malaise [18], as discussed above. This study was based on *in vitro* assays of clonogenic tumour cells. However, the stringent requirements of clonogenic assays cannot usually be met in primary cultures from human tumours. Human tumour *xenografts* maintain the level of drug responsiveness of the source tumours. However, xenografts are unlikely to be of value in individual patients because the time interval between transplantation of the surgical specimen and the results becoming available is too long; moreover the take is low. Nevertheless, xenografts may be useful in combination with short-term *in vitro* assays [50].

3. *Non-clonogenic assays* are being developed and investigated [7]. They provide only an indirect measure of cell survival and must be validated against *in vitro* or *in vivo* clonogenic assays. However, they are important because they overcome the problems that often make clonogenic assays impossible. Treatment with drugs and radiation may take place 1 day after culture is established and the assay is terminated after 2 weeks. The results from the various histological types agree, in general, with clonogenic assays and clinical radio-curability. This is an avenue for research which should be actively explored in view of the considerable variation in the survival at 2 Gy which exists within cells derived from tumours of similar histological types.

One of the problems is that some data [74] strongly suggest that similar variations may also exist within the tumour. In accordance with the concept of tumour progression it has been shown that many tumours contain subpopulations of stem cells with different chemo- or radiosensitivities. Therapy can in some instances select for resistant subpopulations or even induce resistance. The presence and degree of heterogeneity must therefore become an essential part of any test. The problem is further complicated by the interaction which may exist between subpopulations in heterogeneous tumours. These affect growth and metastatic potential and there are data which suggest that they may also have an impact on treatment response *in vivo* [38].

4. *Other assays. Sister chromatid exchanges* which are induced by drugs or radiation are of interest because they may provide an individual measurement of sensitivity for each cell and thus can be used for investigating tumour heterogeneity [7].

Cells with a *micronucleus* are doomed cells and their determination can yield a rough estimate of cell death. After irradiation the number of tumour cells with micronuclei increases [61]. This may be a useful method as suggested by studies with experimental tumours. Unfortunately clinical application at the present time seems difficult.

5. *Identification of biochemical factors* which influence radiosensitivity. Normal cells of a given type are of similar radiosensitivity in most subjects, but there are a few exceptions. Subjects with a genetic defect in the DNA repair system are more radiosensitive (Section 3.3). It has been shown recently that expression of some repair genes, or of oncogenes, may strongly influence the radiosensitivity of the cells [29, 56]. This opens a new avenue for research. Some DNA probes may be used for predictive assays.

Glutathione, a peptide rich in SH groups, is a radioprotector (Section 10.2) and SH groups in cells act as radioprotective agents. The number of SH groups varies during the cell cycle and from one cell line to another; measurement of their concentration may therefore be useful. Intracellular concentration of glutathione is reduced in certain hereditary conditions. It has been shown that this increases cellular radiosensitivity, particularly in anoxic conditions [14]. Radiation resistance in some cell lines made resistant to certain drugs has been attributed to high intracellular glutathione levels; however, there is no difference between the radiosensitivity of pleiotropic drug-resistant cells and that of their parental cell lines despite a two-fold higher glutathione level in the drug-resistant line. There are intracellular sources of SH groups in cells other than glutathione. Moreover there might be small subpopulations with a high glutathione content. Cellular distributions of glutathione levels in tumour specimens should be investigated [40].

Relation between host and tumour [62]

The theory of immune surveillance postulated that the organism was capable of recognizing tumour cells as foreign and of attacking them with T lymphocytes (*killer cells*). This theory suggested that it was not necessary to kill all the tumour cells as the organism could, if it was immunologically active, eliminate the residual cells. This concept was essentially based on work with transplanted tumours whose immunological characteristics are very different from those of the host animal and which for this reason excite an immunological reaction in the recipient animal. In man the existence of immune mechanisms capable of selectively destroying tumour cells has been demonstrated by the occasional success of immunotherapy on certain types of human tumour, in particular melanomas and cancers of the kidney in adults. In this technique certain categories of killer lymphocytes, derived from the patient, are cultivated *in vitro* and activated with interleukin 2 (IL2). They are then reinjected into the patient who also receives massive injections of IL2. Some complete remissions have been obtained in patients presenting with numerous metastases, showing that killer lymphocytes, in particular tumour infiltrating lymphocytes (TIL), can have a therapeutic action when stimulated by IL2 [51]. The side-effects have sometimes been severe, but the occasional successes emphasize the importance of further research on immunological methods involving less toxicity.

Other factors such as age, malnutrition and alcoholism seem to increase the radiosensitivity of normal tissues and thereby to aggravate their response to treatment. Many studies have shown the prognostic value (for local control of the tumour) of the performance index (Karnofsky scale) which is an expression of the general condition of the patient.

The old literature is full of considerations on the effect of radiotherapy on the tumour bed, the stroma. There are, however, few clinical or experimental data. The effect of radiation on the vascular system is undeniable but it develops late and its impact on tumour regression is debatable. It is, however, important to remember that cellular proliferation in capillary vessels supplying tumours is much greater than that in the vessels of normal tissues. The clinical role of these factors has as yet been little studied.

6.4 *Combinations of radiotherapy and chemotherapy* [59]

Microscopic tumour deposits can be destroyed by radiotherapy with moderate doses of the order of 40–45 Gy, but even with these doses the dimensions of the field must be limited to avoid complications. On the other hand chemotherapy is a general treatment but toxicity in normal tissues limits the doses which can be given.

Contribution of CT and RT to the control of the primary tumour

In mice which have received human tumour transplants, the proportion of tumour cells killed by the maximum dose of drug tolerated by the mouse as a single dose, for example that killing 90% of the mice, varies with the drug and the type of tumour; in favourable cases it is about 50% and occasionally exceeds 90%. Radiotherapy has the advantage of greater effectiveness and has an important role in the treatment of large tumours, even those sensitive to chemotherapy (lymphoma, small-cell carcinoma of the lung, etc.). For example, in patients with small-cell lung carcinoma, despite the administration of aggressive modern multidrug CT, a dose of 55 Gy is required in order to reduce the local recurrence rate to below 40% [70]. This dose is necessary even when the induction CT is able to achieve complete remission in most patients, emphasizing the insufficiency of the criteria used to assess the presence of residual tumour. Without RT, a very high rate (>80%) of loco-regional failure has been observed after so-called complete remission.

A simple calculation will illustrate the respective roles of RT and CT in the control of a tumour. Let us consider a tumour of 100 g (10^{11} cells) in which 1% of the tumour cells are clonogenic (10^9 cells) with a D_{50} equal to 2 Gy. As discussed above, the TCD 37 is approximately 60 Gy in 30 fractions. If CT has reduced the number of cells by half, corresponding to a partial remission, the TCD is 58 Gy; it is still 54 Gy if 90% of the tumour cells have been killed, corresponding to a marked regression of the tumour size under CT. It is only when CT has caused a complete remission of the tumour (residual tumour mass smaller than 100 mg) that RT given to eradicate the remaining subclinical disease can be reduced to $20 \times D_{50}$ (40 Gy). If the tumour is radioresistant ($D_{50}=3$ Gy, corresponding to a survival of 63% after a dose of 2 Gy), the corresponding doses are 90, 87, 81 and 60 Gy, respectively. It is easy to see that for radioresistant tumours the TCD can be reduced below the dose tolerated by normal tissues only when CT is able to produce a complete remission in most patients.

In patients with breast cancer, comparison of the incidence of loco-regional recurrence in those treated by surgery alone or by surgery followed by post-operative RT allows one to estimate the efficacy of RT. In order to take into account the indicators which are related to the incidence of local recurrence, such as the histological grade and the number of involved axillary nodes, a multivariate analysis can be carried out. The results show that in over three quarters of the patients, the loco-regional residual disease is controlled by RT (10-year recurrence rates 30% and 6% respectively in patients without or with post-operative RT) [72]. The addition of adjuvant CT further reduces this incidence but its relative effectiveness is limited. In the Danish breast cancer controlled trials [44], the incidence of loco-regional recurrence was slightly, but not significantly, lower in the arm treated by RT plus adjuvant CT than in the arm treated by RT alone (7% versus 12% in premenopausal, 12% versus 17% in postmenopausal patients). In another Danish trial the local recurrence rate was significantly lower in patients treated by RT plus CMF than in patients treated by CT alone (7% versus 24% in premenopausal, 5% versus 25% in postmenopausal patients). In patients with inflammatory breast cancer [52], the 4-year local recurrence rate was significantly higher in patients treated by RT alone (45 Gy plus a boost of 20 Gy to the tumour) than in those treated by RT (45+15 Gy) plus CT (53% versus 32%). However, this local recurrence rate was not further diminished when a more aggressive CT regimen was administered.

These data show that combinations of CT and RT can improve the local control only for those tumours which are both chemosensitive and radiosensitive. When the treatment is initiated with CT, these figures also show that unless the tumour is extremely radiosensitive it is safer to deliver the maximum tolerated radiation dose, in particular when the tumour has not rapidly shrunk under CT.

Timing of the delivery of CT and RT

At least three factors have to be taken into account in the choice of timing: toxic effects, tumour repopulation and the risks of development of chemoresistance and radioresistance.

Toxic effects on normal tissues

The effects of radiation and drugs are additive both on tumours and normal tissues. It had been hoped that administration of drugs during radiotherapy would potentiate the action of radiation on the tumour, but in fact it increases the effect on normal tissues to the same extent and sometimes even more (Chapter 10). Studies are continuing on the radiosensitizing effect of certain drugs such as cisplatin, but in general it seems better to give the two modalities of treatment sequentially. This does not mean that concurrent delivery should be banished, but it is advisable to restrict it to situations in which the cumulative toxic effect on the irradiated critical tissues does not preclude the administration of curative doses of RT and CT. With certain drugs, in particular actinomycin D, additivity of toxic effects is seen even when there is a time interval of several months. Some drugs have a selective toxicity on certain tissues; if these are included in the radiation target volume, serious complications are likely. Particular care is needed for:

Lung:	actinomycin D (Act D), adriamycin (ADM), bleomycin (BL), cyclophosphamide (CP), hydroxyurea (HU), vincristine (VC).
Intestine and colon:	Act D, ADM, BL, BCNU, 5 FU, alkylating agents.
Central nervous system:	methotrexate.
Kidney:	cisplatin.
Bladder:	Act D, ADM, CP.
Liver:	Act D, ADM, CP.

Tumour repopulation

If both CT and RT have to be given sequentially and in full doses, the consequence of this long protraction can be a high level of tumour repopulation [69, 71]. Withers *et al.* [78] pointed out that if CT is given prior to RT, increased repopulation between radiotherapy fractions can then lessen the effect of subsequent RT.

When RT is delivered first, this delays the employment of CT and thus permits further growth of occult metastases located outside the irradiated volume. For example, if the tumour doubling time is equal to 1 month which is a realistic figure for rapidly growing tumours, a delay of 2 months would allow the metastases to become four times larger [71]. This is why, generally, CT is given first; however, RT cannot be delayed too long because CT often has only a limited efficacy on bulky tumours and can even elicit the development of radioresistance. Therefore RT is usually carried out after two to four cycles of CT. At this time, the tumour cells which are still viable undergo an acceleration of their proliferation rate; thus if the pretreatment doubling time is taken to be 1 month, after a few cycles of CT the doubling time may be as short as 6 days. Taking 2 weeks as a conservative estimate, after a 2-month interruption caused by the RT course, the occult metastases located outside the irradiated volume are 16 times larger. Such a marked increase in size of the metastases would considerably lower the efficacy of CT.

In view of the uncertainty about the extent of repopulation, the shortest possible delay between CT and RT is advisable. A compromise must be found between a short delay with the aim of limiting repopulation and a long one required to avoid interaction between drugs and radiation.

Chemoresistance and radioresistance

In patients treated with CT, the main source of failure is the appearance of chemoresistant cells. The rationale of multiple drug CT is to combine drugs without cross-resistance and with independent toxicity. However, when many drugs are used in combination, the individual drug doses must be reduced in order to avoid cumulative toxicity, and some of the drugs are only toxic to vital normal cells without a significant contribution to killing the tumour cells. Thus one should avoid combining drugs which have a high probability of cross-resistance. Moreover, even with the best combination of drugs, drug resistance may develop. This emphasizes the usefulness of other agents with a low probability of cross-resistance, in particular ionizing radiation. For any given drug, there may be a variety of mechanisms by which a cell can become resistant. If these changes occur as isolated defects, the level of resistance is usually relatively low. However, multiple modes of resistance can occur in the same cell, leading to a high level of resistance. Numerous agents that reversibly inhibit DNA synthesis, including most of the cytotoxic agents, can dramatically increase the frequency of gene amplification which is one of the mechanisms associated with the development of resistance [54].

Combination of CT and RT is based on the postulate that there is no cross-resistance between cytotoxic drugs and ionizing radiations. This postulate has been challenged. Hill *et al.* [24] reported that exposure to radiation may induce development of resistance to vincristine. Louie *et al* [32] have developed a series of human ovarian-cancer cell lines, some of which are resistant to doxorubicin, melphalan and cisplatin. Cross-resistance to irradiation was observed in both the cisplatin and melphalan resistant sublines whereas no cross-resistance was observed in the doxorubicin resistant sublines. Mitchell *et al.* [39] and Wallner and Li [73] did not observe any increase of radioresistance in cell lines made chemoresistant to doxorubicin. Thus pleiotropic drug resistance does not necessarily confer radiation resistance. Sklar [56] has shown that the intrinsic radioresistance of one cell line (NIH 3T3) can be markedly increased by the presence of *ras* oncogenes activated by nonsense mutations. Large differences in D_0 (from $0 \cdot 8$ to $2 \cdot 5 \, Gy$) can be caused by adding single genes to these cells. This strongly suggests that some mutations can increase radioresistance without modifying resistance to drugs. However, this does not preclude the existence of alterations to the genome which modify DNA repair and are able to impart both radioresistance and chemoresistance [45]. Early administration of both CT and RT might be the best way to overcome the development of resistance.

Alternating delivery of CT and RT

In order to reconcile the needs for early administration of both agents and for sequential delivery without a long postponement of one of the two modalities, an alternating treatment schedule has been developed in which CT and RT are inter-digitated [70, 71]. This protocol avoids the toxic effects resulting from the concurrent administration of drugs and radiation. Alternating two different treatment modalities with minimal cross-toxicity gives more time for recovery of critical normal tissues after each modality. Furthermore it avoids a long gap in the delivery of CT and shortens the time interval between the various agents. Therefore it limits the role of tumour repopulation and allows a high intensity of treatment. This alternating regimen is consistent with the experimental data produced by Looney [31] and is supported by the results of clinical trials carried out at Villejuif. However, this regimen is of value only in those types of tumour which are both chemosensitive and radiosensitive and in which there is a significant repopulation rate [70, 71] and/or a marked propensity towards an early development of resistance to one of the treatment modalities.

Another aspect of combinations of RT and CT is the irradiation of 'sanctuary sites' into which the drugs do not penetrate well, in particular the central nervous system. Irradiation of the brain to a dose of 24 Gy has transformed the prognosis in acute leukaemia. However, there are significant risks of morbidity after irradiation of the brain combined with intrathecal injection of methotrexate.

References

1. R. Arriagada *et al. Int. J. Radiat. Oncol. Biol. Phys.*, 1985, **11**: 1751–1757.
2. G. W. Barendsen. Intrinsic radiosensitivity of tumor cells, in: *Biological bases and clinical implications of tumor radioresistance* (G. Fletcher, C. Nervi, H. R. Withers, eds), pp. 13–18. Masson, New York, 1983.
3. G. W. Barendsen, J. J. Broerse. Experimental radiotherapy of a rat rhabdomyosarcoma with 15 MeV neutrons and 300 kV X-rays. II. Effects of fractionated treatments, applied five times a week for several weeks. *Eur. J. Cancer*, 1970, **6**: 89–109.
4. H. T. Barkley, G. H. Fletcher. The significance of residual disease after external irradiation of squamous cell carcinoma of the oropharynx. *Radiology*, 1977, **124**: 493–495.
5. H. P. Beck, I. Brammer, F. Zywietz, H. Jung. The application of flow cytometry for the quantification of the response of experimental tumors to irradiation. *Cytometry*, 1981, **2**: 44–46.
6. K. Breur, Growth rate and radiosensitivity of human tumors. *Eur. J. Cancer*, 1966, **2**: 157–188.
7. W. A. Brock, F. L. Baker, P. J. Tofilon. Tumor cell sensitivities to drug and radiation, in: *The prediction of tumor treatment response* (J. D. Chapman, L. J. Peters, H. R. Withers, eds). pp. 139–156. Pergamon Press, Oxford, 1989.
8. A. Charbit, E. P. Malaise, M. Tubiana. Relation between the pathological nature and the growth rate of human tumours. *Eur. J. Cancer*, 1971, **7**: 307–315.
9. V. P. Collins, R. K. Loeffler, H. Tivey. Observations on growth rates of human tumours. *Am. J. Roentgenol*, 1956, **76**: 988–1000.
10. P. J. Dawes. The early response of oral, oropharyngeal, hypopharyngeal and laryngeal cancer related to local control and survival. *Br. J. Cancer*, 1980, **41**, Suppl. IV: 14–16.
11. J. Deacon, M. J. Peckham, G. G. Steel. The radioresponsiveness of human tumours and the initial slope of the cell survival curve. *Radiother. Oncol.*, 1984, **2**: 317–323.
12. J. M. Deacon, P. A. Wilson, M. J. Peckham. The radiobiology of human neuroblastoma. *Radiother. Oncol.*, 1985, **3**: 201–209.
13. J. Denekamp. Tumour regression as a guide to prognosis. A study with experimental animals. *Br. J. Radiol.*, 1977, **50**: 271–279.
14. P. J. Deschavanne, E. P. Malaise, L. Revesz. Radiation survival of glutathione-deficient human fibroblasts in culture. *Br. J. Radiol.*, 1981, **54**: 361–362.
15. S. Dische, M. H. Bennett, M. I. Saunders, P. Anderson. Tumour regression as a guide to prognosis: a clinical study. *Br. J. Radiol.*, 1980, **53**: 454–461.
16. J. Dutreix, M. Tubiana, A. Dutreix. An approach to the interpretation of clinical data on the tumor control probability–dose relationship. *Radiother Oncol.* 1988, **11**: 239–248.
17. J. F. Ensley, J. R. Jacobs, A. Weaver, J. Kinzie, J. Crissman, J. A. Kish, G. Cummings, M. Al-Sarraf. Correlation between response to *cis*-platinum combination and subsequent radiotherapy in previously untreated patients with advanced squamous cell cancers of the head and neck. *Cancer*, 1984, **54**: 811–814.

18. B. Fertil, E. P. Malaise. Inherent cellular radiosensitivity as a basic concept for human tumor radiotherapy. *Int. J. Radiat. Oncol. Biol. Phys.*, 1981, **7**: 621–629.
19. G. H. Fletcher. Basic clinical parameters, in: *Textbook of radiotherapy*, 3rd edn., pp. 180–218. Lea and Febiger, Philadelphia, 1980.
20. G. H. Fletcher, H. D. Suit, C. D. Howe, M. Samuels, R. H. Jesse, R. U. Villareal. Clinical method of testing radiation sensitizing agents in squamous cell carcinoma. *Cancer*, 1963, **16**: 355–363.
21. J. F. Fowler. Potential for increasing the differential response between tumors and normal tissues: can proliferation rate be used? *Int. J. Radiat. Oncol. Biol. Phys.*, 1986, **12**: 641–645.
22. M. Guichard, H. Dertinger, E. P. Malaise. Radiosensitivity of four human xenografts. Influence of hypoxia and cell-cell contacts. *Radiat. Res.*, 1983, **95**: 602–609.
23. A. F. Hermens, G. W. Barendsen. The proliferative status and clonogenic capacity of tumour cells in a transplantable rhabdomyosarcoma of the rat before and after irradiation with 800 rad of X-rays. *Cell Tissue Kinet.*, 1978, **11**: 83–100.
24. B. T. Hill, R. D. H. Whelan, L. K. Hosking, S. A. Shellard, P. Bedford, R. B. Lock. Interactions between antitumor drugs and radiation in mammalian tumor cell lines: differential drug responses and mechanisms of resistance following fractionated X-irradiation or continuous drug exposure *in vitro*. *National Cancer Inst. Monog.*, 1988, **6**: 177–181.
25. M. Hjelm-Hansen, K. Jorgenson, A. P. Anderson, C. Lund. Laryngeal carcinoma — II. Analysis of treatment results using the Ellis model. *Acta Radiol. Oncol. Radiat. Phys. Biol.*, 1979, **5**: 385–407.
26. A. Hliniak, B. Maciejewski, K. R. Trott. The influence of the number of fractions, overall treatment time and field size on the local control of cancer of the skin. *Br. J. Radiol.*, 1983, **56**: 596–598.
27. L. R. Holsti, M. Mantyla. Split course versus continuous radiotherapy. *Acta Oncologica*, 1988, **27**: 153–161.
28. H. Jung, H. P. Beck, I. Brammer, F. Zywietz. Depopulation and repopulation of the R1H rhabdomyosarcoma of the rat after X-irradiation. *Eur. J. Cancer*, 1981, **17**: 375–386.
29. U. Kasid, A. Pfeifer, T. Brennan, M. Beckett, R. R. Weichselbaum, A. Dritschilo, G. E. Mark. Effect of antisense *c-raf-1* on tumorigenicity and radiation sensitivity of a human squamous carcinoma. *Science*, 1989, **243**: 1354–1356.
30. J. B. Little, G. M. Hahn, E. Frindel, M. Tubiana. Repair of potentially lethal radiation damage *in vitro* and *in vivo*. *Radiology*, 1973, **106**: 689–694.
31. W. B. Looney, Special lecture: alternating chemotherapy and radiotherapy. *National Cancer Inst. Monogr.*, 1988, **6**: 85–94.
32. K. G. Louie, B. C. Behrens, T. J. Kinsella, T. C. Hamilton, K. R. Grotzinger, W. M. McKoy, M. A. Winker, R. F. Ozols. Radiation survival parameters of antineoplastic drug-sensitive and resistant human ovarian cancer cell lines and their modification by buthionine. *Cancer Res.*, 1985, **45**: 2110–2115.
33. B. Maciejewski, G. Preuss-Bayer, K. R. Trott. The influence of the number of fractions and overall treatment time on the local tumour control of cancer of the larynx. *Int. J. Radiat. Oncol. Biol. Phys.*, 1983, **9**: 321–328.
34. E. P. Malaise, A. Charbit, N. Chavaudra, P. F. Combes, J. Douchez, M. Tubiana. Change in volume of irradiated human metastases. Investigation of repair of sublethal damage and tumour repopulation. *Br. J. Cancer*, 1972, **26**: 43–52.
35. E. P. Malaise, N. Chavaudra, M. Tubiana. The relationship between growth rate, labelling index and histological type of human solid tumours. *Eur. J. Cancer*, 1973, **9**: 305–312.
36. E. P. Malaise, B. Fertil, N. Chavaudra, M. Guichard. Distribution of radiation sensitivities for human tumor cells of specific histological types. *Int. J. Radiol. Oncol. Biol. Phys.*, 1986, **12**: 617–624.
37. E. P. Malaise, M. Tubiana. Croissance des cellules d'un fibrosarcome expérimental irradié chez la souris C 3H. *C. R. Acad. Sci.*, 1966, **263 D**: 292–295.
38. B. E. Miller, F. R. Miller, G. H. Heppner. Heterogeneities of tumor cell sensitivities: implications for tumor response in: *The prediction of tumor treatment response* (J. D. Chapman, L. J. Peters, H. R. Withers, eds), pp. 227–238. Pergamon Press, Oxford, 1989.
39. J. B. Mitchell, J. Gamson, A. Russo, N. Friedman, J. De Graff, J. Carmichael, E. Glatstein. Chinese hamster pleiotropic multidrug resistant cells are not radioresistant. *National Cancer Inst. Monogr.*, 1988, **6**: 187–191.
40. J. B. Mitchell, A. Russo, J. Carmichael, E. Glatstein. Glutathione as a predictor of tumor response, in *The prediction of tumor treatment response* (J. D. Chapman, L. J. Peters, H. R. Withers, eds), pp. 157–174. Pergamon Press, Oxford, 1989.
41. J. V. Moore, J. H. Hendry, R. D. Hanter. Dose-incidence curves for tumour control and normal tissue injury, in relation to the response of clonogenic cells. *Radiother. Oncol.*, 1983, **1**: 143–157.
42. R. Morrison. The results of treatment of cancer of the bladder — a clinical contribution to radiobiology. *Clin. Radiol.*, 1975, **26**: 67–75.

43. T. Norin, J. Onyango. Radiotherapy in Burkitt's lymphoma: conventional or superfractionated regime. *Int. J. Radiat. Oncol. Biol. Phys.*, 1977, **2**: 399–406.
44. M. Overgaard *et al.* Post mastectomy irradiation in high risk breast cancer patients. *Acta Oncol.*, 1988, **27**: 707–714.
45. R. F. Ozols, H. Masuda, T. C. Hamilton. Keynote address: mechanisms of cross-resistance between radiation and antineoplastic drugs. *National Cancer Inst. Monogr.*, 1988, **6**: 159–165.
46. J. T. Parsons, F. J. Bova, R. R. Million. A reevaluation of split course technique for squamous cell carcinoma of the head and neck. *Int. J. Radiat. Oncol. Biol. Phys.*, 1980, **6**: 1645–1652.
47. J. T. Parsons, T. L. Thar, F. J. Bova, R. R. Million. An evaluation of split-course irradiation for pelvic malignancies. *Int. J. Radiat. Oncol. Biol. Phys.*, 1980, **6**: 175–181.
48. C. Regaud, H. Ferroux. Discordance des effets des rayons X, d'une part dans la peau, d'autre part dans le testicule, par le fractionnement de la dose: diminution de l'efficacité dans la peau, maintien de l'efficacité dans le testicule. *C. R. Soc. Biol.*, 1927, **97**: 431–434.
49. S. Rockwell, E. Frindel, A. J. Valleron, M. Tubiana. Cell proliferation in EMT6 tumors treated with single doses of X-rays or hydroxyurea. I — Experimental results. *Cell Tissue Kinet.*, 1978, **11**: 279–289.
50. E. K. Rofstad. Human tumor xenografts in development of predictive assays of tumor treatment response, in *'The prediction of tumor treatment response'* (J. D. Chapman, L. J. Peters, H. R. Withers eds), pp. 197–216. Pergamon Press, Oxford, 1989.
51. J. A. Rosenberg, P. Spiess, R. Lafreniere. A new approach to the adoptive immunotherapy of cancer with tumor infiltrating lymphocyte. *Science*, 1986, **233**: 1308–1312.
52. J. Rouësse, S. Friedman, D. Sarrazin, H. Mouriesse, T. Le Chevalier, R. Arriagada, M. Spielmann, A. Papacharalambous, F. May-Levin. Primary chemotherapy in the treatment of inflammatory breast carcinoma: a study of 230 cases from the Institut Gustave-Roussy. *J. Clin. Oncol.*, 1986, **4**: 1765–1771.
53. M I. Saunders *et al.* Continuous hyperfractionated accelerated radiotherapy in locally advanced carcinoma of the head and neck region. *Int. J. Radiat. Onc. Biol. Phys.*, 1989, **17**: 1287–1294.
54. R. T. Schimke. Methotrexate resistance and gene amplification. Mechanisms and implications, in: *Accomplishments in cancer research*, J. G. Fortner, J. E. Rhoads, eds), p. 75. J. B. Lippincott, Philadelphia, 1986.
55. W. U. Shipley, J. A. Stanley, G. G. Steel. Tumor size dependency in the radiation reponse of the Lewis lung carcinoma. *Cancer Res.*, 1975, **35**: 2488–2493.
56. M. D. Sklar. The *ras* oncogenes increase the intrinsic resistance of NIH 3T3 cells to ionizing radiation. *Science*, 1988, **239**: 645–647.
57. S. Sobel, P. Rubin, B. Keller, C. Poulter. Tumor persistence as a predictor of outcome after radiation therapy of head and neck cancers. *Int. J. Radiat. Oncol. Biol. Phys.*, 1976, **1**: 873–880.
58. G. C. Steel. *Growth kinetics of tumours*. Clarendon Press, Oxford, 1977.
59. G. C. Steel. The search for therapeutic gain in the combination of radiotherapy and chemotherapy. *Radiother. Oncol.*, 1988, **11**: 31–53.
60. G. C. Steel, J. H. Peacok. Why are some human tumours more sensitive than others? *Radiother. Oncol.*, 1989, **15**: 63–72.
61. C. Streffer, D. Van Beuninger, E. Gross, F. W. Eigler, T. Pelzer. Determination of DNA, micronuclei and vascular density in human rectum carcinomas, in: *The prediction of tumor treatment response* (J. D. Chapman, L. J. Peters, H. R. Withers, eds), pp. 217–226. Pergamon Press, Oxford, 1989.
62. J. E. Talmadge. Immunotherapy of metastatic disease, in: *The prediction of tumor treatment response* (J. D. Chapman, L. J. Peters, H. R. Withers, eds), pp. 239–254. Pergamon Press, Oxford, 1989.
63. K. R. Trott, K. Kummermehr. What is known about tumor proliferation rates to choose between accelerated fractionation or hyperfractionation? *Radiother. Oncol.*, 1985, **3**: 1–9.
64. K. R. Trott, H. von Lieven, J. Kummermehr, D. Skopal, S. Lukas, O. Braun-Falco, A. M. Kellerer. The radiosensitivity of malignant melanoma. II. Clinical studies. *Int. J. Radiat. Oncol. Biol. Phys.*, 1981, **7**: 15–20.
65. K. R. Trott, B. Maciejewski, G. Preuss-Bayer, J. Skolyszewski. Dose-response curve and split-dose recovery in human skin cancer. *Radiother. Oncol.*, 1984, **2**: 123–129.
66. M. Tubiana. The kinetics of tumour cell proliferation and radiotherapy. *Br. J. Radiol.*, 1971, **44**: 325–347.
67. M. Tubiana. Cell kinetics and radiation oncology. *Int. J. Radiat. Oncol. Biol. Phys.*, 1982, **8**: 1471–1489.
68. M. Tubiana. The causes of clinical radioresistance, in: *The biological basis of radiotherapy*, (G. C. Steel, G. E. Adams. M. T. Peckham, eds), chapter 2, pp. 13–33. Elsevier, New York, 1983.
69. M. Tubiana. Repopulation in human tumors. A biological background for fractionation in radiotherapy. *Acta Oncologica*, 1988, **27**: 83–88.

70. M. Tubiana. The combination of radiotherapy and chemotherapy. A review. *Int. J. Radiat. Biol. Phys.,* 1989, **55**: 497–511.
71. M. Tubiana, R. Arriagada, J. M. Cosset. Sequencing of drugs and radiation. *Cancer,* 1985, **55**: 2131–2139.
72. M. Tubiana, D. Sarrazin. The role of post-operative radiotherapy in breast cancer, in *Breast cancer, diagnosis and treatment,* (I. M. Ariel, J. B. Cleary, eds), pp. 280–299. McGraw-Hill, New York, 1987.
73. K. Wallner, G. C. Li. Adriamycin resistance, heat resistance and radiation response in chinese hamster fibroblasts. *Int. J. Radiat. Oncol. Biol. Phys.,* 1986, **12**: 829–833.
74. R. R. Weichselbaum, M. A. Beckett, W. Dahlberg, A. Dritschilo. Heterogeneity of radiation response of a parent human epidermoid carcinoma cell line and four clones. *Int. J. Radiat. Oncol. Biol. Phys.,* 1988, **14**: 907–912.
75. R. R. Weichselbaum, A. Schmit, J. B. Little. Cellular repair factors influencing radiocurability of human malignant tumors. *Br. J. Cancer,* 1982, **45**: 10–16.
76. J. Weininger, M. Guichard, A. M. Joly, E. P. Malaise, B. Lachet. Radiosensitivity and growth parameters in vitro of three human melanoma cell strains. *Int. J. Radiat. Biol.,* 1978, **34**: 285–290.
77. M. V. Williams, J. Denekamp, J. F. Fowler. A review of α/β ratios for experimental tumors: implications for clinical studies of altered fractionation. *Int. J. Radiat. Oncol. Biol. Phys.,* 1985, **11**: 87–96.
78. H. R. Withers, J. M. G. Taylor, B. Maciejewski. The hazard of accelerated tumor clonogen re-population during radiotherapy. *Acta Oncologica,* 1988, **27**: 131–146.

Chapter 7.
Hypoxic cells and their importance in radiotherapy

The effect of oxygen in modifying radiation response has been recognized since the early days of radiobiology [10, 15]. However, it was in 1955 that Thomlinson and Gray [22] suggested that there were hypoxic cells in malignant tumours and that they could be an important factor in local radioresistance. Since then much work has been devoted to this problem. The principal methods used for selective attack on the hypoxic cells include hyperbaric oxygen, hypoxic cell sensitizers and neutrons and other high-LET radiations.

The discovery in 1968 of the phenomenon of tumour reoxygenation by van Putten and Kallman [24] raised doubts about the role of hypoxic cells in radiotherapy. The question arises whether fractionated treatment may not eliminate the hypoxic cells and consequently what is the place of techniques aimed at selective attack on hypoxic cells.

7.1 The oxygen effect

When a population of cells is irradiated with x or γ-rays, under either hypoxic or aerobic conditions, a large difference in radiosensitivity is seen. The *shape* of the survival curve is usually similar but the *dose* needed to reach a given level of survival is multiplied by a factor of about 3 when the cells are irradiated in the absence of oxygen (Figure 7.1). However, some authors have reported a difference in the shape of the curves and in particular a reduction in the shoulder when irradiation is performed under hypoxic conditions [13, 17].

The ratio of doses required for a given biological effect when given under hypoxic or aerobic conditions is called the OER (*oxygen enhancement ratio*). Oxygen is a powerful sensitizing agent. For a given radiation the OER is almost independent of the biological system or the effect considered: survival of mammalian cells, inactivation of bacteria or yeast, inhibition of growth in plants, etc. This is not surprising as oxygen acts on the free radicals (Chapter 2) and therefore has a similar effect whatever the irradiated system.

In all the systems which have been studied (Figure 7.2.), radiosensitivity at first increases quickly with oxygen tension and approaches a plateau when the

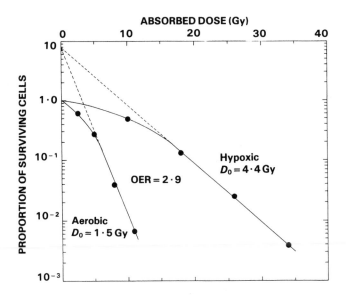

Figure 7.1. Survival curves obtained *in vitro* for mouse mammary EMT6 cells after irradiation by γ-rays under hypoxic or aerobic conditions. The *shape* of the survival curve is the same in the two cases but the *dose* needed to obtain a given surviving fraction is about three times greater under hypoxia. The OER is equal to 2·9 and does not vary with the surviving fraction; oxygen is therefore a simple 'dose modifying factor' (J. Guelette, personal communication).

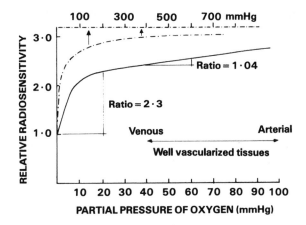

Figure 7.2. Variation of radiosensitivity as a function of the partial pressure of oxygen at the time of irradiation. Radiosensitivity increases with oxygen tension, at first rapidly and then more slowly and tends towards a plateau where it reaches a value about three times greater than that seen under anoxic conditions. At a low oxygen tension (e.g. in some malignant cells) an increase in oxygen tension produces a considerable increase in radiosensitivity. On the other hand in the plateau region (normal well-vascularized tissues) the same increase in oxygen tension has only a small effect on radiosensitivity. The upper curve (broken line) corresponds to the upper scale and the lower line (continuous) to the lower scale which is 10 times smaller. After [4].

oxygen tension exceeds 30 mmHg. The oxygen tension of most normal tissues is similar to that of venous blood or lymph (20–40 mmHg) and normal tissues can therefore be considered as well oxygenated (with a few exceptions such as cartilage).

The OER depends on the LET. For low LET radiations (X- or γ-rays or high energy electrons) the OER is found to be in the region 2·5–3, about 1·6 for fast neutrons used in therapy and close to 1 for α-particles of a few MeV (LET about 150 keV μm^{-1}). We will return to this point later (Section 11.1).

Oxygen must be present *at the time of irradiation* in order to exert its full radiosensitizing power. A small effect may still be seen if oxygen is admitted during the lifespan of the free radicals (a few microseconds) (Figure 2.4).

7.2 The hypoxic cells

The disorded proliferation of malignant cells and the lower rate of growth of blood vessels may lead to an inadequate supply of nutrients and in particular of oxygen. Thomlinson and Gray [22] demonstrated the important consequences of hypoxic cells for radiotherapy. By means of histological sections of human bronchial carcinomas, they observed necrotic zones developing within clusters of tumour cells growing within the stroma (Figure 7.3). There is no necrosis in cell clusters of less than 0·3 mm in diameter but necrosis is always present in clusters greater than 0·4 mm in diameter. In larger tumour masses the zone of central necrosis increases but the thickness of the layer of viable cells remains roughly constant (about 180 μm). Thomlinson and Gray correlated these observations with a study of the diffusing power of oxygen; in tissues with normal metabolism the oxygen tension falls progressively to zero at a distance of about 150–200 μm from the capillary, corresponding exactly to the observed thickness of the layer of viable cells.

Thus it seems that lack of oxygen is responsible for tumour necrosis. Moreover, between the apparently healthy cells close to the capillaries or stroma (some of them in mitosis) and the necrotic zone there must be a region in which the oxygen tension is at a critical level. It is here that the poorly oxygenated but still viable cells must exist (Figure 7.3)†.

Multiplication of cells around the capillaries pushes the hypoxic cells further away, into the necrotic zone. When they are irradiated the hypoxic cells are protected relative to the well-oxygenated cells. Those which have retained their

---

†Consumption of oxygen by respiration of successive layers of tumour cells causes the oxygen tension to diminish with distance from the capillaries towards the necrotic zone. At a large distance from the capillaries the oxygen tension is reduced nearly to zero and the cells are killed or condemned to death. They are no longer of importance. Before falling to zero the oxygen tension diminishes progressively, leading to increased radioresistance of the cells when the oxygen tension falls below 10 mmHg; only a small number of cells lie within this layer.

To simplify the presentation we will speak of the 'hypoxic cells' as though they form a single compartment characterized by a single value of radiosensitivity. The hypoxic cells which are important in radiotherapy are therefore those which have retained their proliferative capacity (which can be demonstrated *in vitro* and may be responsible for recurrence *in vivo*) and which exist in conditions of hypoxia such that their radiosensitivity is reduced by a factor of up to 3.

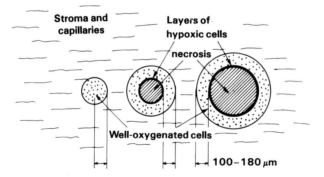

Figure 7.3. To illustrate the development of hypoxic cells in malignant tumours.
Left: initially there is a small group of malignant cells which multiply in the stroma
containing capillaries. No necrosis is seen when the diameter of the group of cells is less
than about 300 μm.
Centre: necrosis at the centre of the group of cells is always seen when its diameter
exceeds about 400 μm. There is inadequate diffusion of oxygen into the central part. *Right:*
with growth of the tumour mass the central zone of necrosis becomes larger but the
thickness of the surrounding layer of apparently viable cells remains roughly constant
(about 180 μm). It would seem therefore that the cells are able to survive and multiply only
when the distance from the stroma and the capillaries remains less than about 180 μm.
This distance corresponds to the diffusing power of oxygen in tissues. The hypoxic cells
are to be found at the interface between the layer of viable cells and the zone of necrosis
(allowing for the gradient of oxygen tension, the hypoxic cells occupy only a few layers).
After [22].

clonogenic capacity can then start to proliferate as soon as they are placed in
better conditions.

The existence of hypoxic cells has been demonstrated in most experimental
tumours (Table 7.1). The method used for determining the percentage of hypoxic
cells present in a tumour is shown schematically in Figure 7.4. Analysis of the
survival curve of the malignant cells irradiated *in vivo*, i.e. in their normal
environment, shows that there are two populations of differing sensitivity. For
example, the survival curve obtained for a lymphosarcoma irradiated *in vivo*
has a biphasic shape indicating the existence of two populations of cells of which
one has a value of D_0 three times that of the other. These can be identified with
the hypoxic and well-oxygenated compartments.

The results obtained on the existence of hypoxic cells in experimental
tumours can presumably be extrapolated to man. Moreover necrotic zones are
seen in histological sections of human tumours. Unfortunately there is little
information about the percentage of hypoxic cells in human tumours.

7.3 Tumour reoxygenation

The presence of even a small proportion of hypoxic and therefore radioresistant
cells in a malignant tumour represents an important factor in the response to
radiation, precluding any hope of sterilization at least if radiation is applied as
a single dose (Figure 7.5). With fractionated irradiation, if the compartments of
hypoxic and well-oxygenated cells behave independently (without exchange),
the hypoxic cells would remain a factor controlling radioresistance. In these

Table 7.1 Percentage of hypoxic cells in experimental tumours.

Type of tumour	Percentage of hypoxic cells
F/CBA sarcoma	>50
Lymphosarcoma of Gardner	1
Adenocarcinoma MTG-B	21
Sarcoma KHT/C3H	14
Rhabdomyosarcoma BA111/2	15
Epidermoid carcinoma D	18
Mammary carcinoma/C3H (250 mm³)	>20
(0·6 mm³)	0·2
Mammary carcinoma/C3H	7
Osteosarcoma C22LR	14
Fibrosarcoma RIB5	17
Fibrosarcoma KHT	12
Carcinoma KHJJ	19
Sarcoma EMT6	35
Mammary carcinoma/C3H (female)	1
(male)	17
Sarcoma F/CBA (*in situ*)	<10
(excised)	50
Squamous carcinoma G (intradermal)	< 1
(subcutaneous)	>46
'MT' anaplastic/WHT (*in situ*)	>80
(excised)	5
Carcinoma DC	10–30
Carcinoma RH	2–25
Carcinoma NT/CBA	7–18
Carcinoma S	< 0·01
Carcinoma S (rapid growth)	1–30
Sarcoma FA	30–70
Sarcoma BS2	5–25

After [4].

circumstances, how is it possible to explain the radiocurability of certain groups of tumours observed clinically?

Fate of the hypoxic cells after irradiation

Van Putten and Kallman [11, 24] followed the variation in the percentage of hypoxic cells in a tumour after different regimes of irradiation. With the techniques described above, these authors found a proportion of 14% of hypoxic cells in a mouse sarcoma before irradiation. After irradiation (four or five fractions of 1·9 Gy), they measured almost the same percentage of hypoxic cells as before irradiation (Table 7.2), whereas a much larger proportion was to be expected as the hypoxic cells are three times more radioresistant than the aerobic ones. This result shows that a certain number of cells which had been hypoxic subsequently became aerobic. This phenomenon of *reoxygenation* is rapid and was complete in 24 h in the experiment described. In addition Kallman and Bleehen [12], working with the same tumour, found that the proportion of hypoxic cells was only 20% when examined 6 h after a dose of 10 Gy which should have allowed only the hypoxic cells to survive.

Because of their importance in radiotherapy these studies have been repeated

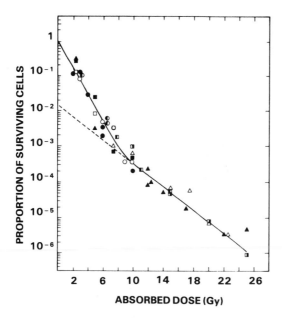

Figure 7.4. Survival curve of a population of cells from a mouse lymphosarcoma. The subcutaneous solid tumour was irradiated *in vivo*. The survival of cells was evaluated by the method of cloning *in vitro* (see Figure 4.3). The resulting survival curve (continuous line) is biphasic. The first part corresponds to survival of the well-oxygenated fraction of the population ($D_o = 1 \cdot 1$ Gy). The second part of the curve corresponds to the survival of the hypoxic fraction ($D_o = 2 \cdot 6$ Gy). By extrapolating the second part of the survival curve back to the ordinate axis (dotted line) the fraction of hypoxic cells is obtained. This technique makes it possible to determine the proportion of hypoxic cells in different conditions and in particular at different times after irradiation.
After [16].

with different tumours (Figure 7.6). Large variations of both the importance and the time course of reoxygenation have been seen from one tumour to another. For some tumours (those with a rapid growth rate?) fractionation alone succeeded in overcoming the handicap represented by the presence of hypoxic cells. For others (e.g. the osteosarcoma studied by Kallman [11] and van Putten and Kallman [24]), reoxygenation would be too slow and, during daily fractionated irradiation, the fraction of hypoxic cells would become steadily greater, precluding any hope of local sterilization of the tumour by X-rays or γ-rays. In 1967 Thomlinson [19] proposed a model of the variation of the percentage of hypoxic cells in an irradiated tumour (Figure 7.7).

Extrapolation of these findings to clinical radiotherapy is hazardous as transplanted experimental tumours are often poor models of spontaneous human tumours. It is, however, likely that tumour reoxygenation also has an important role in explaining the success of radiotherapy of human tumours. Nevertheless, the studies with hyperbaric oxygen and hypoxic cell radiosensitizers suggest that reoxygenation does not completely eliminate the hypoxic cells in every clinical situation. This justifies the efforts made to attack selectively the hypoxic cells.

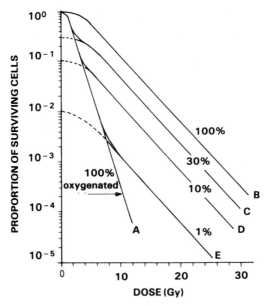

Figure 7.5. Diagram to illustrate the role of even a small proportion of hypoxic cells in the radioresistance of a tumour to *a single dose of radiation*. A: survival curve of a population of well-oxygenated cells. B: survival curve of this population under hypoxic conditions (taking OER=3). The biphasic curves C, D, E correspond to populations containing respectively, 30, 10 and 1% of hypoxic cells. The hypoxic cells give survival curves parallel to B, but leaving the origin at values of $0\cdot3, 0\cdot1$ and $0\cdot01$ respectively; the well-oxygenated cells behave in the same way as curve A. With low doses the response of a mixed population is determined by the well-oxygenated cells. Beyond the points of inflection of the biphasic curves (about 3, 4 and 8 Gy for the three cases considered) the hypoxic cells become determinant.

Normal tissues which are well oxygenated behave in the same way as curve A. If the dose per fraction is increased beyond the point of inflection of a biphasic curve the normal cells are killed preferentially. This dose therefore represents the absolute limit of the dose per fraction which one should deliver. These doses are much lower than those required to reduce the surviving fraction to a small enough level for tumour sterilization. The same situation appertains with fractionated irradiation if reoxygenation does not take place.
After [24].

The mechanisms of reoxygenation

The mechanisms of tumour reoxygenation are poorly understood. During fractionated irradiation extended over several weeks, to some extent 'the tumour returns along its natural history' and the mechanisms which led to the appearance of hypoxic cells are reversed. Thus the tumour regression seen after a few weeks of treatment leads to improved blood perfusion of the residual tumour, once the killed cells and cellular debris have been eliminated. Also reduction of tumour volume relieves tissue compression and so improves blood flow [21]. However, disintegration and lysis of the 'killed' cells (in the sense of 'reproductive death', Section 4.1) does not occur until the following mitosis. This suggests that, in general, reoxygenation will be faster in tumours with intense proliferation and slower in more slowly growing tumours.

Tumour regression requires at least several days and cannot explain the rapid reoxygenation seen in some animal tumours. Also, for continuous irradiation at low dose rate extended over several days, reoxygenation cannot be explained by tumour regression during treatment. As the effectiveness of brachytherapy requires the elimination of hypoxic cells (whatever may be the mechanism) there must be some rapid reoxygenation.

One possible mechanism is migration of the hypoxic cells towards the well-oxygenated zones. In the representation of Figure 7.3, where the hypoxic cells are localized in a thin layer, a movement over a distance of a few cell diameters would be enough to reoxygenate a hypoxic cell. Another hypothesis explains the presence of hypoxic cells and reoxygenation by local perturbations in the disorganized blood supply of the tumour, leading to fluctuating acute hypoxia. It is also possible that the cells surrounding the capillaries consume less oxygen after irradiation, increasing the quantity of oxygen available and thereby improving the transport of oxygen to the zone of hypoxic cells.

Table 7.2 Variation in the percentage of hypoxic cells after irradiation of a mouse sarcoma.

Radiation schedule	Interval of time after the last fraction (h)	Percentage of hypoxic cells
Controls	—	15
1 fraction of 10 Gy	1	32
	6	20
	12	20
5 fractions of 1·9 Gy (24-h intervals)	72	18
4 fractions of 1·9 Gy (24-h intervals)	24	14

After [12, 24].

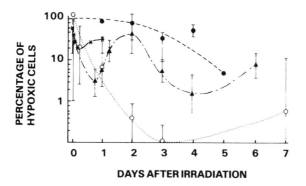

DAYS AFTER IRRADIATION

Figure 7.6. Variation in the percentage of hypoxic cells in several tumours as a function of the time after irradiation:
○, in a mouse mammary carcinoma, reoxygenation is rapid and complete: 3 days after irradiation the percentage of hypoxic cells is lower than that seen before irradiation;
*, for a transplantable mouse sarcoma, reoxygenation is not complete by 24 h;
▲, for rat fibrosarcoma RIB5 there is at first a rapid reoxygenation. However, the proportion of hypoxic cells increases again at 2 days and then falls to about 5% at 3 and 4 days;
●, for a mouse osteogenic sarcoma reoxygenation is very slow. Comparison of the different curves shows that the time course and extent of reoxygenation varies over a wide range from one tumour to another.
After [20].

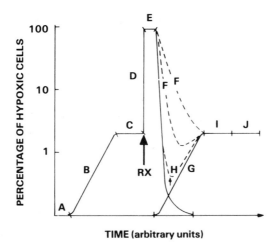

TIME (arbitrary units)

Figure 7.7. Model illustrating the variation in the percentage of hypoxic cells in a tumour. The percentage of hypoxic cells is shown as a function of time; there is no scale on the abscissa as the diagram is only schematic.

A. At the beginning, the tumour consists of only a small number of cells and none are hypoxic (Figure 7.3).

B. The hypoxic cells appear as soon as the tumour volume exceeds a certain size.

C. The percentage of hypoxic cells is assumed to reach a plateau which depends on the nature of the tumour and its localization, etc. The level of this plateau is variable (e.g. see Table 7.1 for experimental tumours in animals).

D. After irradiation the percentage of hypoxic cells increases almost instantaneously because of their greater radioresistance in comparison with that of the well-oxygenated cells. It rises to a value which is dose dependent reaching almost 100% after a large dose (e.g. 10 Gy).

E. The percentage of hypoxic cells remains constant for a certain time (blockage of progression through the mitotic cycle, see Section 5.1).

F. For the reasons discussed (earlier in this chapter) the percentage of hypoxic cells diminishes.

G. The surviving cells begin to multiply again leading (as in B) to the formation of hypoxic cells.

H. The percentage of hypoxic cells passes through a minimum. The value of this minimum and the time at which it occurs vary with the type of tumour. This minimum may or may not be lower than the percentage of hypoxic cells before irradiation. This represents the best moment at which to deliver the following fraction.

I. The proportion of hypoxic cells returns to the pre-irradiation level.

After [19].

Tumour reoxygenation and radiotherapy

In the absence of further experimental information, the consequences of tumour reoxygenation can only be evaluated theoretically. We will consider the two extreme hypotheses (Figure 7.8):

1. Tumour reoxygenation does not take place: the compartment of hypoxic cells must be considered independently.
2. Before each dose fraction, reoxygenation returns the percentage of hypoxic cells to the level existing before the previous fraction.

In the first case the hypoxic cells become the determining factor after a few fractions and sterilization of the tumour is unlikely. In the second case the proportion of hypoxic cells does not increase and they always represent a small fraction of the malignant population; they have little effect on the results of treatment.

In practice it is likely that there are large variations of reoxygenation in human tumours. Reoxygenation *certainly* occurs in curable tumours; it *may occur to some extent* in radioresistant tumours. Finally, if the degree of reoxygenation depends on the nature of the tumour, it equally depends on the fractionation and total time of treatment. It is therefore important not to abandon, without good reason, fractionation schedules which have been proved to have clinical value.

7.4 *Methods of selectively attacking the hypoxic cells*

Given the uncertainty surrounding the role of hypoxic cells in radiotherapy, it seems logical to try methods aimed at attacking them selectively.

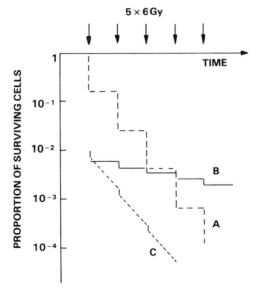

Figure 7.8. **Practical consequences of tumour reoxygenation in fractionated radiotherapy. The surviving fraction of the well-oxygenated malignant cells (99%, curve A, large dashes) and of the hypoxic cells (1%) have been calculated as a function of time. Curve B (solid line) indicates the survival of the hypoxic cells *in the complete absence of reoxygenation;***
curve C (small dashes) shows the result when reoxygenation returns the proportion of hypoxic cells to the *level existing before the previous dose fraction.* In the first case (B) the hypoxic cells quickly become the determining factor and compromise the radiocurability of the tumour. In the second case (C), the hypoxic cells remain a small proportion of the viable population of the tumour. The oblique segments (curve C) represent the passage of surviving hypoxic cells into the oxygenated compartment. The calculations were made for a fractionated irradiation consisting of five sessions of 6 Gy each. After each session the surviving fraction of the oxygenated component is taken as 15% and of the hypoxic component as 70%.
After [8].

Hyperbaric oxygen (HBO)

The first method to be used consists of administering oxygen under several atmospheres, with the patient in a high pressure tank, in order to saturate the blood plasma and thereby to extend the limits of the oxygenated zone around the capillaries to include the hypoxic cells [3]. Because of the high gradient of oxygen tension around the capillaries it is necessary to increase the oxygen tension in the capillaries by 40–60 mmHg in order to increase by 45–80 μm the radius in which the oxygen tension will be, for example, greater than 12 mmHg. Oxygen pressures of 3 atm. have been used, the maximum which the patient can tolerate without anaesthetic.

Use of hyperbaric oxygen is beset by many difficulties. To begin with, it is not certain whether the oxygen dissolved at high pressure in the plasma really reaches the hypoxic tumour cells (Figure 7.9). Secondly, although most normal tissues are well oxygenated and consequently not affected by an increase in oxygen tension (Figure 7.2), it is possible that some, particularly cartilage, could be sensitized by hyperbaric oxygen. Finally, the method involves several practical problems: convulsions due to oxygen, complications in the lungs and ears due to the high pressure, claustrophobia, danger of fire and explosion, difficulties of beam alignment when the patient is exposed in the oxygen tank, and the need in certain cases for a general anaesthetic. It has been shown that one can obtain the same effectiveness but with less risk by using a mixture of 95% O_2 plus 5% CO_2 at 1 atm (carbogen). The CO_2 acts as a vasodilator.

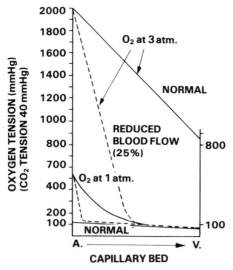

Figure 7.9. Diagram to illustrate the variation in oxygen tension along the capillaries under different conditions:
(i) The patient breathes air at normal pressures;
(ii) The patient breathes oxygen at 1 or 3 atm;
(iii) As (ii) but with a 25% reduction in blood flow (broken lines). A moderate reduction in blood flow to a large extent abolishes the advantage of hyperbaric oxygen. In this respect it is known that vascular perfusion of malignant tumours is often poor (insufficient vascular development, stasis, compression), and that an increase in oxygen tension may lead to vasoconstriction.
After [6].

Table 7.3 Hyperbaric oxygen in the treatment of stage III cancer of the uterine cervix (therapeutic trial of the Medical Research Council).

Centre	Number of patients	Number of fractions	Oxygen (%)	Air (%)
			5 year survival	
Portsmouth	37	6	42	17
Oxford	23	10	46	8
Glasgow	127	20	50	37
Mount Vernon	56	27	39	28
			Local control at 5 years	
Glasgow			87	60
Mount Vernon			76	50
			Serious intestinal complications	
			12	4

After [25].

Although the use of hyperbaric oxygen has been abandoned, it is essential to assess the clinical results obtained in order to clarify the role played by hypoxic cells in radiotherapy.

Two therapeutic trials of the effect of hyperbaric oxygen have been performed at Cardiff on tumours of the head and neck. In the first trial the total doses were 35–45 Gy given in 10 fractions over 3 weeks, i.e. with doses per fraction of 3·5–4·5 Gy. We have seen earlier in this chapter that a beneficial effect of oxygen is to be expected with large doses per fraction; in fact, in this trial a significant improvement was seen in the rate of local control, with a small increase in the number of complications. In the second trial [9], the patients treated in air were given a more conventional regime of 64 Gy in 30 fractions over 6 weeks, or 2·1 Gy per fraction. Treatment in hyperbaric oxygen still gave better results than treatment in air, with few complications on either side (four in HBO and two in air). Local control at 5 years improved from 40 to 60% and survival from 30 to 56% ($P<0·02$). Nearly all the improvement occurred in patients with T2 and T3 tumours and there was little effect in T4 patients. Thus the second trial demonstrates that tumour reoxygenation under air-breathing conditions is not complete even with 30 fractions.

The results of another randomized trial organized by the Medical Research Council in Great Britain using hyperbaric oxygen in the treatment of cancer of the uterine cervix (stage III) are also instructive (Table 7.3). For the two centres which used daily fractionation (Glasgow and Mount Vernon) there was a highly significant improvement in the rate of local control, together with an increase in the fraction of survivors at 5 years (at the limit of statistical significance). On the other hand, in the centres which used only a small number of fractions (6–10 fractions), the better results seen in the group treated under hyperbaric oxygen were due essentially to the poor quality of the results in the group who were treated in air (the importance of fractionation has been discussed in Chapter 6).

The results of about 15 therapeutic studies with hyperbaric oxygen, particularly those obtained using daily fractionation, show that for certain categories of tumour the hypoxic cells do play a role in radiotherapy, even if this role is modest and is not always easy to demonstrate. Moreover these results confirm clinical observations indicating that anaemic patients respond less well to radiotherapy and that their response can be improved after transfusion for correcting the anaemia [7, 2]. We will return to this point at the end of this section.

Another way of supplying more oxygen to the tumour consists of injecting oxygen carriers into the blood circulation. Perfluorochemicals are of particular interest since they are known to absorb large amounts of oxygen and to release it quickly in tissue, particularly in a low pH environment. They can absorb more than 40% of their volume of oxygen whereas plasma will dissolve only 2%. A dose of 15 mg kg^{-1} is well tolerated. To achieve a significant increase in the oxygen blood concentration (normally 20% in volume) the subject must breathe an enriched atmosphere, usually carbogen (95% O_2 + 5% CO_2). A therapeutic gain has been demonstrated in animal tumours [18].

Tourniquet hypoxia

Instead of increasing the radiosensitivity of the hypoxic tumour cells to the level of the well-oxygenated cells, one might reduce the radiosensitivity of the well-oxygenated cells of normal tissues to the level of the hypoxic tumour cells. For tumours in a limb this can be done by placing a tourniquet above the tumour. This technique has been tried in the clinic, particularly for osteosarcomas of the limbs [23]. To obtain the same reaction in normal tissue it was confirmed that the dose had to be increased by a factor of about 3 (the value of the OER).

Hypoxic cell sensitizers

Certain drugs selectively increase the radiosensitivity of hypoxic cells and reduce or even abolish the difference in radiosensitivity between oxygenated and hypoxic cells. The drugs available today are toxic at the doses required (see Chapter 10), which limits their effectiveness.

High-LET radiation

The therapeutic value of neutrons and other high-LET particles is due to their OER being lower than that of X- or γ-rays; the potential therapeutic gain is equal to the ratio of the OER values.

However, the differences in the biological effects of high- and low-LET radiation are not limited to the OER. Intracellular repair and variations in radiosensitivity around the cell cycle are less important with high-LET radiation. We will return to this question in Chapter 11.

Haemoglobin level

Finally it is useful to recall some clinical observations showing the importance of the haemoglobin level. Anaemic patients respond less well to radiotherapy and they are usually transfused before treatment. However, even when the haemoglobin level remains within normal limits, it may still influence the

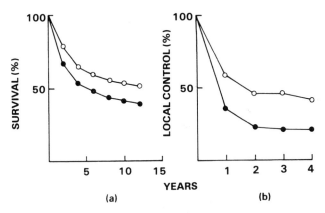

Figure 7.10. Influence of haemoglobin level on response to radiotherapy. (a) Actuarial survival curves for patients suffering from cancer of the uterine cervix (stages II B and III) and presenting with a haemoglobin level above (o) or below (•) 12 g% during treatment [2] (b) Local control at 4 years for male patients suffering from extensive cancer of the hypopharynx and presenting with a haemoglobin level above (o) or below (•) 14·5 g% [14].

response to treatment [1]. Bush *et al.* [2] followed the fate of patients treated by radiotherapy for cancer of the uterine cervix (stage II B or III): survival was significantly better in the group presenting with a haemoglobin level > 12 g% (Figure 7.10a).

The Medical Research Council's study on the effect of hyperbaric oxygen in patients with locally advanced tumours of the uterine cervix were discussed above (Table 7.3). Thirty eight of these patients presented with severe anaemia (<10 g% Hb) and needed transfusion before treatment, 15 were randomized to hyperbaric oxygen and over 90% of them achieved local tumour control, whereas of the 23 randomized to treatment in air only 20% were locally controlled. Moreover, the patients who were transfused and treated under hyperbaric oxygen responded better than those, also treated under hyperbaric oxygen, who did not need transfusion [5].

The study of Overgaard *et al.* [14] on advanced tumours of the pharynx showed that local control without recurrence was longer in the patients whose haemoglobin level was greater than 14·5 g%. In addition, while misonidazole gave a general improvement in response, the benefit was particularly marked in the patients whose haemoglobin level was above normal.

These results, together with others, confirm the importance of hypoxic cells in the response to radiotherapy and suggest that it is possible to improve results by increasing the haemoglobin level.

References

1. G. E. Adams, I. J. Stratford, I. Ahmed, P. W. Sheldon. Some new developments in tumour radiosensitization. *Third international meeting on progress in radio-oncology*, Ed. K. H. Karcher. ICRO (Vienna) 1987 pp. 81–88.
2. R. S. Bush, R. D. T. Jenkin, W. E. C. Allt, F. A. Beale, H. Bean, A. J. Dembo, J. F. Pringle. Definitive evidence for hypoxic cells influencing cure in cancer therapy. *Br. J. Cancer*, 1978, **37**, Suppl. III: 302–306.

3. I. Churchill-Davidson, C. A. Foster, G. Wiernik, C. D. Collins, N. C. D. Pizey. D. B. L. Skeggs, P. R. Purser, The place of oxygen in radiotherapy. *Br. J Radiol.*, 1966, **39**: 321–331.
4. J. Denekamp. Does physiological hypoxia matter in cancer therapy? in: *The biological basis of radiotherapy* (G. C. Steel, G. E. Adams, M. J. Peckham, eds.), pp. 139–155. Elsevier, Amsterdam, 1983.
5. S. Dische, P. J. Anderson, R. Sealy, E. R. Watson. Carcinoma of the cervix, anaemia, radiotherapy and hyperbaric oxygen. *Br. J. Radiol.*, 1983, **56**: 251–255.
6. W. Duncan A. H. W. Nias. *Clinical radiobiology*. Churchill Livingstone, Edinburgh, 1977.
7. J. C. Evans, P. Bergsjo. The influence of anemia on the results of radiotherapy in carcinoma of the cervix. *Radiology*, 1965, **84**: 709–717.
8. J. F. Fowler. La Ronde — radiation sciences and medical radiology (The second Klaas Breur memorial lecture). *Radiother. Oncol.*, 1983, **1**: 1–22.
9. J. M. Henk. Late results of a trial of hyperbaric oxygen and radiotherapy in head and neck cancer: a rationale for hypoxic cell sensitizers? *Int. J. Radiat. Oncol. Biol. Phys.*, 1986, **12**: 1339–1341.
10. H. Holthusen. Beitrage zur Biologie der Strahlenwirkung. *Pflüger's Arch. Ges. Physiol.*, 1921, **187**: 1–24.
11. R. F. Kallman. The phenomenon of reoxygenation and its implications for fractionated radiotherapy. *Radiology*, 1972, **105**: 135–142.
12. R. F. Kallman, N. M. Bleehen. Post-irradiation cyclic radiosensitivity changes in tumours and normal tissues. *Proceedings of the symposium on dose rate in mammalian radiobiology*. Oak Ridge, Tenn., 1968. (D. G. Brown et al., eds.), pp. 20.1–20.23. Springfield, Va: CONF-680410, CFSTI, 1968.
13. B. Littbrand, L. Revesz. The effect of oxygen on cellular survival and recovery after irradiation. *Br. J. Radiol.*, 1969, **42**: 914–924.
14. J. Overgaard, S. H. Hansen. A. P. Anderson, M. Hjelm-Handsen, K. Jorgensen, K. Sandberg, J. Rygard, R. H. Jensen, M. Peterson, Misonidazole as an adjuvant to radiotherapy in the treatment of invasive carcinoma of the larynx and the pharynx. *Third international meeting on progress in radio-oncology*, Ed. K. H. Karcher. ICRO (Vienna) 1987 pp. 137–147.
15. E. Petry, Zur Kenntnis der Bedingungen der biologischen Wirkung der Röntgenstrahlen. *Biochem. Zeitschr.*, 1923, **135**: 353–383.
16. W. E. Powers, L. J. Tolmach. A multicomponent X ray survival curve for mouse lymphosarcoma cells irradiated *in vivo*. *Nature*, 1963, **197**: 710–711.
17. L. Revesz. B. Littbrand. Variation of the relative sensitivity of closely related neoplastic cell lines irradiated in culture in the presence or absence of oxygen. *Nature*, 1964, **203**: 742–744.
18. S. Rockwell. Use of perfluorochemical emulsion to improve oxygenation in a solid tumour. *Int. J. Radiat. Oncol. Biol. Phys.*, 1985, **11**: 97–103.
19. R. H. Thomlinson. Oxygen therapy — Biological considerations, in: *Modern trends in radiotherapy* (T. J. Deeley, C. A. P. Wood, eds.), vol. 1, pp. 52–72. Butterworths Scientific Publications, London, 1967.
20. R. H. Thomlinson. Time and dose relationships in radiation biology as applied to radiotherapy. In *Proceedings of N.C.I.-A.E.C. conference*, Carmel, California U.S.A.E.C. Catalogue n° BNL-50203 (C57). Springfield, Va: U.S. Dept. of Commerce, 1969.
21. R. H. Thomlinson. Hypoxia and tumours. *J. Clin. Path.*, 1977, **30**, Suppl. (Roy. Coll. Path.), *11*: 105–113.
22. R. H. Thomlinson, L. H. Gray. The histological structure of some human lung cancers and the possible implications for radiotherapy. *Br. J. Cancer*, 1955, **9**: 539–549.
23. H. A. S. van den Brenk. The oxygen effect in radiation therapy. *Curr. Top. Radiat. Res.*, 1969, **5**: 197–254.
24. L. M. van Putten, R. F. Kallman. Oxygenation status of a transplantable tumour during fractionated radiation therapy. *J. Natl. Cancer Inst.*, 1968, **40**: 441–451.
25. E. R. Watson, K. E. Halnan, S. Dische, M. I. Saunders, I. S. Cade, J. B. McEwen, G. Wiernik, D. J. D. Perrins, I. Sutherland. Hyperbaric oxygen and radiotherapy: a Medical Research Council trial in carcinoma of the cervix. *Br. J. Radiol..*, 1978, **51**: 879–887.

Chapter 8.

Time and fractionation in radiotherapy

Treatment with radiation can be given in various ways as a function of time. In external beam therapy the dose is usually given in daily fractions extending over several weeks. The number of sessions and the dose per session define the *fractionation* and the time interval between the first and last session defines the *overall time*. Very occasionally (e.g. in contact therapy) the treatment is given in a single session lasting a few minutes. In brachytherapy (curietherapy) the radiation is usually given continuously over a period of a few days.

The biological effect depends on the distribution of dose as a function of time and fractionation. It is reduced when the number of fractions or the overall time are increased; consequently the dose needed to obtain a given effect (the *isoeffect dose*) must be increased.

The importance of these factors depends on the tissue and the effect considered. Consequently, when two tissues are exposed to the same irradiation, the fractionation and overall time may lead to a differential effect, i.e. a modification in the response of one tissue relative to the other.

This differential effect is of the utmost importance in radiotherapy as the choice of fractionation and overall time makes it possible to reduce the consequences of irradiation on normal tissues. Optimization of the fractionation and time is the objective of many ongoing studies.

8.1. Standard fractionation and its variations in practice

Treatment with radiation was first given in the early years of the present century using a single, or at most a few, treatment sessions. The aim was to deliver a dose which could be tolerated by the normal tissues (in practice, the skin) in as short a time as could be achieved with the apparatus available. With the exception of moderately sized skin tumours the therapeutic results were poor.

Later clinical experience has shown (Chapter 6) that when the treatment is given in 20 or 30 fractions extended over a period of 4–6 weeks, the effect on the tumour can be greatly increased without exceeding the tolerance of normal tissues. Nowadays radiobiological knowledge makes it possible to interpret the role of fractionation and overall time on biological effects and to understand the mechanisms of a differential effect between two tissues.

Division of the dose into many *fractions* allows partial repair of the damage inflicted at each fraction and leads to relative protection of the cells which are able to accumulate and repair the damage effectively (Figure 8.2). Extension of the *overall time* of the treatment allows the surviving cells to multiply and favours the tissues in which proliferation is most rapid.

In addition to cellular repair and repopulation, fractionation and extension in time allow reoxygenation of hypoxic cells to take place (Section 7.3) and lead to changes in the distribution of cells in the cell cycle, both of which influence the final biological effect.

All these mechanisms also play a role in *irradiation at low dose rate* as in brachytherapy, and in irradiations extending over a very long period of time which have to be considered in radiation protection.

Radiotherapy is usually given in a standard schedule (conventionally 5 fractions of 2 Gy per week) up to a total dose which is determined by clinical experience, depending on the histology of the tumour and on the site and extent of the target volume. However, there are several circumstances in which it is necessary to consider the effects of fractionation and overall time.

1. The treatment regime used may differ from one centre to another or depending on the type of tumour. Thus it may be necessary to compare two treatments with different irradiation parameters whose relative biological effects are not immediately obvious (e.g. $30 \times 2\,Gy = 60\,Gy$ in 6 weeks and $15 \times 3\,Gy = 45\,Gy$ in 4 weeks).
2. One may wish for various reasons to modify the standard treatment regime, e.g. to accelerate or slow down the treatment or because the treatment has been temporarily interrupted. It is then necessary to correct the total dose originally prescribed in order to take account of this modification.
3. Finally, one may wish to improve certain therapeutic results by using different values of fractionation or total time which one hopes will be more effective against the tumour. The total dose must then be adjusted in order not to exceed the tolerance of the normal tissues.

For all these problems it is necessary to establish the relation between the isoeffect dose and the two parameters, fractionation and time. In spite of many clinical studies, the formulae which have been proposed to represent this relation are still uncertain and valid only within certain limits.

8.2. *Effects of fractionation and time: historical development*

Relation between isoeffect dose and treatment regime

The systematic study of clinical data presented by Strandqvist in 1944 [54] is a historic reference. His aim was to establish the relation between the isoeffect dose and the time factor, both for acute reactions of skin and for cure of epitheliomas. This study was concerned only with treatment given at the rate of 5 fractions per week; the two factors, the number of fractions (N) and the time (t) in days, are then connected by $N = 5t/7$ and the study leads to a single parameter.

The method used by Strandqvist, which has been taken up again in many similar studies, is as follows. On a diagram whose coordinates represent the total dose (D) and the duration of treatment (t), each clinical case is represented by a point. For a given effect, e.g. desquamation of the skin, the clinical cases are separated into those in which the effect occurs and those in which it does not and the best line is drawn to separate the two groups of points: in this way the isoeffect curve is obtained for the biological effect considered. The results analyzed by Strandqvist are shown in Figure 8.1a. Within the range of values of t (or N) considered, the isoeffect curves on log–log coordinates are compatible (within the modest precision of the available data) with straight lines corresponding to the relation $D=k\times t^n$. Their slope n (equal to $0\cdot22$) is the same for all the effects studied (various degrees of skin reaction and cure of epithelioma); there appears to be no differential effect. These results suggest that whatever the prolongation of treatment, the dose corresponding to cure of the tumour is greater than the dose causing moist desquamation and lower than the dose resulting in skin necrosis.

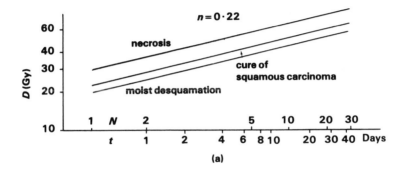

(a)

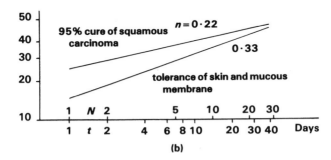

(b)

Figure 8.1. Isoeffect dose as a function of the duration of treatment. The curves were established for irradiations given as 5 fractions per week. The number of fractions (N) and total time (t) are therefore connected $(N=5t/7)$. The curves correspond to the expression $D=kt^n$, and on logarithmic coordinates are straight lines of slope n.
(a) Curves of Strandqvist [54]: for the effects indicated the slope n of the curves is the same $(0\cdot22)$.
(b) Curves of Cohen [7]: the slope is greater for skin or mucosal 'tolerance' $(n=0\cdot33)$ than for 95% cure of squamous carcinoma $(n=0\cdot22)$. There is a differential effect between the two end points which depends on the total time of treatment.

Demonstration of a differential effect

In 1960 the same type of study was undertaken by Cohen [7] based on a large number of published results. For the treatment of squamous epitheliomas with 5 fractions per week for various times, the isoeffect curves are sufficiently precise to show that the slope for skin tolerance ($n=0\cdot33$) is greater than that for cure of 95% of the tumours ($n=0\cdot22$). The dose needed for cure of the tumour is equal to the tolerance dose when the treatment is given in 30 fractions over 6 weeks; for shorter treatments, cure requires a dose greater than tolerance. The study of Cohen brought to light a differential effect connected with the treatment time but did not distinguish the separate roles of fractionation and total time.

Separation of the parameters fractionation and time

In 1967 Ellis [20, 21] proposed a formula whose aim was to allow corrections to be made easily in clinical practice. His work was based on the data of Cohen and he aimed to separate the roles of the number (N) of fractions and the total time (t) which govern the isoeffect dose. He expressed the isoeffect dose for normal tissues by the relation known as the NSD formula (nominal standard dose):

$$D=(\text{NSD})\times N^{0\cdot24}t^{0\cdot11}$$

The NSD formula does not claim to represent a biological law; Ellis presented it as a method for practical calculation and indicated in particular that the formula could not be applied when the number of fractions N is lower than 4. The NSD does not represent the equivalent dose for a single fraction ($N=1, t=1$). To emphasize the arbitrary character of this quantity, Ellis proposed to give it a particular unit, the *ret*, corresponding to a rad (cGy) as the unit of dose.

The reasoning which led to the NSD concept is based on hypotheses whose validity is debatable. Moreover, the practical use of this formula has been disputed. We will discuss its limitations in the following paragraphs.

The Ellis formula rests on two principal hypotheses:

1. *For the tumour the time factor is negligible* (i.e. there is little cell proliferation during treatment). The increase in isoeffect dose with increasing duration of treatment is due to *fractionation*. The isoeffect dose given by the expression $D=kt^{0\cdot22}$ on Cohen's graph should more logically be expressed with the factor $N=(5t/7)$, i.e. $D=k(7N/5)^{0\cdot22}$. For the usual values of N this can be represented as $D=kN^{0\cdot24}$ (isoeffect dose for tumour).

2. *For skin and mucosa N has the same value as for epithelioma.* This implies that the corresponding cell survival curve has the same form and that there is no differential effect between tumour and normal tissue connected with the *fractionation*.

   The difference in slopes of the isoeffect doses for the two effects (that is $0\cdot33-0\cdot22=0\cdot11$) is therefore attributed to cell proliferation taking place in normal tissue. This gives the *time factor* $t^{0\cdot11}$ where t is measured in days.

Ellis emphasized that the NSD formula can be applied only to irradiations corresponding to the *tolerance of normal tissues*. For the usual target volumes this corresponds to an NSD close to 1800 ret, a value which can vary a little with the size of the field and the personal feeling of the radiotherapist as to what reaction is 'tolerable'.

Ellis expected that the NSD formula would apply to *late reactions* in all normal tissues, on the hypothesis that these reactions result from damage to the same cells (fibroblasts or capillary endothelium) in all types of tissue. In fact the clinical data on which the formula was based relate mainly to early reactions. Radiobiological experiments (Section 8.3) and clinical experience [2, 24, 25, 41] have shown that late reactions are more severe for a small number of fractions than is indicated by the NSD formula. In the next section we will discuss the differences which have now been established between the effects of fractionation on early and late reactions in normal tissues.

Other formulae have been derived to facilitate the use of NSD, particularly for irradiations whose regime is changed during treatment: *Time Dose Factor* (TDF) [44], *Cumulative Radiation Effect* (CRE) [40]. The criticisms of the fundamental bases and the numerical coefficients of NSD apply equally to these formulae.

Recent radiobiological data enable a rational analysis to be made of the relation between the isoeffect dose and the number of fractions and overall time and make it possible to assess the empirical formulae given above which were established from clinical data.

8.3. *Experimental data and radiobiological interpretation of the differential effects of fractionation*

We have seen in Chapter 4 that the survival curve of a homogeneous population of cells makes it possible to determine the proportion of survivors after a fractionated irradiation given in N fractions of dose d and to establish the variation as a function of N or d of the isoeffect dose ($D=Nd$) which leads to a given survival S.

The isoeffect dose increases as the dose per fraction is reduced and tends towards a maximum value when d is so small that the survival curve cannot be distinguished from its initial tangent. The increase in isoeffect dose depends on the shape of the survival curve; *fractionation produces a differential effect* between two cell populations when their survival curves have *different shoulders* (Figure 8.2). Reduction in the dose per fraction confers relative protection on the population for which there is a greater increase in isoeffect dose. The isoeffect dose increases more rapidly when the shoulder on the survival curve is more marked — i.e. when it has a greater curvature — and when the slope of the initial tangent is smaller.

In the *linear–quadratic model* (Section 4.3), the surviving fraction after a single dose D is given by the relation

$$s=e^{-(\alpha D+\beta D^2)}$$

The coefficient α indicates the initial slope of the survival curve and the coefficient β characterizes its curvature. The increase in isoeffect dose when the dose per fraction is reduced depends on the ratio α/β. It is greater when this ratio

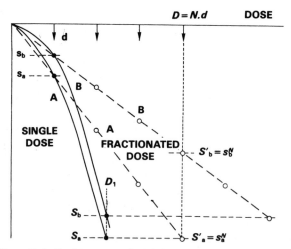

Figure 8.2. Differential effect connected with fractionation. The figure represents the survival curves of two cell lines, A and B. The surviving fractions are S_a and S_b for a single dose D_1 and s_a and s_b for a dose d (per fraction). N fractions of dose d lead to a surviving fraction for population A

$$S'_a = S_a \text{ for } D = Nd$$

i.e. $D = Nd$ is an isoeffect dose equivalent to the single dose D_1. For the population B, the surviving fraction $S'_b > S_b$ and the isoeffect dose equivalent to D_1 is greater than $N.d$. Fractionation gives a greater degree of protection to the population B than to A. A small difference between the survival curves is amplified by fractionation, since

$$S'_b/S'_a = (s_b/s_a)^N$$

For example, if for $d = 2$ Gy, $s_a = 0.4$ and $s_b = 0.5$, for $N = 30$ fractions

$$S'_b/S'_a = 800$$

is smaller, i.e. when the curvature of the survival curve is more marked. The surviving fraction s for a dose per fraction d is given by

$$-\log s = \alpha d + \beta d^2$$

and for N fractions the final surviving fraction is (Section 4.5)

$$S = s^N \text{ or}$$
$$-\log S = -N \log s = N(\alpha d + \beta d^2)$$
$$= Nd\,(\alpha + \beta d)$$

where Nd represents the total dose D.
The same surviving fraction S can be obtained with N' fractions of dose d'

$$-\log S = N'd'\,(\alpha + \beta d')$$

and the ratio of isoeffect doses is given by

$$\frac{N'd'}{Nd} = \frac{\frac{\alpha}{\beta} + d}{\frac{\alpha}{\beta} + d'}$$

For given values of d and d' this ratio depends only on α/β: e.g. if the dose per fraction is changed from $d=2$ Gy to $d'=5$ Gy, the isoeffect dose is reduced to 80% if $\alpha/\beta=10$ Gy and to 57% if $\alpha/\beta=2$ Gy.

Values of the ratio α/β have been determined from *in vitro* survival curves (Section 4.4) and for several tissues *in vivo*. They show considerable variation, which explains why the effect of fractionation varies from tissue to tissue (Chapter 5).

Cell survival curves cannot as a rule be determined for normal tissues or human tumours. However, it is not essential to know the shape of the cell survival curve in order to evaluate the isoeffect dose. It can be determined for any observable effect, such as animal lethality or functional alteration of an organ, skin reaction, tumour sterilization etc., by assessing the doses needed to produce a given effect by two regimes of irradiation using different numbers of fractions. The effect of total time can be eliminated by comparing two irradiations given over the same time, on the assumption that cell proliferation is the same and that the difference between the isoeffect doses is due only to the difference in fractionation (Section 4.5).

For example, 50% mortality has been seen in mice given abdominal irradiation over a period of 10 days with 10 fractions of $3 \cdot 3$ Gy or 20 fractions of $1 \cdot 8$ Gy. This equivalence: $10 \times 3 \cdot 3$ Gy $= 20 \times 1 \cdot 8$ Gy is correct whatever the total time. If the time is increased (e.g. 20 days instead of 10) the biological effect is reduced (mortality 25%) because of cellular repopulation, but in the same way for each fractionation regime. To obtain 50% mortality with treatment over 20 days, experiments have shown that the number of fractions must be increased in the same proportion, $12 \times 3 \cdot 3$ Gy $= 24 \times 1 \cdot 8$ Gy.

This experimental study establishes the ratio of isoeffect doses for $3 \cdot 3$ and $1 \cdot 8$ Gy per fraction. By repeating with different doses per fraction one can construct the isoeffect curve relating to fractionation alone, independent of cellular proliferation (Section 4.5).

When the dose per fraction is reduced from d to d', the isoeffect dose increases from $D(=Nd)$ to D' $(=N'd')$ and the relative increase D'/D has a single value independent of the number of fractions, i.e. of the level of effect considered. On the other hand, an increase in the number of fractions from N to N' has a different consequence on the isoeffect dose, depending on whether the doses per fraction are small or large (Table 8.1). It is more informative when specifying the fractionation to refer to the dose per fraction rather than to the number of fractions.

Isoeffect curves as a function of the dose per fraction have been obtained experimentally for various biological effects. They show considerable differences depending on the effect considered (Figure 8.3). From these curves one can determine the correction factor to apply to the dose when the dose per fraction is changed from d to d'. If, for two different end points, the isoeffect curves have different forms, a change in fractionation introduces a differential effect.

Analysis of the available radiobiological data indicates that there are two classes of isoeffect curve corresponding to early and late effects in the tissues studied [56,68,71]. For *early effects* in skin (dry or moist desquamation), intestinal mucosa (cell survival measured by cloning *in vivo* and lethality after abdominal irradiation) and rat testis, the curves (Figure 8.4) increase slowly as the dose per fraction d is reduced and approach their maximum values when d

Table 8.1. **Isoeffect dose for different numbers of fractions.** *S* is the surviving fraction of cells, *d* is the dose per fraction. Each line in the table shows two irradiations (*D*=*N*×*d* and *D'*=*N'*×*d'*) giving the same surviving fraction of cells. The cell survival curve is that of mouse intestinal stems cells [62]. The survival after each fraction (*d* and *d'*) is shown by the values *s* and *s'* given in the table in parentheses. It is assumed that there is no cellular proliferation during irradiation.
When the dose per fraction is reduced from 4 to 2·2 Gy the isoeffect dose is increased by 10% for all values of *N*, i.e. for all final surviving fractions *S*. When the number of fractions *N* is increased from 3 to 6, the increase in the isoeffect dose depends on the final surviving fraction of cells; it is 30% for *d*=10 Gy and 10% for *d*=4 Gy.

S	N×d=D	N'×d'=D'	D'/D
2·2×10⁻⁶	3×10 Gy=30 Gy (s=0·013)	6×6·45 Gy=38·7 Gy (s'=0·114)	1·3
3·9×10⁻²	3× 4 Gy=12 Gy (s=0·338)	6×2·2 Gy=13·2 Gy (s'=0·581)	1·1
2·2×10⁻⁶	12× 4 Gy=48 Gy	24×2·2 Gy=52·8 Gy	1·1

becomes less than about 2 Gy. Also, the relative variation of isoeffect dose as a function of the dose per fraction is much the same for these biological effects, so that a modification of fractionation does not induce any differential action.

Curves relating to *late effects* (Figure 8.5) have been obtained for skin (fibrosis and contraction), lung, kidney, spinal cord and capillaries. The variation of isoeffect dose with dose per fraction is greater than for the curves of Figure 8.4 and the curves continue to rise when *D* is reduced below 2 Gy.

Thus fractionation has more important consequences for late effects than for early reactions. This provides a coherent explanation of the complications seen clinically after treatment with reduced fractionation (2 or 3 fractions per week) and doses per fraction which are greater than the conventional value of 2 Gy [24, 25]. If the total dose is adjusted according to the isoeffect curve for early reactions, the late complications are more severe than with the standard regime of fractionation. In terms of cell survival curves, this difference in isoeffect curves suggests that the 'shoulder' on the survival curve is greater and the initial slope of the curve smaller or the ratio α/β is smaller, for the cells responsible for late effects than for those which give rise to early reactions.

The tissues in which early reactions have been studied (epidermis, intestinal mucosa, seminiferous epithelium etc.) are hierarchical tissues (Section 5.1) with rapidly renewing maturing cells; their isoeffect curves have very similar shapes. Tissues showing late reactions are often of the flexible type with a low cell turnover rate and their isoeffect curves also present a certain similarity of shape, suggesting that similar types of cell are responsible in all the tissues (e.g. fibroblasts or capillary endothelial cells). The isoeffect curves are not however so closely parallel as would be expected on this hypothesis, but experimental studies of late reactions are generally difficult and not very precise. Barendsen [1] distinguishes late reactions in the nervous system due to demyelinization from damage in tissues composed of highly differentiated cells with a very low rate of renewal (lung, kidney, vascular system etc.). In this last group fractionation plays a particularly important role, suggesting a very large capacity for accumulation and repair of cellular damage after small doses.

If the isoeffect curve is known it is possible to deduce the correction to be applied to the total dose *D* for a change in dose per fraction *d*, i.e. to answer one

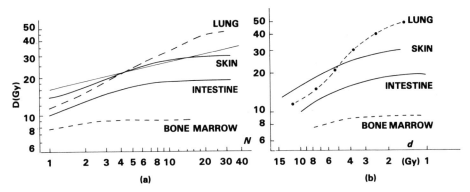

Figure 8.3. Isoeffect dose as a function of fractionation. The tissues and biological effects considered are:
(1) tolerance of bone marrow, determined by 50% lethality at 30 days in mice after total body irradiation [19];
(2) early tolerance of the intestinal mucosa, determined by the 50% lethal dose in mice after abdominal irradiation [62];
(3) early skin reaction in humans: dry desquamation [18];
(4) lung tolerance determined by the 50% lethal dose in mice after thoracic irradiation [17].
(a) The curves represent the variation in isoeffect dose as a function of the number of fractions N; over a certain range they approximate to a function of the form kN^n. For skin and intestine the exponent n has the value $n=0.24$ proposed by Ellis. It has a greater value for lung and a smaller value for bone marrow. To eliminate the time factor the curves have been established for a constant time.
(b) The curves represent the variation of isoeffect dose D as a function of the dose per fraction d (d increases towards the left to keep the same general shape of the curve as in the more conventional presentation as a function of N [56]).
The curves for skin and intestine are superimposable by a vertical shift; the relative increase in dose with reduction in the dose per fraction is the same for skin desquamation in man and early tolerance of intestinal mucosa in mice, i.e. fractionation has the same effect for both reactions. The general slope of the curve is greater for lung and smaller for bone marrow.

of the practical questions in radiotherapy. For this purpose it is convenient to give it a mathematical expression. A straightforward idea is to check whether the formulae for cell survival can provide a satisfactory fit to the experimental isosurvival results. Cohen and Creditor [8] used the combined single target single hit plus multi target single hit model (Section 4.3). The *linear–quadratic* model gives a simpler mathematical expression with a satisfactory fit to the experimental results.

The ratio α/β can be deduced from measurements of isoeffect doses in the following way. The cell survival after a dose d is given by

$$s=e^{(-\alpha d+\beta d^2)}$$

After N equal fractions, the surviving fraction S is given by

$$S=s^N=e^{-N(\alpha d+\beta d^2)}$$

Assuming that an isoeffect corresponds to a constant value of S,

$$N(\alpha d+\beta d^2)=A \text{ (constant)}$$

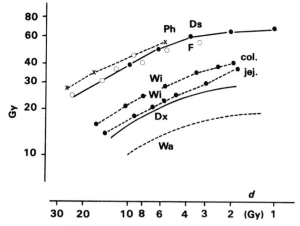

Figure 8.4. Isoeffect dose as a function of fractionation. Early reactions of rapidly renewing tissues.
Skin (mouse): F—Fowler *et al.* [26] Ds—Douglas *et al.* [13];
Human skin: Dx—Dutreix *et al.* [18];
Intestine: Wi—Withers *et al.* [67]; Wa—Wambersie *et al.* [62]; *Oesophagus:* Ph—Phillips *et al.* [47].
For all the reactions represented, the increase in isoeffect dose as the dose per fraction *d* is reduced is relatively slow and the isoeffect dose seems almost to reach a maximum value when *d* is <2 Gy. The similarity of the curves in the logarithmic representation indicates that the relative increase in isoeffect dose, when the dose per fraction *d* is reduced to *d'*, is the same for all the effects (e.g. the total dose is multiplied by 1·3 when the dose per fraction is reduced from 5 to 2 Gy).

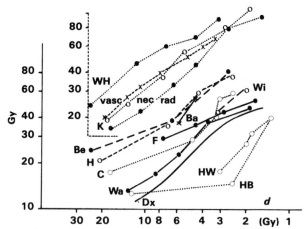

Figure 8.5. Isoeffect dose as a function of fractionation. Late reactions.
Skin: Wi—Withers *et al.* [70], Be—Berry *et al.* [3], H—Hopewell *et al.* [33], Ba—Bates and Peters [2];
Lung: Wa—Wara *et al.* [65], F—Field *et al.* [23], Dx—Dutreix and Wambersie [17];
Kidney: C—Caldwell [6], HB—Hopewell and Berry [32], HW—Hopewell *et al.* [33];
Central Nervous System (for ease of reading the graph the ordinate scale has been shifted upward for this series of curves): K—van der Kogel [59], [rad (radiculitis), nec (necrosis), vasc (vascularization)], WH—White and Hornsey [66].
For these effects the variation in isoeffect dose with dose per fraction is much greater than for the early reactions (Figure 8.4): e.g. for lung the total dose is multiplied by 2 when the dose per fraction is reduced from 5 to 2 Gy.

or $$\alpha D+\beta Dd=A$$

where $D=Nd$

and $$1/D=\alpha/A+\beta d/A$$

Hence if $1/D$ is plotted against d a straight line should be obtained. Figure 8.6 shows some results for acute skin reactions in mice obtained by Douglas and Fowler [12] who originated this method. Up to 64 equal fractions were given in times up to 8 days, short enough to prevent cellular repopulation. The close fit to a straight line confirms the validity of the linear–quadratic model over the range of doses used, from 1 to 23 Gy per fraction. The intercept on the ordinate axis, when $d=0$, is $1/D=\alpha/A$. The slope of the line is β/A. The ratio α/β is therefore given by intercept/slope. The intercept on the abscissa, when $1/D=0$, is given by $\alpha/\beta=-d$. It is more accurate to calculate α/β from the ratio intercept/slope. This experiment gave $\alpha/\beta=10\cdot4$ Gy.

The actual values of α and β can be estimated if there is independent information on the cell survival curve for the cells responsible for the acute skin reaction. Survival curves for the clonogenic cells in mouse epidermis have been measured by several teams (Section 4.2). Douglas and Fowler fitted their results to one of these curves to deduce the value of the constant A, and hence to estimate α and β.

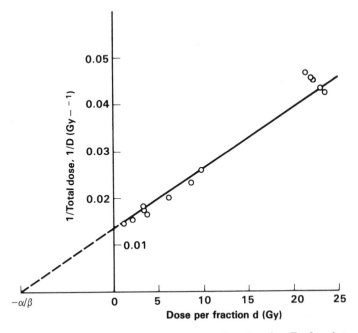

Figure 8.6. $1/D$ plotted against d for acute skin reactions in mice. Each point represents an isoeffect dose for a different number of fractions. From 1 to 64 fractions were used in total times up to 8 days, a short enough period to prevent repopulation from influencing the result. The slope is proportional to β. The intercept on the ordinate axis is proportional to α. The intercept on the abscissa gives a value of d equal to $-\alpha/\beta$. Redrawn from [12].

As a rule α/β is large (7–15 Gy) for early reactions of normal tissues and low (1–7 Gy) for late reactions, corresponding to the different slopes of the dose–effect relations shown in Figures 8.4 and 8.5. Thames and Hendry [55] have reviewed the information available on α/β for early and late reactions in normal tissues; Table 8.2 is taken from their compilation. The actual values of α and β, also from their compilation, are given in Table 8.3. The values of α are similar for early and late reactions but β is larger for late than for early reactions. This is to be expected as β reflects the capacity of the cells for repair and the initial curvature of the survival curve.

For tumours, α and β can be estimated readily from survival curves of tumour cells measured *in vitro*. Estimates from isoeffect curves *in vivo* are more difficult because of the effects of hypoxia and reoxygenation. It is essential that the clonogenic tumour cells should be of uniform sensitivity; this can be approached by clamping the tumour to render all the cells hypoxic or by making them all effectively aerobic with high-pressure oxygen or large doses of misonidazole. These approaches cannot be used with human patients, whose tumours are, in

Table 8.2. Estimates of α/β for normal tissues, X-and γ-rays.

	α/β (Gy)
Early reactions	
Skin (desquamation)	9·4–21
Hair follicles (epilation)	
Anagen	7·7
Telogen	5·5
Lip mucosa	7·9
Jejunum	7·1
Colon	8·4
Testis	13·9
Spleen	8·9
Late reactions	
Spinal cord (paralysis)	
Cervical	2·5–3·4
Lumbar	4·1–5·2
Brain (LD 50/10 months)	2·1
Eye (cataracts)	1·2
Kidney	
Rabbit	0·4
Mouse	1·6–4·1
Bladder	7·2–7·8
Lung (LD 50/pneumonitis)	2·1–4·3
Bowel	3·0–5·0
Dermis/subcutis	*c.* 1·5
Total body irradiation	
(LD 50/1 year)	5·1

After [55].

Table 8.3. Estimates of α and β for the cells responsible for early and late reactions.

	10α (Gy^{-1})	100β (Gy^{-2})
Early	0·3–1·3	0·1–0·8
Late	0·6–2·3	2·2–6·4

After [55].

any case, very heterogeneous. Table 8.4 gives values of these parameters obtained from survival curves of human tumour cells measured *in vitro*. It shows that α/β is usually similar to values for early reactions in normal tissues and greater than those for late reactions. The same conclusion can be drawn from studies of animal tumours irradiated *in vivo* where most values of α/β are in the range 9–30 Gy [55]. There are, however, a few tumours and tumour cell lines for which α/β is similar to the values found for late reactions in normal tissues.

The α/β model is convenient for predicting the reactions of different tissues, but it must not be regarded as having absolute significance as the linear–quadratic model does not give a perfect description of survival curves. Evidence has been found that in some circumstances the model is not correct, in particular when the dose per fraction is very small ($<0\cdot5$ Gy) [36]. As with other models it should be used only within certain limits.

For *squamous carcinomas*, the isoeffect curves (Figure 8.1) for cure and skin desquamation are parallel. In Cohen's diagram their slopes show a small difference, but this may be connected with the total treatment time which in these studies was proportional to the number of fractions. Finally, a large number of therapeutic trials made with varying doses per fraction have shown no evidence of a significant differential effect between the response of squamous carcinomas and the acute reactions of skin and mucosa.

For a given effect on squamous carcinoma, the early reactions of skin and mucosa are therefore almost constant whatever the fractionation, whereas late reactions become less severe as the dose per fraction is reduced.

For other types of tumour there are few clinical data or cell survival curves. The results obtained with melanomas show large differences in the shapes of the survival curves [43] and in particular in the initial slope. This corresponds

Table 8.4. Parameters of the cell survival curves from different human tumours cultivated *in vitro*. The table gives examples of the values of α and β.†

	$\alpha\times10$ (Gy^{-1})	$\beta\times100$ (Gy^{-2})	α/β (Gy)
Melanomas (8 cases)	1·37	5·37	2·5
	5·55	10·5	5·3
	2·78	3·15	8·8
	2·77	1·52	18
Colorectal adenocarcinoma	1·48	6·84	2·2
	2·04	4·11	5
Squamous carcinoma of the neck	1·72	7·96	2·2
	3·16	5·64	5·6
	2·69	2·95	9
	3·19	2·88	11
Glioma	0·86	3·94	2·2

Distribution of the values of α/β for the 40 tumours studied

α/β (Gy)	2–4	4–6	6–10	10–20	>20
Number of cases	8	7	8	7	10

†High values of α/β have also been observed for medulloblastoma, osteosarcoma, tumours of the pancreas and small cell carcinoma of the bronchus. The values of α and β for different animal tumours were given in Table 4.2.
After [22].

with the great variety in clinical response of this type of tumour after conventional irradiation with about 2 Gy per fraction. These results suggest that fractionation may have a protective effect on certain melanomas. One clinical study [34] has suggested a therapeutic advantage of relatively large doses per fraction. Although disputed by other authors, this seems confirmed by a study of Overgaard *et al.* [45] indicating $\alpha/\beta = 2\cdot5$ Gy.

It is therefore not impossible that the ratio α/β may be very small for some types of tumour and that fractionation may protect them against the effect of radiation. Thus in rare cases use of many small doses per fraction to obtain a given effect on the tumour might necessitate a total dose which is much greater than that required with large doses per fraction; this would result in more severe early reactions than after larger doses per fraction. Nevertheless, taking account of the fact that 'tolerance' is essentially a function of late reactions, it is doubtful whether a reduction in the number of fractions can have any therapeutic advantage. This will only occur if the protection afforded by fractionation is greater for the tumour than for the late reactions in normal tissue, a situation which has not been proved for the tumours studied until now. Most attempts to use more than 2 Gy per fraction have led to unfavourable results and sometimes to clinical catastrophes [52].

Remarks

The ratio α/β represents the relative importance for cell killing of the events whose probability is proportional to dose (αD) and those whose probability is proportional to the square of the dose (βD^2). It governs the *variation in isoeffect dose* as a function of fractionation, but it has no direct relation with the surviving fraction, i.e. the *radiosensitivity*, which is a function of the absolute values of α and β.

For therapeutic irradiations it is logical to relate 'radiosensitivity' to the cell survival corresponding to the usual dose per fraction (2 Gy). For doses of this order the term αD is more important than the term βD^2 (if α/β is greater than 2 Gy which is usually the case), so that 'radiosensitivity' to normal radiotherapy is essentially connected with the absolute value of the coefficient α which, for human tumours, varies between $0\cdot1$ and 1 Gy^{-1} [22].

8.4. *The effect of overall treatment time*

When the *overall time* of a fractionated course of irradiation is increased, the radiation effect may be reduced due to cellular repopulation between the fractions. To obtain a given effect with a constant number of fractions N the dose per fraction d must be increased: the isoeffect dose increases with total time, but a *differential effect* may appear if mitotic activity varies in different tissues.

Numerous radiobiological studies relate to irradiations given in two fractions on cells *in vitro*. We have seen (Section 4.5) that when the interval i between the two fractions is increased, the total dose necessary to obtain a given surviving fraction varies in a complex way due to:

(i)   intracellular repair of sublethal and potentially lethal damage;

(ii) synchronization; and

(iii) cell proliferation.

With conventional fractionation, the treatment time has little influence on the first two mechanisms since the interval between fractions is long enough to allow almost complete repair of the reparable intracellular damage and synchronization is less marked in tissue than in cells in culture. In addition, synchronization becomes blurred during irradiation given as many fractions. The increase in the isoeffect dose is therefore due essentially to cellular repopulation.

Most radiobiological studies *in vivo* have been made on early effects in skin and mucosa. Figure 8.7 represents the variation of isoeffect dose for the intestinal mucosa. The isoeffect dose increases steadily with the total time; the increase tends to slow down as the duration is extended, suggesting a reduction of mitotic activity.

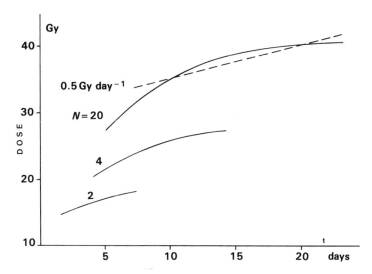

Figure 8.7. Variation of the isoeffect dose as a function of time. The biological effect considered is tolerance of mouse intestinal mucosa, determined by the LD 50 after abdominal irradiation. For each curve the number of fractions (*N*) is constant. With conventional fractionation and overall times of 2–4 weeks, the total dose must be increased by approximately 0·5 Gy per additional day.
After [61].

The cell kinetics of mouse skin show a more complex variation (Figure 8.8). During a fractionated irradiation containing 5 fractions per week each of 3 Gy, Denekamp [11] has shown that cell multiplication begins at the ninth day, increases to the end of the fourth week, the dose necessary to compensate for cell multiplication increasing progressively to 1·3 Gy per day, and then becomes slower in the fifth week (0·2 Gy per day) (Figure 8.8a).

For desquamation of human skin irradiated with 2 fractions of 8–10 Gy with a variable interval, a latent period of about 1 week has been seen, followed by an

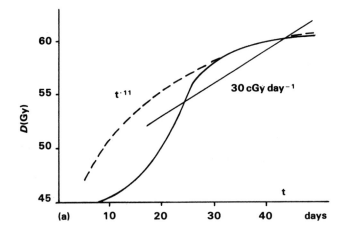

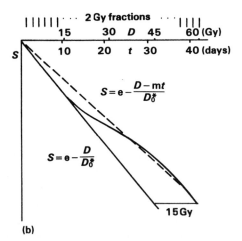

Figure 8.8. Role of overall time on acute reactions in skin.
(a) Increase in the isoeffect dose as a function of overall time.
(i) The continuous curve corresponds to the experimental data of Denekamp [11] for mouse skin. During fractionated irradiation, cell proliferation begins after a latent period of 10 days, is strongly stimulated for 2 weeks and then slows down.
(ii) The straight line represents an additional dose of 30 cGy per day to allow for cell proliferation.
(iii) The dashed curve represents the variation corresponding to the function $t^{0.11}$ in the NSD formula (Section 8.2).
(b) Role of cell proliferation on the number of cells during fractionated irradiation.
(i) In the absence of proliferation the survival curve would be an exponential ($S' = e^{-D/D^*_0}$). (D_0^* = effective mean lethal dose — Section 4.5),
(ii) After an initial latent period, cell proliferation is stimulated leading to a downward bending of the survival curve and later becomes slower.
(iii) Dashed line — survival curve on the assumption of constant cell multiplication, equivalent to a reduction in the dose by a constant amount (m) per day.

increase in the isoeffect dose of $0 \cdot 2$ Gy per day during the following 2 weeks and then of $0 \cdot 1$ Gy per day after the third week†. For the mucosa of the buccal cavity [15], during fractionated irradiation with 3×3 Gy per week, mucositis reaches a maximum in the second week and declines during the third week, suggesting that cell multiplication more than compensates for cell killing caused by the radiation.

These clinical and experimental findings make it possible to show schematically the changes in the fraction of surviving cells responsible for early reactions in the skin during fractionated irradiation (Figure 8.8b).

Cell proliferation thus depends on the dosimetric factors which control the speed and degree of cellular depletion (dose per fraction, dose per day and total dose) and varies with the elapsed time; it also depends on the organization of the tissue and its renewal kinetics. Correction to the dose for a change in total time cannot be very exact. However, an approximation is acceptable as this correction is usually small, much less than the correction needed for a change in the number of fractions (Table 8.5).

Table 8.5. Isoeffect doses for desquamation in pig skin. This study showed that the isoeffect dose increased much more when the *number of fractions* was increased from 1 to 20 than when the *overall time* was increased from 5 to 28 days with a constant number of fractions ($N=5$).

$N \times d$	t days	D(Gy)		
1×20 Gy	1	20		
5×6 Gy	5	30		
$20 \times 2 \cdot 5$ Gy	28	50	} 15 Gy	} 5 Gy
5×7 Gy	28	35		

After [27]

The most common problem in radiotherapy is how to allow for a small change in total time or an unintended interruption in treatment or a split-course regime. A correction which is clinically satisfactory is obtained by giving an additional dose per day to allow for the increased time (Figure 8.8). The accepted value for early reactions of the skin and mucosa in the head and neck is $0 \cdot 3$ Gy per day (for 2–3 Gy per fraction). If the overall time is increased by 2 weeks the total dose should be increased by about 4 Gy. This correction can be applied to interruptions of treatment up to a period of 3 weeks [16]. It cannot be applied for a very extended treatment exceeding 10 weeks. The problem of subsequent re-irradiation will be discussed later (Section 8.7). For short treatments of less than one week the actual duration has no importance as there is little cellular multiplication during this period and the correction would in any case be small.

---

†The increase in dose necessary to compensate for a prolongation of the overall time depends on the size of the fractions. In the case considered, the indicated value corresponds to the dose increase for the two fractions; for instance, if the time interval is increased from 10 to 15 days, the additional dose is $5 \times 0 \cdot 2$ Gy$=1$ Gy; thus 2×8 Gy in 10 days is equivalent to $2 \times 8 \cdot 5$ Gy in 15 days. If the additional dose is delivered with small fractions, it should be approximately three times larger (ratio of slopes of the cell survival curve at 8 Gy and at a small dose): for instance 2×8 Gy in 10 days is equivalent to 2×8 Gy$+3 \times 1$ Gy in 15 days.

For early intestinal reactions where the cell kinetics are rapid, the increase of tolerance is $0\cdot5$ Gy per day for normal periods of treatment (Figure 8.7). In this tissue, stimulation of proliferation takes place rapidly and the latent period is reduced to about 2 days. It is prudent to limit this correction for cell multiplication to a total of 20 Gy for the usual conditions of radiotherapy.

For tissues with slow cell turnover responsible for late effects, the role of total time is reduced. For the lung an additional dose of $0\cdot1$ Gy per day has been proposed by Field [23]; for the central nervous system Van der Kogel *et al.* [60] have observed no increase in tolerance with overall time, at least up to 8 weeks.

In summary the total time probably has little effect for the critical normal tissues in which late effects occur. It is important mainly for early reactions such as those in skin, mucosa and haemopoiesis; its effect on late effects in these tissues is probably small.

It used to be thought that a long overall time leads to a favourable differential effect between normal tissue reactions and tumour control. This assumption may be valid for many tumours when *early reactions* in normal tissues are considered, suggesting that cell proliferation in skin and mucosa stimulated by irradiation is more active than in the tumour. However, it has been revised in recent years (see Chapter 6) and shortening the treatment may be advisable in some situations [69].

8.5. *Hyperfractionation*

Hyperfractionation means the use of a larger number of fractions in the same total time. It is necessary to give more than one fraction per day but the dose per fraction is reduced. Alternatively the dose per fraction and the number of fractions can be kept the same and the total time reduced; this is known as accelerated fractionation.

The first trials of these methods used 4–8 fractions per day. Recent clinical and experimental data suggest that an interval of 3 or 4 h between fractions is rather too short for complete repair of sublethal and potentially lethal damage in many tissues and that an interval of 6–7 h is preferable [72]. Nowadays most studies are limited to 2 or 3 fractions per day [46, 51, 57, 64].

Hyperfractionation makes it possible to change the fractionation and the overall time independently. In one EORTC trial a conventional treatment of 70 Gy in 7 weeks given at the rate of 5×2 Gy per week was compared with 2 fractions per day of $1\cdot15$ Gy, 5 days per week to a total dose of $80\cdot5$ Gy in 7 weeks. The preliminary results suggest that the acute reactions were more severe but the late reactions the same with an increased effect on the tumour [58].

The aim of accelerated fractionation is to carry out the irradiation in as short a period as possible in order to limit the detrimental effect of tumour repopulation. However, the choice of the optimal period should also take into account repopulation in normal tissues, in particular skin and mucosa [64] (see Chapters 5 and 6).

In the regime proposed by Saunders *et al.* [51], in order to achieve the greatest advantage of accelerated irradiation, treatment is given 3 times each day for 12 consecutive days without a rest period. The total tumour dose is 50·4 Gy. The treatment was well tolerated in a series of patients with bronchial and head and neck tumours. The preliminary results are promising and justify the design of a controlled study comparing conventional and accelerated regimes.

If the total time and the dose per fraction are kept constant, hyperfraction-ation enables the radiation treatment to be concentrated into a smaller number of treatment days. This is particularly useful when radiotherapy is combined with chemotherapy, hyperthermia or radiosensitizing drugs.

Thus hyperfraction makes it possible to use treatment schedules very different from the conventional one of 5 fractions of 2 Gy per week. These schedules require that treatments are given at unconventional times (during the evening and night for 3 fractions per day with intervals of 6–7 h) and during the weekend if the shortest possible overall time is needed. Controlled clinical trials are now under way which should help to identify the tumours for which unconventional fractionation confers a therapeutic advantage. In the mean-while conventional regimes of treatment should be retained for most patients in order to avoid the risks of untoward reactions (so often seen in previous trials of new methods) and severe disturbance to the work of the department.

8.6. *Treatment at low dose rate*

Low dose rate brachytherapy by interstitial and intracavitary techniques is well known to be an effective method of radiotherapy. Several factors may be adduced to explain the success of this method:

(i)   a selected group of tumours is treated by brachytherapy; they are of limited volume and often have a good prognosis;

(ii)   the irradiated volume is smaller than in external beam radiotherapy and the dose falls off quickly at the periphery of the target volume; conse-quently there is an increased tolerance, allowing the tumour dose to be increased;

(iii) the dose rate is low.

To evaluate the relative importance of the last two factors, two types of clinical study have been undertaken:

1. External beam treatment at low dose rate using telecobalt equipment with low activity sources [48].

2. Inversely, brachytherapy with very high activity sources. In this way the treatment can be given with schedules similar to those of external radio-therapy but with the spatial dose distribution provided by brachytherapy [37].

Continuous irradiation at low dose rate involves a number of radiobiological factors. The two most important are repair of sublethal damage and cellular repopulation, but they are not sufficient for interpretation of all the results and other factors have to be considered.

Repair of sublethal damage

Reduction of dose rate leads to an increase in cell survival owing to repair of sublethal damage (Section 4.5) taking place during irradiation. With very low dose rates cell death is due solely to directly lethal events whose effects are independent of dose rate. In practice this situation is reached when the dose rate is lower than $1\,Gy\,h^{-1}$.

The isoeffect dose increases with reduction in dose rate and therefore with lengthening of the period of irradiation. For example (Figure 8.9), the LD 50/5 of mice after abdominal irradiation increases from $12 \cdot 4\,Gy$ for a short irradiation to 19 Gy for a continuous irradiation of 6 h and to 22 Gy for 14 h $(1 \cdot 57 Gy\,h^{-1})$. This last value is equal to the LD 50 for fractionated irradiation with doses per fraction of the order of 2 Gy. This relation between isoeffect dose and dose rate can therefore be interpreted as being due only to repair of sublethal damage.

The variation in isoeffect dose as a function of dose rate differs from one tissue to another. These differences are connected essentially with the relative contributions of sublethal and lethal lesions to cell death after acute irradiation, i.e. to the shape of the cell survival curve (Figure 4.13). For lung tolerance determined by the LD 50 at 200 days after thoracic irradiation, Hill [30] found a value of $10 \cdot 5$ Gy for acute irradiation and 21 Gy for continuous irradiation over $7\,h\,(3\,Gy\,h^{-1})$. This variation is greater than that for intestinal mucosa, which is in agreement with the difference seen between the two tissues for the variation in isoeffect dose as a function of the dose per fraction (Figure 8.5).

The range of dose rates in which the main variation of isoeffect dose is observed depends on the rate of repair expressed by the repair half-time T_{r}

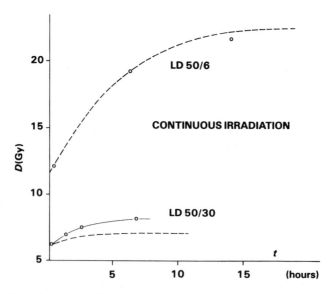

Figure 8.9. Variation in isoeffect dose as a function of the length of continuous irradiation. For the intestine (LD 50 at 6 days in mice [63]), the variation seen is that expected from the repair of sublethal damage on the assumption that the half-time of repair is 1 h. For the bone marrow (LD 50 at 30 days in mice [19]), the increase in isoeffect dose (continuous line) is greater than would be expected from repair of sublethal damage (dashed line).

(Section 4.5). At a given dose rate more sublethal injury is repaired if the repair is fast, e.g. $T_r = 0 \cdot 5\,h$, than if it is slow, e.g. $T_r = 1 \cdot 5\,h$. Experimental determinations of T_r values for various tissues have led to conflicting results ([55], Table 3.6) but there is a trend for a correlation between the rate of repair and the capacity for cell proliferation.

A given biological effect can be achieved with a single irradiation at low dose rate or with a series of acute irradiations (fractions) given at high dose rate. Assuming that the limiting cell survival curve for low dose rates is the same as that for a large number of very small fractions with full repair of sublethal damage between each, and ignoring cell repopulation, Liversage [42] has proposed a formula relating the total time (t) of the protracted irradiation to the number of fractions, the total dose being the same in each case.

$$N = \frac{\mu t}{2\{1 - (1 - e^{-\mu t})/\mu t\}}$$

where $\mu = 0 \cdot 693/T_r$ and N is the number of high dose-rate fractions. This expression has been confirmed experimentally [9, 53].

In curietherapy $t \gg T_r$. Thus $\mu t \gg 1$ and $N \approx \mu t/2$. For instance, if $T_r = 1\,h$, 60 Gy in 6 days brachytherapy is equivalent to $N = 0 \cdot 693 \times 6 \times 24/2 = 50$ fractions, each of which must be $1 \cdot 2\,Gy$ to deliver 60 Gy.

The equivalent treatment given at $5 \times 2\,Gy$ per week can be derived by calculating the correction to the total dose for the change in dose per fraction using the linear-quadratic model and adding sufficient dose to compensate for the additional time.

Cellular proliferation during irradiation

When the irradiation is extended over a long enough time in comparison with the renewal time of the tissue, cell mortality is in part compensated by proliferation and the isoeffect dose increases with the period of irradiation. For most normal tissues and tumours it is doubtful whether proliferation plays a significant role when the continuous irradiation is limited to a few days. The clinical experience of Pierquin *et al.* [49] has shown that for mucosa and squamous carcinoma the isoeffect dose does not vary appreciably for irradiation times between 3 and 9 days.

For rapidly renewing tissues, proliferation plays a more important role and may compensate for cell killing when the dose rate is less than a 'critical' value; this amounts to 4 Gy per day (about $0 \cdot 2\,Gy\,h^{-1}$) for rat intestine [50] and $0 \cdot 5–1\,Gy$ per day for haemopoietic bone marrow [4]. The critical dose rate is increased for the more rapidly renewing tissues.

Effects of continuous irradiation on cell kinetics

The role of cellular proliferation is complicated by the effects of irradiation on cell kinetics. A number of mechanisms play a role and their effects may be opposed (Chapter 5):

(i)   mitotic delay;

(ii) changes in the distribution of cells in different phases of the cycle;
(iii) stimulation of proliferation;
(iv) changes in the length of cell transit times in different compartments of hierarchical tissues.

Experimental studies have shown the importance of these mechanisms. They are probably the cause of the variations in isoeffect dose which cannot be interpreted by repair and cell proliferation.

For example, the increase in isoeffect dose for acute reactions of human skin with irradiation times up to 10 h (dose rate $1 \cdot 6$ Gy h^{-1}) is less than would be expected from cellular repair alone [14]; on the other hand, for daily irradiations of 8 Gy (at $0 \cdot 9$ Gy h^{-1}) repeated for 3 days, the isoeffect dose has the same value as for a fractionated irradiation with small doses per fraction. For irradiation times which do not exceed 10 h the skin therefore seems to show an increase in radiosensitivity which may be due to accumulation of the cells in a radiosensitive phase. Accumulation in G_2 (Table 5.1) has been seen during continuous irradiation (at $0 \cdot 75$ Gy h^{-1}) for rat rhabdomyosarcoma [38] and for bone marrow cells [28]; it may help to explain an increase in radiosensitivity. These findings may be related to the results of Frindel *et al.* [28] for the NCTC tumour: after acute irradiation and irradiation at $0 \cdot 5$ Gy h^{-1}, the survival curves (*in vitro-in vivo*) are almost the same (up to 12 Gy) and show a considerable shoulder.

On the other hand, for 30 day lethality in mice due to bone marrow failure after total body irradiation, it is known [22] that for a dose rate of 2 Gy h^{-1} the increase in isoeffect dose is greater than would be expected from intracellular repair alone. Frindel *et al.* [28] found that cell density in bone marrow was the same after 12 Gy in 24 h ($0 \cdot 5$ Gy h^{-1}) as after an acute irradiation of $5 \cdot 5$ Gy. The reduction in dose rate has a protective effect on the bone marrow, which cannot be entirely explained either by intracellular repair which is relatively small in this biological system nor by cell multiplication for the short time under consideration. The additional mechanism involved may be related to the complex regulation systems of cell proliferation and differentiation in the various cell compartments (Section 5.3).

Reoxygenation during continuous irradiation

We have seen earlier in this chapter that reoxygenation of hypoxic tumour cells occurs between treatments during fractionated irradiation. This phenomenon is fast enough to take place during irradiation at low dose rate. Radiobiological experiments have shown that reoxygenation is almost complete at a dose rate of 1 Gy h^{-1}. Thus, in a mixed population the proportion of hypoxic cells remains constant during irradiation. When this proportion is small the survival curve for the mixed population is close to that of the well-oxygenated cells, as is the case in fractionated irradiation. Reoxygenation may be the reason for the observations [28, 31, 39] showing that in certain experimental tumours the survival curve at low dose rate is close to that found with acute irradiation (Figure 8.10).

Thus low dose rate and fractionation have comparable consequences on repair of sublethal injury and reoxygenation. The two modalities of irradiation differ

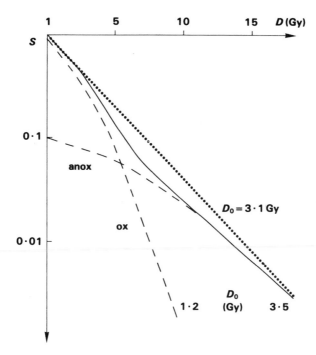

Figure 8.10. Survival curve at low dose rate for a mixed population. The population is assumed to contain 10% of hypoxic cells. The dashed lines show the survival curves of the two components for an acute irradiation. The continuous line shows the survival curve of the total population. The survival curve after low dose rate irradiation is shown (dotted) on the assumption that it corresponds to the initial slope of the curve for the well-oxygenated cells after acute irradiation, i.e. that there is complete reoxygenation during the low dose rate irradiation. With this hypothesis it appears that the surviving fraction after a given dose may be almost the same for exposures at low dose rate as for acute exposures.

in the overall time which is a few days in curietherapy and several weeks in fractionated irradiation. As we have seen, this reduction in time has little effect on slowly renewing tissues which give rise to late reactions (see earlier in this chapter), whereas it can increase the effect on the tumour. The two modalities may, however, have different effects on cell kinetics and the distribution of cells in the cycle but the experimental results do not enable general conclusions to be drawn.

8.7. Re-irradiation

After irradiation with a dose great enough to cause permanent injury, re-irradiation involves serious risks of necrosis. Exhaustion of the capacity for tissue regeneration slows down or prevents healing.

However, a few months after an irradiation which has left no observable sequelae the early tolerance of skin and mucosa return almost to their initial values. Clinical experience shows that after re-irradiation the reactions of skin and mucosa are similar to those for the first irradiation. In mice which have survived abdominal irradiation to about 10 Gy, a second irradiation given a few months later shows that the LD 50/7 has the same value as for animals which had not previously been irradiated.

Nevertheless, certain experimental studies show a residual effect of the first irradiation. For early skin reactions in mice, the residual damage has been found to be equivalent to 10% of the original dose 6–10 months after a dose of 20–30 Gy [10, 29]. In patients, as in animal experiments, the bone marrow never recovers its initial tolerance to radiation or drugs and the number of stem cells remains reduced a year after irradiation (Section 5.3).

There is little experimental information on residual damage in those tissues in which late effects are observed. In experimental animals slow repair has been noticed but for clinical conditions the data are scarce and inconclusive. Brown and Probert [5] found, for deformation of the mouse paw after doses of 10×3 Gy and 10×5 Gy, that there was residual damage equivalent, respectively, to 20% and 40% of the dose. Hunter and Stewart [35] studied 15 patients who were re-irradiated on the neck 15–50 years after the first irradiation which in seven cases had left marked sequelae. The second irradiation was given with doses of $21 \cdot 5$–50 Gy on a field of about 5×10 cm^2; the early skin reaction was that expected after a first irradiation and in five patients who survived a further 2 years no late complication was seen.

Skin and mucosa can therefore withstand re-irradiation at a much later time over a relatively small area; but in practical radiotherapy a safe rule is to limit a second dose to about 30 Gy after an extended irradiation to high dose. The decision about a second irradiation with curative intent must take into account the likely risks which depend on the volume to be treated and its anatomical content. Curietherapy has advantages for making up a curative dose over small volumes.

References

1. G. W. Barendsen. Dose fractionation, dose rate and isoeffect relationships for normal tissue response. *Int. J. Radiat. Oncol. Biol. Phys.*, 1982 **8**: 1981–1997.
2. T. D. Bates, L. J. Peters. Dangers of the clinical use of the NSD formula for small fraction numbers. *Br. J. Radiol.*, 1975, **48**: 773.
3. R. J. Berry, G. Wiernik, R. J. S. Patterson, J. W. Hopewell. Excess late subcutaneous fibrosis after irradiation of pig skin consequent upon the application of the NSD formula. *Br. J. Radiol.*, 1974, **47**: 277–281.
4. N. M. Blackett, P. J. Roylance, K. Adams. Studies of the capacity of bone marrow cells to restore erythropoiesis in heavily irradiated rats. *Br. J. Haematol.*, 1964, **10**: 453–467.
5. J. Brown, J. C. Probert. Early and late radiation changes following a second course of irradiation. *Radiology*, 1975, **115**: 711–716.
6. W. L. Caldwell. Time–dose factors in fatal post-irradiation nephritis, in: *Cell survival after low doses of radiation: theoretical and clinical implications* (T. Alper, ed.), pp. 328–332. John Wiley and Son, Bristol, 1975.
7. L. Cohen. Clinical radiation dosage II. *Br. J. Radiol.*, 1949, **22**: 706–713.
8. L. Cohen, M. Creditor. Iso-effect tables and therapeutic ratios for epidermoid cancer and normal tissue stroma. *Int. J. Radiat. Oncol. Biol. Phys.*, 1983, **9**: 1065–1071.
9. R. G. Dale. The application of the linear–quadratic dose effect equation to fractionated and protracted radiotherapy. *Br. J. Radiol.*, 1985, **58**: 515–528.
10. J. Denekamp. Residual damage in mouse skin, five or eight months after irradiation. *Radiology*, 1975, **115**: 191–195.
11. J. Denekamp. Changes in the rate of repopulation during multifraction irradiation of mouse skin. *Br. J. Radiol.*, 1973, **46**: 381–387.
12. B. G. Douglas, J. F. Fowler. The effect of multiple small doses of X-rays on skin reactions in the mouse and a basic interpretation. *Radiat. Res.*, 1976, **66**: 401–426.

13. B. G. Douglas, J. F. Fowler, J. Denekamp, S. R. Harris, S. E. Ayers, S. Fairman, S. A. Hill, P. W. Sheldon, F. A. Stewart. The effect of multiple small fractions of X-rays on skin reactions in the mouse, in: *Cell survival after low doses of radiation: theoretical and clinical implications.* (T. Alper, ed.) pp. 351–361. John Wiley and Son, Bristol, 1975.
14. J. Dutreix, A. Sahatchiev. Clinical radiobiology of low dose-rate radiotherapy. *Br. J. Radiol.*, 1975, **48**: 846–850.
15. J. Dutreix, M. Tubiana, A. Wambersie, E. Malaise. The influence of cell proliferation in tumours and normal tissues during fractionated radiotherapy. *Eur. J. Cancer*, 1971, **7**: 205–213.
16. J. Dutreix, A. Wambersie. Facteurs temps dans les réactions précoces de la peau humaine. *J. Radiol. Electrol.*, 1975, **57**: 813–816.
17. J. Dutreix, A. Wambersie. Isoeffect total dose as a function of the number of fractions for skin, intestine and lung, in: *Conference on the time dose relationships in clinical therapy* (W. L. Caldwell, D. D. Tolbert, eds), pp. 21–30. University of Wisconsin, 1975.
18. J. Dutreix, A. Wambersie, C. Bouhnik. Cellular recovery in human skin reactions: application to dose fraction number overall time relationship in radiotherapy. *Eur. J. Cancer*, 1973, **9**: 159–167.
19. J. Dutreix. A. Wambersie, M. Loirette, G. Boisserie. Time dose factors in total body irradiation. *Pathol. Biol.*, 1979, **27**: 365–369.
20. F. Ellis. Fractionation in radiotherapy, in: *Modern trends in radiotherapy* (T. J. Deeley, C. A. P. Woods eds), vol. 1, pp. 34–51. Butterworths, London, 1967.
21. F. Ellis. Dose, time and fractionation. A clinical hypothesis. *Clin. Radiol.*, 1969, **20**: 1–6.
22. B. Fertil, E. Malaise. Inherent cellular radiosensitivity as a basic concept for human tumor radiotherapy. *Int. J. Radiat. Oncol. Biol. Phys.*, 1981, **7**: 621–629.
23. S. B. Field, S. Hornsey. Y. Kutsutani. Effects of fractionated radiation on mouse lung and a phenomenon of slow repair. *Br. J. Radiol.*, 1976, **49**: 700–707.
24. G. H. Fletcher, H. T. Barkley. Present status of the time factor in clinical radiotherapy. Part 1 — The historical background and the recovery exponents. *J. Radiol. Electrol.*, 1974, **55**: 443–450.
25. G. H. Fletcher, H. T. Barkley, L. J. Shukowski. Present status of the time factor in clinical radiotherapy. Part II — The Nominal Standard Dose Formula. *J. Radiol. Electrol.*, 1974, **55**: 745–751.
26. J. F. Fowler, J. Denekamp, C. Delapeyre, S. R. Harris, P. W. Sheldon. Skin reactions in mice after multifraction X-irradiation. *Int. J. Radiat. Biol.*, 1974, **25**: 213–223.
27. J. F. Fowler, M. A. Morgan, J. A. Silvester, D. K. Bewley, B. A. Turner. Experiments with fractionated X-ray treatment of the skin of pig. I — Fractionation up to 28 days. *Br. J. Radiol.*, 1963, **36**: 188–196.
28. E. Frindel, G. M. Hahn, D. Robaglia, M. Tubiana. Responses of bone marrow and tumor cells to acute and protracted irradiation. *Cancer Res.*, 1972, **32**: 2096–2103.
29. J. H. Hendry, I. Rosenberg, D. G. Greene, J. G. Stewart. Re-irradiation of rat tails to necrosis at six months after treatment with a "tolerance" dose of X-rays or neutrons. *Br. J. Radiol.*, 1977, **50**: 567–572.
30. R. P. Hill. Response of mouse lung to irradiation at different dose rates. *31st Annual Meeting Radiation Research Society.* Salt Lake City, 18–22 April 1982, Abstract Bi-2, p. 29.
31. R. P. Hill, R. S. Bush. The effect of continuous or fractionated irradiation on a murine sarcoma. *Br. J. Radiol.*, 1973, **46**: 167–174.
32. J. W. Hopewell, R. J. Berry. The predictive value of the NSD system for renal tolerance to fractionated X-irradiation in the pig. *Br. J. Radiol.*, 1974, **47**: 679–686.
33. J. W. Hopewell, J. L. Foster, C. M. A. Young, G. Wiernik. Late radiation damage to pig skin. *Radiology*, 1979, **130**: 783–788.
34. S. Hornsey. The relationship between total dose number of fractions and fraction size in the response of malignant melanoma in patients. *Br. J. Radiol.*, 1978, **51**: 905–909.
35. R. D. Hunter, J. G. Stewart. The tolerance to re-irradiation of heavily irradiated human skin. *Br. J. Radiol.*, 1977, **50**: 573–575.
36. M. C. Joiner. The dependence of radiation response on the dose per fraction, in: *The scientific basis of modern radiotherapy*, BIR report No. 19, pp. 20–26, 1989.
37. C. A. F. Joslin, W. E. Liversage, N. W. Ramsay. High dose rate treatment moulds for after loading techniques. *Br. J. Radiol.*, 1969, **42**: 108–112.
38. H. B. Kal, G. W. Barendsen. Effects of continuous irradiation at low dose rate on a rat rhabdomyosarcoma. *Br. J. Radiol.*, 1972, **45**: 279–283.
39. H. B. Kal, G. W. Barendsen. The OER at low dose rates. *Br. J. Radiol.*, 1976, **49**: 1049–1051.
40. J. Kirk, W. M. Gray, R. Watson. Cumulative radiation effect. Part I — Fractionated treatment regimes. *Clin. Radiol.*, 1971, **22**: 145–155.
41. J. P. Le Bourgeois, H. Bouhnik. Importance du fractionnement dans la radiothérapie de la maladie de Hodgkin. *J. Radiol. Electrol.*, 1976, **57**: 828–830.
42. W. E. Liversage. A general formula for equating protracted and acute regimes of radiation. *Br. J. Radiol.*, 1969, **42**: 432–440.

43. E. P. Malaise, J. Weininger, A. M. Joly, M. Guichard. Measurements *in vitro* with three cell lines derived from melanoma, in: *Cell survival after low doses of radiation: theoretical and clinical implications.* (T. Alper, ed.), pp. 223–225. John Wiley and Son, Bristol, 1975.

44. C. G. Orton, F. Ellis. A simplification in the use of the NSD concept in practical radiotherapy. *Br. J. Radiol.*, 1973, **46**: 529–537.

45. J. Overgaard, M. Overgaard, P. V. Hansen, H. von der Maase. Some factors of importance in the radiation treatment of malignant melanomas. *Radiother. Oncol.*, 1986, **5**: 183–192.

46. L. J. Peters, K. K. Ang, H. D. Thames Jr. Accelerated fractionation in the radiation treatment of head and neck cancer. *Acta Oncologica*, 1988, **27**: 185–194.

47. T. Phillips, L. W. Margolis. Radiation pathology and the clinical response of lung and esophagus, in: *Frontiers of Radiation Therapy and Oncology* (J. M. Vaeth, ed.), vol. 6, pp. 254–273. Karger, Basel, 1972.

48. B. Pierquin. L'effet différentiel de l'irradiation continue (ou semi-continue) à faible débit des épithéliomas épidermoïdes. *J. Radiol. Electrol.*, 1970, **51**: 533–536.

49. B. Pierquin, D. Chassagne, F. Baillet, Ch. Paine. Clinical observations on the time factor in interstitial radiotherapy using Iridium 192. *Clin. Radiol.*, 1973, **24**: 506–509.

50. H. Quastler, J. R. M. Bensted, L. F. Lamerton, S. M. Simpson. Adaptation to continuous irradiation: observations on the rat intestine. *Br. J. Radiol.*, 1959, **32**: 501–512.

51. M. I. Saunders, S. Dische, J. F. Fowler, J. Denekamp, E. P. Dunphy, E. Grosch, D. Fermont, R. Ashford, *et al.* Radiotherapy employing three fractions on each day of twelve consecutive days. *Acta Oncologica*, 1988, **27**: 163–167.

52. K. Singh. Two regimes with the same TDF but different morbidity used in the treatment of stage III carcinoma of the cervix. *Br. J. Radiol.*, 1978, **51**: 357–362.

53. G. C. Steel, J. D. Down, J. H. Peacock, T. C. Stephens. Dose rate effects and the repair of radiation damage. *Radiother. Oncol.*, 1986, **5**: 321–331.

54. M. Strandqvist. Studien über die kumulative Wirkung der Röntgenstrahlen bei Fraktionierung. *Acta Radiologica*, 1944, suppl. 55: 1–300.

55. H. D. Thames, J. H. Hendry. *Fractionation in radiotherapy.* Taylor and Francis, London, 1987.

56. H. D. Thames, H. R. Withers, L. J. Peters, G. H. Fletcher. Changes in early and late radiation responses with altered dose fractionation: implications for dose-survival relationships. *Int. J. Radiat. Oncol. Biol. Phys.*, 1982, **8**: 219–226.

57. K. R. Trott, J. Kummermehr. What is known about tumour proliferation rates to choose between accelerated fractionation or hyperfractionation? *Radiother. Oncol.*, 1985, **3**: 1–9.

58. W. van den Bogaert, E. van der Scheuren, J. C. Horiot, G. Chaplain, G. Arcangeli, D. Gonzales, V. Svoboda. The feasibility of high-dose multiple daily fractionation and its combination with anoxic cell sensitizers in the treatment of head and neck cancer. *Int. J. Radiat. Oncol. Biol. Phys.*, 1982, **8**: 1649–1655.

59. A. J. Van der Kogel. Radiation tolerance of the rat spinal cord. Time–dose relationships. *Radiology*, 1977, **122**: 505–509.

60. A. J. Van der Kogel, H. A. Sissingh, J. Zoetelief. Effects of X-rays and neutrons on repair and regeneration in the rat spinal cord. *Int. J. Radiat. Oncol. Biol. Phys.*, 1982, **8**: 2095–2097.

61. A. Wambersie, J. Dutreix, J. Gueulette. Isoeffect total dose for intestinal tolerance in mice as a function of fraction number and overall time. *Int. J. Radiat. Biol.*, 1976, **29**: 576.

62. A. Wambersie, J. Dutreix, J. Gueulette, J. Lellouch. Early recovery for intestinal stem cells, as a function of the dose per fraction, evaluated by survival rate after fractionated irradiation of the abdomen of mice. *Radiat. Research*, 1974, **58**: 498–515.

63. A. Wambersie, J. Dutreix, M. R. Stienon-Smoes, M. Octave-Prignot. Influence du débit de dose sur la tolérance intestinale chez la souris. *J. Radiol. Electrol.*, 1978, **59**: 315–322.

64. C. C. Wang. Accelerated fractionation, in: *Innovations in radiation oncology research* (H. R. Withers, L. J. Peters, eds), pp. 239–243. Springer-Verlag, Heidelberg, 1987.

65. W. M. Wara, T. L. Phillips, L. W. Margolis, V. Smith. Radiation pneumonitis: a new approach to the derivation of time dose factors. *Cancer*, 1973, **32**: 547–552.

66. A White, S. Hornsey. Radiation damage to the rat spinal cord: the effect of single and fractionated doses of X-rays. *Br. J. Radiol.*, 1978, **51**: 515–523.

67. H. R. Withers, A. M. Chu, B. O. Reid, D. H. Hussey. Response of mouse jejunum to multifraction radiation. *Int. J. Radiat. Oncol. Biol. Phys.*, 1975, **1**: 41–52.

68. H. R. Withers, K. A. Mason. The kinetics of recovery in irradiated colonic mucosa of the mouse. *Cancer*, 1974, **34**: 896–903.

69. H. R. Withers, J. M. G. Taylor, B. Maciejewski. The hazard of accelerated tumor clonogen repopulation during radiotherapy. *Acta Oncologica*, 1988, **27**: 131–146.

70. H. R. Withers, H. D. Thames, B. L. Flow, K. A. Mason, D. H. Hussey. The relationship of acute to late skin injury in 2 and 5 fraction/week X-ray therapy. *Int. J. Radiat. Oncol. Biol. Phys.*, 1978, **4**: 591–601.

71. H.R. Withers, H.D. Thames, L.J. Peters. Differences in the fractionation response of acutely and late responding tissues, in: *Progress in radio-oncology II* (K.H. Kärcher, H.D. Kogelnik, G. Reinartz, eds), pp. 287–296. Raven Press, New York, 1982.
72. H.R. Withers. Biologic basis for altered fractionation schemes. *Cancer*, 1985, **55**: 2086–2095.

Bibliography

T. Alper (ed.). *Cell survival after low doses of radiation: theoretical and clinical implications*. John Wiley, Bristol, 1975.

W.L. Caldwell, D.D. Tolbert (eds). *Proceedings of the Conference on the time–dose relationships in clinical therapy*. University of Wisconsin, 1975.

L.F. Fajardo (ed.). *Pathology of radiation injury*. Masson, New York, 1982.

G.H. Fletcher, C. Nervi, H.R. Withers (eds). *Biological bases and clinical implications of tumor radioresistance*. Masson, New York, 1983.

M. Friedman (ed.). *The biological and clinical basis of radiosensitivity*. Charles C. Thomas, Springfield, 1974.

P. Rubin, G.W. Casarett. *Clinical radiation pathology* (2 vols). Saunders, Philadelphia, 1968.

Chapter 9.
Hyperthermia

Hyperthermia is the best known physical agent which modifies radiosensitivity; its use in the treatment of cancer is of great interest. In this chapter hyperthermia is considered in relation to radiobiology and their combined use in radiotherapy. Only an outline treatment is given; more complete accounts, particularly with respect to technical and biological factors, appear in the bibliography to this chapter.

The therapeutic use of hyperthermia antedates the discovery of ionizing radiation. It originated from observations made in the middle of the 19th century of rare cases of spontaneous regression of tumours in patients suffering from a very high fever. This led to attempts at treatment by artificial induction of fever or an increase in temperature localized to the tumour. The results have been variable and difficult to analyze. Technical difficulties and lack of a biological rationale hindered development of the method and the discovery of ionizing radiation led to its almost total eclipse.

Study of the biological effects of hyperthermia were actively taken up again about 1960, making use of the scientific methodology employed in radiobiology together with new techniques of heating and measurement of temperature.

Total body hyperthermia in man can be achieved by immersion in hot water or paraffin or with heated clothing. Localized hyperthermia can be obtained by various techniques depending on the thickness and depth of the tumour. The use of infra-red radiation or direct contact with heated material such as water produces very superficial heating which is useful only for experiments with small animals or samples *in vitro*. For clinical use, local or regional heating must be given to larger and deeper volumes and can be performed by diathermy techniques using electric currents, electromagnetic waves or ultrasound.

The distribution of temperature results from the equilibrium established at each point between the heat deposited by the heating equipment, exchanges of heat by conduction in the tissues and loss of heat through circulating blood. The achievement of uniform heating over a limited volume raises difficult technical problems, increasing with the depth of the tumour, which have hindered the clinical use of hyperthermia. Nevertheless the method continues to be of interest as it has a firm biological basis established by many experimental studies demonstrating the lethal effect of hyperthermia on cells and the sensitization of tissues to radiation and chemotherapy.

9.1 *Lethal effects of hyperthermia on cells*

The lethal effect of hyperthermia on cell cultures or tissues *in vivo* is easily demonstrated. It occurs with temperatures of 42°C and above, considerably lower than the temperature at which biological media coagulate (Figure 9.1). The cell survival curves [S(t)], at a given temperature normally show a shoulder suggesting that cell death is due, at least in part, to the accumulation of sublethal lesions, analogous to cell death due to the accumulation of radiation-induced sublethal lesions.

The effect increases with temperature and the time during which it is applied. For a given effect the two parameters are connected; an increase in temperature of 1°C is compensated by a reduction in the period of application by a factor of about 2.

There are several biological mechanisms which may be at the origin of cell death. An increase in temperature modifies the structure of the lipoproteins composing the membranes, leading to disturbance of their physiological function. There is also denaturation of thermolabile proteins. Both mechanisms, involving membranes and enzymes, may play a part in the modification of ionic gradients and metabolic reactions which are observed.

At the temperatures under consideration there is no direct damage in DNA and chromosome aberrations are not seen. Enzymatic changes may affect the synthesis and repair of DNA but they do not seem to have lethal consequences. The lesions induced by heat are not of the same nature as those due to radiation.

There is a large variation in sensitivity with the phase of the cell cycle: sensitivity is high in S phase, the opposite of the effect of ionizing radiation, emphasizing the different mechanisms of action of the two agents.

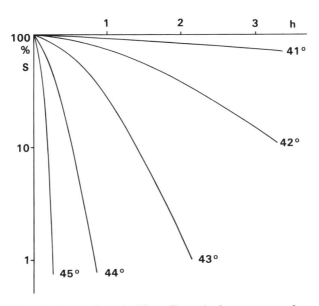

Figure 9.1. Cell killing by hyperthermia. The cell survival curves are schematic only and represent the mean of several experimental studies. Cell killing depends on the temperature and the time during which it is applied. Above 42°C an increase of 1°C produces the same survival if the time of heating is reduced by a factor of about 2.

Effects in tissues

Figure 9.2 shows the relationship between temperature and the time of heating to produce a given effect in a number of normal tissues and tumours, assessed *in situ*. The slope of the lines is similar in all cases; the form of the relationship is the same as that established by Arrhenius between temperature and the rate of chemical reactions. There is a wide variation in absolute sensitivity to heat but no consistent difference between normal tissues and tumours. The most sensitive system shown in Figure 9.2 is weight loss of the testis and the least sensitive necrosis and burns in skin. Spermatogonia are particularly sensitive to heat, as they are to radiation (see Section 5.3).

There is a difference in the time of appearance of the reactions after heat and radiation. For the latter, reactions are delayed, usually by periods of a few weeks, depending on the cell kinetics as reproductive death of irradiated cells occurs at a subsequent mitosis. After hyperthermia reactions develop much sooner, often in less than 24 h.

Experiments *in vitro* have shown that thermosensitivity is increased when cells are poorly nourished, e.g. in dense culture, impoverished media or hypoxia. A reduction in pH also increases mortality. These are the normal conditions in regions of tumours poorly perfused by blood and containing hypoxic and radioresistant cells; thus hyperthermia and radiation act on tumours in a complementary fashion. Reduced tumour blood floww also causes a greater increase in temperature in tumours than in well-perfused normal tissues. The difference is accentuated by vasodilation which appears in the normal capillaries about 10 min after the beginning of heating. Moreover, the new blood vessels in the tumour seem particularly sensitive to hyperthermia

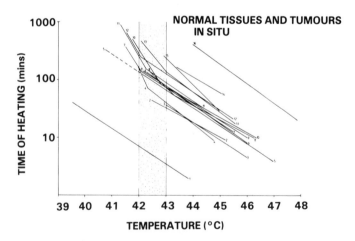

Figure 9.2. Relationship between the time of heating and temperature for a given level of damage in a range of normal tissues and tumours *in situ*: (1) mouse testis weight loss. (2) rat tumour 9L, heated *in vivo*, assayed *in vitro*; (3) mouse jejunum LD_{50}; (4) mouse jejunum, 50% loss of crypts (5) mouse sarcoma 180, majority cure; (6) baby rat tail, 50% necrosis; (7) mouse ear skin, 50% necrosis; (8) rat skin epilation; (9) baby rat tail, 5% stunting; (10) baby rat tail (whole tail necrosis); (11) mouse tumour C3H/Tif regrowth; (12) mouse tumour F(Sal) (TCD_{50}); (13) mouse foot skin epilation; (14) mouse skin, feet and legs; (15) mouse tumour C3H, 50% cures; (16) pig and human skin necrosis and cutaneous burns.
From [4] with permission of the author and publisher.

which induces capillary emboli; this may be the direct cause of much cell death. The progressive reduction in blood flow in the course of repeated treatment with hyperthermia may increase the selective heating of the tumour.

Induced thermotolerance

An exposure to heat normally leads to a reduction in sensitivity to a second exposure. This effect develops during the first few hours following heating and slowly disappears when the cells or tissue are kept at physiological temperatures.

Figure 9.3 shows an example of thermotolerance measured in the rat tail, using necrosis as the end point. In the absence of pre-treatment, 32 min at 44·5°C produces the specified level of effect. After a pre-treatment at 43°C for 30 min which produces no visible damage on its own, the tissue becomes more resistant to a second application of heat. The maximum resistance in this experiment was reached at 10 h, when 140 min at 44·5°C was needed to produce the specified effect. Thermal resistance dies away gradually over about 1 week.

The extent of thermotolerance depends on the effectiveness of the pre-treatment. It varies between different cells and tissues and the maximum degree of thermotolerance usually requires an increase in heating time by a factor between 2 and 5. Its maximum extent cannot be increased by repeated treatment. There is no clear difference between normal tissues and tumours in the extent or timing of thermal tolerance. In cancer treatment, the effects of thermotolerance can be largely avoided by giving only one or two treatments per week.

If there is a heterogeneous distribution of temperature, the thermotolerance varies from one region to another of the treated volume and these regions have differing sensitivities to a second exposure given a few days later. This might

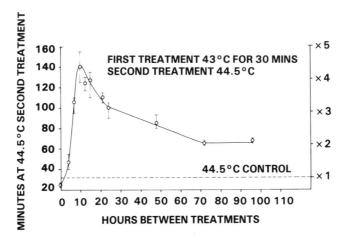

Figure 9.3. Thermotolerance in the rat tail following 43°C for 30 min, tested by measuring the time required to cause a given level of necrosis at 44.5°C at various intervals after the initial treatment. The full line at the bottom shows the effect in the absence of prior treatment.
From [4] with permission of the author and publisher.

reduce the heterogeneity of the total effect but might equally make it worse as thermotolerance in the regions receiving the greatest heating in the first treatment may have almost no response to the second.

9.2 Radiosensitization by hyperthermia

In addition to a direct damaging effect, hyperthermia enhances the effects of irradiation. This is a true case of synergistic action. A moderate exposure to heat such as 42°C for 1 h, causing no observable tissue reaction on its own, will nevertheless sensitize tissues to irradiation. The reaction occurs at the same time as it would have done in the absence of hyperthermia.

The degree of radiosensitization is expressed by the TER (Thermal Enhancement Ratio):

$$TER = D_{ph}/D_{th}$$

the ratio of the doses producing the same effect at a physiological temperature (D_{ph}) and at the hyperthermic temperature (D_{th}).

The TER depends on the temperature, the period of heating and the time interval between heat and radiation. It is greatest when irradiation and hyperthermia are simultaneous. There is considerable variability in TER values among normal tissues and tumours but no consistent difference between the two. Figure 9.4 shows the range of TER values observed when heat and radiation are applied simultaneously or with a minimum time interval. The TER rises steadily with the thermal exposure and the response of tumours seems even more varied than that of normal tissues.

When heat and irradiation are separated by a few hours the TER is reduced. When heat is given after irradiation there seems to be a difference between the response of normal tissues and tumours [4, 7] (Figure 9.5). This provides a

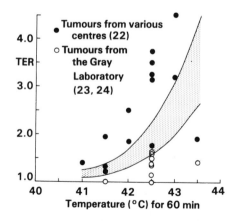

Figure 9.4. Thermal enhancement ratio for tumours and normal tissues as a function of temperature for 1 h heating. The two curves indicate the range of values for normal tissues. The data points refer to various experimental tumours. From [4] with permission of the author and publisher.

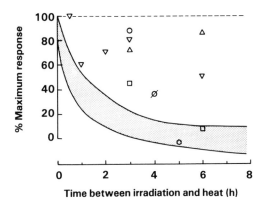

Figure 9.5. The decay of thermal enhancement of X-ray damage by heat given after irradiation. The shaded area indicates the range for normal tissues. Symbols and the broken line indicate values for different rodent tumours. From [4] with permission of the author and publisher.

rationale for sequential application, with heat given 4 h or more after irradiation. Some clinical studies have confirmed the advantage of sequential rather than quasi-simultaneous administration [4].

There is some indication that thermotolerance also reduces thermal sensitization, but to a lesser extent than for direct thermal damage.

There seem to be several mechanisms of radiosensitization which may be different depending on whether hyperthermia is given before or after irradiation. Ben-Hur *et al.* [1] have shown that heat inhibits the repair of radiation induced lesions; but heating 8–12 h after irradiation still has some sensitizing effect at a time when the repair of radiation induced lesions is already complete.

The response of hypoxic cells to a combination of radiation and hyperthermia is controversial. Some studies have shown an increased TER under hypoxia, i.e. a reduction in OER by hyperthermia, but this finding has not been confirmed in other studies.

9.3 Chemosensitization by hyperthermia

Hyperthermia increases the cytotoxicity of various chemotherapeutic agents. The effect appears at relatively low temperatures (40°C) and becomes very important at 42°C (Figure 9.6).

There are various mechanisms of action:

(i)   for adriamycin there is an increase in intracellular concentration, due to modification of the properties of the membrane by hyperthermia;

(ii) for bleomycin, sensitization is due at least in part to inhibition of repair of the chemically induced lesions;

(iii) the biochemical environment of the cells is an important factor and sensitization is more marked in conditions of low pH, low oxygenation and poor nutrient supply.

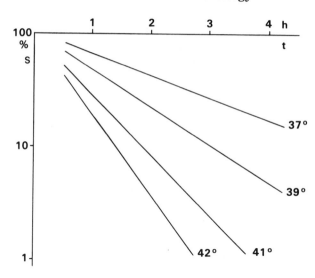

Figure 9.6. **Chemosensitization by hyperthermia. Cell killing by many chemotherapeutic drugs is greatly increased by hyperthermia. Cell survival curves are shown as a function of time of heating in the presence of 5 mg/l thiotepa (after [5]).**

The cytotoxicity of nitro-imidazoles, used as hypoxic-cell radiosensitizers (Section 10.3), is strongly influenced by temperature. The cytotoxicity of these compounds for hypoxic cells is moderate at 37°C and becomes important at 42–45°C while their cytotoxicity remains almost zero for well-oxygenated cells. It is likely that other compounds which do not affect cells at 37°C may become toxic at increased temperatures due to greater penetration through the cell membranes.

9.4 Therapeutic applications

Although the biological effects of hyperthermia are well established, its value in the treatment of human cancer is still uncertain.

Total body hyperthermia is little used. Its biological basis is different from that of localized hyperthermia because the temperatures which can be tolerated (about 41°C) are usually insufficient to cause cell death or to induce significant radiosensitization or chemosensitization. Its toxicity is serious, particularly for the liver and heart. Nevertheless interesting results have been reported, particularly for lymphomas and osteosarcomas [6, 8].

For tumours in the limbs (melanomas, osteosarcomas), regional hyperthermia can be achieved by extra-corporeal circulation of heated blood [2].

Most clinical trials are concerned with localized hyperthermia. When it is possible to achieve a temperature greater than 42°C, tumour regression after 6–10 applications of 1 h each occurs in about 30% of the cases. In general, hyperthermia on its own has only a temporary effect on the tumour and complete regression is exceptional, perhaps owing to difficulties in achieving a uniformly raised temperature in the entire population of tumour cells. This is a difficult problem for deeply-sited tumours. There may also be lack of uniformity on a microscopic scale due to the effect of blood flow. The increase in temperature of cells close to the small vessels is limited by cooling due to the circulating blood. In spite of these problems, hyperthermia often produces a useful degree of tumour regression and relief of pain is appreciable in one third of the cases.

Combination of hyperthermia with radiotherapy seems to be a more promising treatment. Owing to the difficulties of heating deep-seated tumours, most studies have been carried out on superficial disease such as breast tumours and melanomas. Usually 20–30 Gy is given in two fractions of 2–5 Gy per week (to avoid the effect of thermotolerance)[9]. Overgaard[7] has reviewed 24 trials of this kind; in every case the rate of complete response was increased by adjuvant use of hyperthermia. The actual rate of complete response varied widely, most being in the range 30–90%. This variation is due both to the types of tumour treated and to the conditions of heating. The response rate is correlated with the temperature attained and approaches 100% for minimum temperatures greater than 43°C.

Most of these studies have been performed by external irradiation. The combination of hyperthermia with brachytherapy is very effective: both heating and irradiation can be given interstitially by using the guides for iridium needles as electrodes. This enables a high and uniform temperature to be achieved in the volume of the implant. A dose of 30–40 Gy delivered after an application of 44°C for 45 min often produces a lasting disappearance of the tumour [3]. There have been promising results in patients suffering from local recurrence in an irradiated area, a situation which precludes the delivery of a further high dose of radiation.

In spite of favourable experimental and clinical results, the outlook for hyperthermia combined with radiotherapy is still uncertain. It enables the radiation dose to be reduced, which seems *a priori* desirable when the target volume is large or when the sequelae of previous irradiation prevent a second high dose treatment. But there will be no therapeutic advantage unless the combination of hyperthermia with radiation has a smaller effect on the normal tissues than on the tumour.

Overgaard[7] has reconsidered the principles of combined hyperthermia and radiotherapy in the light of experimental and clinical results. Heat has a particularly marked cytotoxic effect on certain components of the tumour such as hypoxic cells which are relatively radioresistant. Hyperthermia and radiation can be considered to have different cellular targets and their combination has the advantage of complementary action. In addition, some tumours have relatively poor blood perfusion and reach higher temperatures than well-perfused normal tissues. Selectivity between tumour and normal tissue may also be achieved by giving hyperthermia several hours after irradiation (Figure 9.5). Treatments with hyperthermia must be separated by several days to avoid the effects of thermal tolerance. It is usual to give 1 or 2 treatments per week. At the present time the principal problem in the treatment of large or deep-seated tumours is that of achieving a uniformly increased temperature throughout the tumour. Thus the future of hyperthermia in clinical oncology depends on the development of better equipment for heating and for measurement of the temperature reached.

References

1. E. Ben-Hur, M. M. Elkind, B. V. Bronk. Thermally enhanced radioresponse of cultured chinese hamster cells: inhibition of repair of sublethal damage and enhancement of lethal damage. *Radiat. Res.*, 1974, **58**: 38–51.
2. R. Cavalière, F. Di Filipo, G. Miricca, *et al.* Hyperthermia and chemotherapy by regional perfusion for tumours of the extremities, in: *Biomedical thermology* (M. Gautherie, E. Albert), pp. 775–792. Alan Liss, New York, 1982.
3. J. M. Cosset, J. Dutreix, J. Dufour, *et al.* Combined interstitial hyperthermia and brachytherapy. *Int. J. Radiat. Oncol. Biol. Phys.*, 1984, **10**: 307–312.
4. S. B. Field. Hyperthermia in the treatment of cancer. *Phys. Med. Biol.*, 1987, **32**: 789–811.
5. H. A. Johnson and M. Pavelec. Thermal enhancement of trio-TEPA cytotoxicity. *J. Nat. Cancer Int.*, 1973, **50**: 903–908.
6. H. C. Nauts. Bacterials pyrogens: beneficial effects on cancer patients, in: *Biomedical Thermology* (M. Gautherie, E. Albert, eds). pp. 687–696. Alan Liss, New York, 1982.
7. J. Overgaard. The current and potential role of hyperthermia in radiotherapy. *Int. J. Rad. Oncol. Biol. Phys.*, 1989, **16**: 535–545.
8. R. T. Pettigrew. Cancer therapy by whole body heating. *Proceedings Int. Symposium on Cancer Therapy by Hyperthermia and Radiation* (M. Wizenberg, J. E. Robinson, eds.), pp. 282–288. Baltimore, Am. College Radiology Press, 1975.
9. J. Van Der Zee, G. C. Van Rhoon, J. L. Wike-Hooley, H. S. Rheinhold. Clinically derived dose effect relationship for hyperthermia given in combination with low dose radiotherapy. *Br. J. Radiol.*, 1985, **58**: 243–250.

Bibliography

L. J. Anghileri, J. Robert. *Hyperthermia in cancer treatment* (3 vols.). CRC Press, Inc., Boca Raton, Florida, 1986.

G. Arcangeli, F. Mauro. *Hyperthermia in radiation oncology.* Masson, Milan, 1980.

L. A. Dethlefsen, W. C. Dewey. *Cancer therapy by hyperthermia, drugs and radiation.* Washington, NCI Monograph 61, 1982.

S. B. Field, C. Franconi (Eds). Physics and technology of hyperthermia. Martinus Nijhoff, Dordrecht, 1987.

S. B. Field. Cellular and tissue effect of hyperthermia and radiation, in: *The biological basis of radiotherapy* (G. Steel, M. Peckham, eds.), pp. 287–303. Elsevier, Amsterdam, 1983.

M. Gautherie, E. Albert. *Biomedical thermology.* Alan R. Liss, New York, 1982.

G. M. Hahn. *Hyperthermia and cancer.* Plenum Press, New York, 1982.

J. Overgaard. *Hyperthermic oncology.* Taylor and Francis, Philadelphia, London, 1984.

Chapter 10.
Chemical modifiers of radiosensitivity

The effects of radiation can be increased or reduced by various chemical substances called radiosensitizers or radioprotectors, according to their action. Their mechanisms of action have been considered in Chapter 2.

Radiosensitizers have been studied intensively because of their possible application in radiotherapy. In the past the main interest of radioprotectors has been for application in the military field and in space; however, more interest is now being shown in their possible use in radiotherapy.

10.1 Radiosensitizers other than oxygen

Radiosensitization will be considered in terms of cell death and the resulting effects on tissues. Ideally the sensitizer has no lethal effect on its own, but at a given dose of radiation the presence of the radiosensitizer reduces the proportion of surviving cells (Figure 10.1a). The sensitization is expressed by the sensitizer enhancement ratio (SER), analogous to the oxygen enhancement ratio (OER). $SER = D/D_m$, the ratio of the doses needed to obtain a given effect in the absence (D) and in the presence (D_m) of the sensitizer. This definition can be used for any observable effect, even if it cannot be measured in numerical terms.

If the sensitizer has a toxic effect on its own, this complicates the demonstration and even more the measurement of any synergistic effect. Modification of the surivial curve $S(D)$ by chemical pre-treatment can result from several mechanisms which are considered in Figure 10.1b.

In addition, chemical pretreatment may modify the survival curve either because of a selective lethal effect on subpopulations of resistant cells, e.g. cells in S phase, or because of synchronization. In this case the lethal effect of radiation can be increased if the cells are synchronized in a radiosensitive phase of the cycle, without any change in their intrinsic radiosensitivity. In fact this phenomenon has never been observed in patients.

The most important true radiosensitizer is oxygen. Chapter 7 was devoted to it because of its importance and its significance in radiotherapy. It has no toxic effect on cells at the concentration attained in tissue. Oxygen acts during the initial physico-chemical stages of radiation action. It must be present during irradiation even if this is very short. Some other substances, particularly

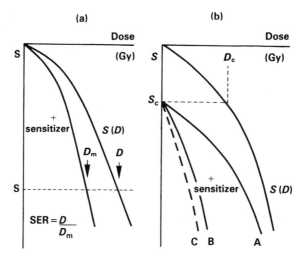

Figure 10.1. Effect of a radiosensitizer on survival curves.
(a) The sensitizer enhancement ratio (SER) is defined as the ratio of doses needed to obtain a given surviving fraction without (D) or with (D_m) the radiosensitizer.
(b) If the radiosensitizer is itself toxic, a change in the survival curve may not imply true sensitization. In this case the cells receive chemical pre-treatment which on its own leads to a surviving fraction S_c. If the cells are then irradiated with increasing doses D, the survival curve may take various shapes, as follows:
A. The curve A has the same shape as $S(D)$; it is formed from $S(D)$ by a simple vertical shift. In this case the mechanisms of cell death are totally independent and there is no interaction.
B. Curve B corresponds to the part of $S(D)$ beyond S_c; it is formed from $S(D)$ by a horizontal shift. In this case the chemical agent is a true radiomimetic: the effect of the chemical pre-treatment is the same as that of an irradiation to dose D_c leading to the surviving fraction S_c; the condition of the population of surviving cells, in particular with regard to the sublethal lesions, is the same as after a dose D_c. The effect of irradiation to dose D after chemical pre-treatment is therefore the same as for irradiation to dose $D_c + D$. There is a simple addition of the effects of the two agents which have the same action. If the interval of time between the pre-treatment and irradiation is increased, one would expect, as with two fractions of irradiation, that curve B would shift towards curve A.
C. A synergistic effect or true radiosensitization is demonstrated only if the surviving fraction is below that given by curve B; inversely, radioprotection if the surviving fraction is greater than given by curve A. In many cases the curve lies between A and B which neither excludes nor demonstrates a synergistic action.

sensitizers of hypoxic cells, have biochemical and radiobiological properties similar to those of oxygen.

Most of the other radiosensitizers operate by their action on DNA [20]. They may:

modify the structure of DNA in such a way as to make it more sensitive to the action of radiation;
inhibit the repair of sublethal damage produced by irradiation;
inhibit DNA synthesis.
Only the first two of these represent true radiosensitization.

The structure of DNA can be modified by incorporation of a halogenated pyrimidine, which is an analogue of thymine: 5-bromo (or chloro-, iodo-, fluoro-) deoxyuridine (BrdU, CldU, IdU, FdU).

The configuration of the halogenated pyrimidines is sufficiently close to that of thymine to allow their substitution during DNA synthesis (Chapter 3, Figure 3.27); a similar substitution is possible with cytosine. It has been found with bacteria and later with mammalian cells that substituted DNA is sensitized to the action of radiation (Table 10.1 and Figure 3.28).

Radiosensitization by halogenated pyrimidines depends on their incorporation into DNA. This increases with the number of cell cycles. One might therefore hope for a greater incorporation of BrdU into tumour cells which are in rapid proliferation than into the cells of normal tissue. A differential radiosensitizing effect between a mouse sarcoma and skin has been shown by Brown *et al.* [9]. Clinical studies have been made with BrdU on tumours of the head and neck and brain tumours [4]. The results have not been encouraging, perhaps because of the mitotic stimulation in normal tissues during fractionated irradiation (Chapter 5); in fact some toxicity has been seen for the bone marrow and intestine.

Table 10.1 Radiosensitization by 5-BrdU. Hamster cells cultured for 6 days in the presence of BrdU at the concentration C.

C(μm)	O	0·05	0·2	0·5	1
Dose (Gy) for $S=10^{-3}$	12·4	11·5	9·8	8·2	6·7
SER	1	1·08	1·27	1·52	1·86

After [22].

Several substances inhibit DNA repair. This effect has been shown for caffeine [10], cytosine arabinoside (Ara-C), aphidicolin and other specific inhibitors of DNA polymerase. Inhibition of DNA repair eliminates the shoulder of the survival curve as the lesions which are normally sublethal and reparable in a few hours become lethal when they are fixed (Figure 4.9). Repair-deficient mutant cell lines show little radiosensitization.

A number of chemotherapeutic agents (such as actinomycin D, bleomycin, adriamycin, 5-fluoro-uracil) (Table 10.2) reduce the shoulders of survival curves when their concentrations are high enough to cause appreciable cell mortality. Under these circumstances it is difficult to distinguish true radiosensitization, due to inhibition of repair, from apparent radiosensitization which is really only an additive effect discussed above (Figure 10.1b). In addition certain substances (5-fluoro-uracil) are particularly toxic for cells in S phase, leading to an apparent radiosensitization by selection.

Table 10.2 Sensitizer enhancement ratio (SER) for some normal tissues with different cytotoxic drugs.

	Dose (mg kg^{-1})	Oesophagus	Lung	Intestine
Actinomycin D	0·75	1·6	1·6	1·2
Bleomycin	3	1·14	0·91	
Cis. Platinum	13	1·49		1·3
Vincristine	0·5	0·98	1·17	0·95
Adriamycin	8			1·15
5 fluoro-uracil	140			1·2
Methotrexate	700			0·9

After [25]

In summary, it has not been established whether the substances currently used in chemotherapy lead to true radiosensitization. However, platinum complexes cause a marked radiosensitization of hypoxic cells, at concentrations which have no effect on the radiosensitivity of oxygenated cells. In any case, even without any synergistic effect, radiotherapy and chemotherapy act in a complementary fashion, justifying their combination in treatment [34, 37].

10.2 Radioprotectors

Mechanism of action

The possibility of reducing the biological effects of irradiation by chemical substances was demonstrated in 1949 by animal experiments showing that the LD50 was considerably increased by administration of glutathione or cysteamine. The possible value of radioprotectors led to the development of pharmacological substances whose toxicity is low enough to enable them to be used clinically [33]. Moreover cells contain natural aminothiols which have some protective power and modify the biological effects of irradiation.

We have seen (Section 2.4) that the protective action of cysteamine and glutathione is attributed to the capture of OH. radicals by sulphydryl groups (– SH). The mechanism of action is complicated by interaction with oxygen; this is due either to competition between the fixation by – SH and O_2 of the radiolysis products of water, or to inactivation of the toxic products created by O_2. The effect of the radioprotector is smaller when irradiation is given under anoxic conditions; it is also reduced with increasing LET, i.e. when the contribution of O_2 to the biological effect is reduced [29].

In general, a protective substance must be easily oxidized by the radiolysis products of water, OH., $O_2H.$, H_2O_2, but it must not be easily oxidized by O_2 which is normally present in biological media. These characteristics occur in a group of molecules with a linear structure containing a few carbon atoms with an amine group, – NH_2, at one end and a sulphurated group at the other (Table 10.3). With one of these drugs (WR 2721) an enhancement of the rejoining of DNA strand breaks has been observed, implying that an increased capacity for cellular repair may play a role in the protective effect.

The protective effect is expressed by the dose modifying factor (DMF) by which the dose must be multiplied to obtain a given biological effect after administration of the radioprotector (Table 10.4).

For oxygenated cells, the survival curve with the radioprotector tends towards the survival curve in anoxic conditions, i.e. the DMF is close to the

Table 10.3 Principal types of radioprotector in current use.

	– H thiols
$NH_2 – (C– ... – C) – S$	– SO_3H thiosulphate
(amino-)	
	– PO_3H phosphoro-thioate
	– SR disulphur
Ex.: cysteamine	$NH_2 – CH_2 – CH_2 – SH$
cystamine	$NH_2 – CH_2 – CH_2 – S$ ⌉
	$NH_2 – CH_2 – CH_2 – S$ ⌋

Table 10.4 Dose modifying factors (DMF). Protector: WR 2721 (NH$_2$ (CH$_2$)$_3$ NH CH$_2$ CH$_2$ SPO$_3$ H$_2$).

Site	DMF†	C‡
Bone marrow	2·4–3	3·5
Liver	2·7	5·3
Skin	2·0–2·4	3·3
Intestine	1·4–2·0	3·9
Kidney	1·5	0·1
CNS	1·0	

† After [38].
‡ After [26].
C, concentration relative to concentration in blood (mice).

OER, suggesting that the radioprotector counteracts the effects of O$_2$ but is unable to suppress them completely at usable concentrations.

For anoxic cells, the effect of radioprotectors is much smaller and the DMF is only a little greater than 1. Nevertheless the fact that it is greater than 1 shows that the radioprotector has an effect independent of its interaction with O$_2$.

The role of radioprotectors which are normally found in biological media has been demonstrated by Revesz *et al.* [28] and Deschavannes *et al.* [12] in subjects presenting with a congenital condition characterized by an intracellular deficiency of glutathione. These cells do not show an oxygen effect, i.e. their radiosensitivity is not reduced in hypoxic conditions. This suggests that the glutathione present in normal cells has a radioprotective effect if the concentration of O$_2$ is very low (900 ppm) but that it cannot counteract the effect of O$_2$ at normal concentration. In cells deficient in glutathione, oxygen exerts its full effect at a very low concentration, i.e. when the cells are hypoxic; the addition of an artificial radioprotector (cysteamine 20 mM) gives the same reduction in biological effect as it does in normal cells under hypoxic conditions. Moreover it has been shown that the content of glutathione in cells varies during the cell cycle in a manner corresponding to the variations of radiosensitivity (Section 4.4). Compounds able to react with thiol groups can cause a depletion of natural intracellular aminothiols or a reduction of their activity. *In vitro* they increase cellular radiosensitivity. Their effectiveness *in vivo* is small, probably because of metabolic instability.

Clinical applications of radioprotectors have been limited by their toxicity: nausea, vomiting, diarrhoea, hypotension, somnolence, etc. Nevertheless, the more recent products do give appreciable protection at concentrations which are well tolerated.

After administration by mouth or injection, the degree of protection is variable and depends on the tissue considered (Table 10.4). It depends on the concentration in the tissue; this is high in liver and very low in the central nervous system. However, the correlation is not very strict. The pharmacokinetics vary depending on the product. The time to reach maximum protection and the duration of protection are also variable and are in the range 15 min to 3 h.

Applications

Radioprotectors act only if they are present at the time of irradiation. They cannot therefore be used to reduce the effect of accidental external irradiation. Their applications in the military field and in space are limited to certain instances where irradiation can be foreseen, e.g. fallout from a nuclear explosion or solar flares. For use in a planned intervention after a civil or military accident (e.g. in a reactor) the protector must not interfere with consciousness. This raises difficult problems as most radioprotectors induce somnolence; a mixture of compounds may be more effective.

In radiotherapy they may be useful for total-body and half-body irradiation, in order to reduce the effect of irradiation on the bone marrow; usually there seems to be a greater protective effect on this tissue than on others (see Table 10.4).

For localized irradiation, radioprotectors would be of interest only if they had a selective action on normal tissues. Studies on experimental tumours have shown that they are less well protected than normal tissues, due to the small concentration reached in the tumour, which may be attributed to poor perfusion of blood. Another favourable characteristic for radiotherapy is the absence of protection for anoxic cells.

Application in radiotherapy depends on the development of products with low toxicity, allowing repeated administration of effective quantities of radioprotector during a course of fractionated irradiation [21].

10.3 Hypoxic cell sensitizers

The role of oxygen in the biochemical and biological effects of radiation is largely due to its interaction with the radicals produced during the radiolysis of water (Chapters 2 and 7). This action is of a physico-chemical nature and is connected with the affinity of the oxygen molecule for electrons. In 1963, Adams and Dewey [2] suggested that other electron-affinic molecules should have a similar action. Experiments *in vitro* have confirmed the correlation between radiosensitization of hypoxic cells and the electron-affinity of derivatives of quinones, acetophenones and nitrofuran, but the possibility of clinical use of these substances is very limited because of their toxicity or their instability in the living body.

In 1973 [1] attention was focused on derivatives of imidazole, in particular on metronidazole, a common pharmaceutical (Flagyl) whose pharmacological properties were well understood.

Experiments with cells *in vitro* [18] showed that, at a concentration of 10 mM, metronidazole:

(i) has no lethal effects on oxygenated cells and does not affect their radiosensitivity;
(ii) increases the radiosensitivity of hypoxic cells. With γ-rays the SER is equal to $1 \cdot 7$, the OER being reduced from 3 to $1 \cdot 8$; with neutrons the OER is reduced from $1 \cdot 5$ to $1 \cdot 25$ (SER$=1 \cdot 2$).

Animal experiments have confirmed that metronidazole, in doses without any observable pathological effect, produces radiosensitization of normal tissues which have been rendered artificially hypoxic. A study on a mouse mammary carcinoma [5] showed an increase in the therapeutic effect, the dose of radiation needed to obtain 50% tumour control being reduced from 40 to 31 Gy after administration of metronidazole ($2 \cdot 5$ g kg^{-1}).

A clinical study on patients suffering from glioblastoma [35] showed a prolongation of life in patients who had received metronidazole at a dose of 6 g m^{-2} of body surface 4 h before each fraction of irradiation. However, in order to reduce the number of administrations of the drug, the irradiation was given in 9 fractions of $3 \cdot 3$ Gy over 18 days; the results of irradiation alone given under these conditions were inferior to those obtained with a conventional fractionation scheme and the metronidazole only compensated for the unfavourable effect of the reduced number of fractions. A second trial [36] undertaken with standard fractionation of 58 Gy in 30 fractions over 6 weeks no longer showed any advantage of metronidazole.

The next drug to be tried was misonidazole which, in the series of nitro-imidazoles, shows a particularly great affinity for electrons [3]. *In vitro* experiments have confirmed a large sensitization of hypoxic cells; at a concentration of 10 mM (2 mg ml^{-1}), the SER is close to the OER (Figure 10.2). Experiments on the skin of mice [11] (Figure 10.3), made hypoxic by nitrogen breathing for 35 s before irradiation, showed an SER of $2 \cdot 2$ for misonidazole at $1 \cdot 5$ g kg^{-1} given 7–12 min previously, which is only a little less than the OER ($2 \cdot 5$–$2 \cdot 8$).

For mouse mammary tumours the dose needed to obtain 50% control is reduced from 44 to 24 Gy by administration of misonidazole at 1 g kg^{-1} [31] (Figure 10.4). As one might expect from the phenomenon of reoxygenation (Section 7.3), the effect is reduced with fractionated irradiation [32]: when the radiation doses are adjusted to give the same effect on the skin, the rate of tumour control without sensitizer increases with fractionation whereas after administration of misonidazole it remains almost constant. Misonidazole increases the tumour control rate from 0 to 50% for a single dose of 25 Gy, from

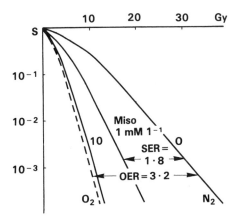

Figure 10.2. **Radiosensitizing effect of misonidazole on anoxic cells; hamster cells *in vitro*. At a concentration of 10 mM (2 mg ml^{-1}) the radiosensitivity of anoxic cells is close to that of oxygenated cells, i.e. the SER for anoxic cells is close to the OER. After [16].**

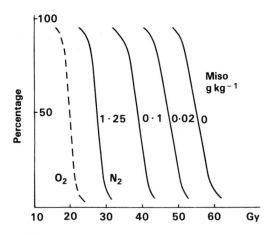

Figure 10.3. Radiosensitizing effect of misonidazole *in vivo* on mouse skin. The full lines represent the percentage of clones obtained in the skin of nitrogen-breathing mice as a function of the radiation dose, after administration of misonidazole with the dosage shown. The broken curve corresponds to normal oxygenation. After [11].

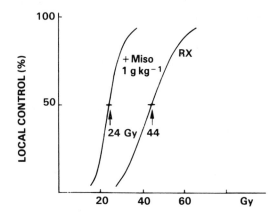

Figure 10.4. Therapeutic effect of misonidazole on mammary tumours in mice. After [23, 31, 32].

25 to 50% for 5 fractions of 8·7 Gy and has no appreciable effect with 15 fractions.

In addition to radiosensitization, nitro-imidazoles have a lethal effect on hypoxic cells. This effect is increased with hyperthermia (Section 9.3), raising the possibility of using nitro-imidazoles in combination with hyperthermia as a chemotherapeutic agent which is relatively selective for the hypoxic cells. The cytotoxic effect on the tumour can be enhanced by using vasodilating drugs (hydralazine) which reduce blood flow in the tumour and increase tumour hypoxia (up to 100% in some experimental tumours), with a lesser effect on normal tissues. The vasodilators also increase the tumour toxicity of melphalan with a small increase in systemic cytotoxicity. Various methods of combining them with sensitizers, chemotherapeutic drugs and radiation have been suggested for clinical applications [17]. Severe tumour hypoxia can also be induced by modifiers of the oxyhaemoglobin association curve in order to reduce its affinity for oxygen.

Clinical use of misonidazole began in 1974 [13, 15]. After oral administration, the concentration in serum reaches a maximum between 2 and 4 h and diminishes over a period of 10–15 h. The maximum concentration is about 50 mg l^{-1} for a dose of 1 g m^{-2} of surface area or 30 mg kg^{-1} weight. Its concentration in normal tissues is close to the concentration in blood whereas in tumours it is very variable, from 10 to 90% of the blood concentration.

The doses usable in the clinic are limited by gastrointestinal and neurological toxicity. Convulsions have occurred after high doses. With lower doses, toxicity takes the form of peripheral neuropathy affecting mainly the sensory nerves: tingling sensations, painful cramps and loss of sensitivity to vibration. The frequency of neuropathy depends on the dose used: 30% for 12 g m^{-2}, 80% for 15 g m^{-2}, which limits the acceptable dose to about 10 g m^{-2}. If the total acceptable dose is divided into many fractions the blood concentration cannot reach the level necessary for a significant radiosensitization of the hypoxic cells. Some radiotherapists have opted for a treatment regime of less than 10 fractions with a dose of misonidazole before each. If one wishes to retain the therapeutic advantage of small doses per fraction (Section 8.3) and the multiple phases of reoxygenation which occur with conventional fractionation, the administration of misonidazole must be limited to only a part of the course of irradiation. Use of several fractions per day makes it possible to reduce the number of treatment days and to reconcile small doses of radiation per fraction with the presence of the radiosensitizer at each treatment [6, 19]. With two or three fractions separated by a few hours on each treatment day, almost complete repair of sublethal damage can be expected together with considerable reoxygenation. The pharmacokinetics of misonidazole make it possible to give these fractions after each dose of drug during the time when the serum concentration is close to the maximum [13].

Therapeutic trials of misonidazole have given conflicting results [7, 13, 24, 27]. Nevertheless one third of the trials in tumours of the head and neck did have a favourable conclusion, which justifies a continuation of clinical studies aimed at identifying the best conditions of use [8, 14].

Clinical use of hypoxic-cell radiosensitizers is limited by their toxicity. Pharmacological research is continuing in several directions in order to reduce their toxicity and increase their effectiveness [13]. The neurotoxicity seems to be connected with the lipophilic characteristic of the product, which has much less effect on its intracellular uptake. This should be reduced with less lipophilic drugs. The partition coefficient between octanol and water, which expresses the relative affinity of lipids and water, is high for misonidazole (0·43) and very low (0·02) for the more hydrophilic derivatives of the imidazoles which can, however, still cross cell membranes. Pharmacokinetics also play a role since toxicity is related to the time profile of the blood concentration and is reduced when elimination is fast. The 'area under the curve' is relevant for toxicity whereas the efficacy is related to the tissue concentration at the moment of irradiation. Two particularly promising drugs, etanidazole (SR 2508) and pimonidazole (Ro 03-8799) are under clinical evaluation.

Another line of research is chemical protection against the neurotoxicity of misonidazole. This possibility was revealed by the observation of reduced neurotoxicity in patients receiving a steroid (dexamethasone) in the course of treatment. A certain number of other substances have shown a protective effect *in vitro* on the toxicity of misonidazole without reducing its effectiveness as a radiosensitizer.

Radiosensitization and toxicity are not directly related, an encouragement into research towards more effective drugs. Derivatives of imidazole with greater electron affinity than that of misonidazole have been identified, and have shown themselves to be more effective *in vitro*. Their toxicity *in vivo* has not yet been evaluated.

Electron affinity is a characteristic determining the effectiveness of hypoxic-cell sensitizers. However, some highly electro-affinic compounds which are very efficient *in vitro* have no effect *in vivo* because of their high metabolic reactivity. Furthermore, certain compounds have been found to possess a markedly greater effectiveness, both *in vitro* and *in vivo*, than would be expected from their electron affinity. This effectiveness can be due to a high intracellular concentration or to selective binding to DNA. Studies are continuing on derivatives with cytotoxic properties, particularly those containing alkylating groups; some of these give a sensitization equal to that of misonidazole with a concentration 10 times lower, but study of their toxicity is not yet complete.

There is also interest in combinations of sensitizers having different types of toxicity (e.g. pimonidazole and etanidazole) enabling their sensitizing action to be added without exceeding general tolerance.

Intratumour injection of the sensitizer may be a means of reducing its general toxicity and clinical studies have given encouraging results [30].

Clinical studies of hypoxic-cell sensitizers have generated less interest during recent years as their practical effectiveness has not been demonstrated, whereas their toxic effects are well established. However, there is continuing interest connected on the one hand with new pharmacological developments and on the other with identification of the tumours in which hypoxic cells are an important factor in therapeutic failure.

References

1. G. E. Adams. Chemical radiosensitization of hypoxic cells. *Br. Med. Bull.*, 1973, **29**: 48–53.
2. G. E. Adams, D. L. Dewey. Hydrated electrons and radiobiological sensitization. *Biochem. Biophys. Res. Commun.*, 1963, **12**: 473–477.
3. G. E. Adams, I. R. Flockart, C. E. Smithen, J. J. Strafford, F. Wardman, M. E. Watts. Electron-affinic sensitization VIII. A correlation between structures, one electron reduction potentials and efficiencies of nitroimidazoles as hypoxic cells radiosensitizers. *Radiat. Res.*, 1976, **67**: 9–20.
4. M. A. Bagshaw, R. L. Doggett, S. C. Smith. Intra-arterial 5-bromodeoxyuridine and X-ray therapy. *Am. J. Roentgenol.*, 1967, **99**: 889–894.
5. A. C. Begg, P. W. Sheldon, J. L. Foster. Demonstration of radiosensitization of hypoxic cells in solid tumours by metronidazole, *Br. J. Radiol.*, 1974, **47**: 399–404.
6. W. van den Bogaert, E. van der Schueren, J. C. Horiot, *et al.* The feasibility of high-dose multiple daily fractionation (MDF) and it combination with anoxic cell sensitizers in the treatment of head and neck cancer. A pilot study of the EORTC Radiotherapy Group. *Int. J. Radiat. Oncol. Biol. Phys.*, 1982, **8**: 1649–1655.
7. J. M. Brown. Clinical trials of radiosensitizers: what should we expect? *Int. J. Radiat. Oncol. Biol. Phys.*, 1984, **10**: 425–429.
8. J. M. Brown. Hypoxic cell radiosensitizers: what next? *Int. J. Radiat. Oncol. Biol. Phys.*, 1989, **16**: 987–993.
9. J. M. Brown, D. R. Goffinet, J. E. Cleaver, R. F. Kallman. Preferential radiosensitization of mouse sarcoma relative to normal skin by chronic intra-arterial infusion of halogenated pyrimidine analogs. *J. Natl. Cancer Inst.*, 1971, **47**: 75–89.
10. J. Calkins. A method of analysis of radiation response based on enzyme kinetics. *Radiat. Res.*, 1971, **45**: 50–62.
11. J. Denekamp, B. D. Michael, J. R. Harris. Hypoxic cell radiosensitizers: comparative tests of some electron affinic compounds using epidermal cell survival *in vivo*. *Radiat. Res.*, 1974, **60**: 119–132.
12. P. J. Deschavanne, J. Midander, M. Edgren, A. Larsson, E. P. Malaise, L. Revesz. Oxygen enchancement of radiation induced lethality is greatly reduced in glutathione deficient human fibroblasts. *Biomedicine*, 1981, **35**: 35–37.
13. S. Dische. Chemical sensitizers for hypoxic cells: a decade of experience in clinical radiotherapy. *Radioth. Oncol.*, 1985, **3**: 97–115.
14. S. Dische. Hypoxic cell sensitizers: clinical developments. *Int. J. Radiat. Oncol. Biol. Phys.*, 1989, **16**: 1057–1060.
15. S. Dische, A. J. Gray, G. D. Zanelli. Clinical testing of the radiosensitizer Ro-07-0582 II. Radiosensitization of normal and hypoxic skin. *Clin. Radiol.*, 1976, **27**: 159–166.
16. J. F. Fowler, G. E. Adams, J. Denekamp. Radiosensitizers of hypoxic cells in solid tumours. *Cancer Treat. Rev.*, 1976, **3**: 227–256.
17. M. Guichard. Chemical manipulations of tissue oxygenation for therapeutic purpose. *Int. J. Radiat. Oncol. Biol. Phys.*, 1989, **16**: 1125–1130.
18. E. J. Hall, L. Roizin-Towle. Hypoxic sensitizers: radiobiological studies at the cellular level. *Radiology*, 1975, **117**: 453–457.
19. J. C. Horiot, A. Nabid, G. Chaplain, S. Jampolis, W. van den Bogaert, E. van der Schueren, G. Arcangeli, D. Gonzales, V. Svoboda, H. P. Hamers. Clinical experience with multiple fractions per day (MFD) in the radiotherapy of head and neck carcinoma. *J. Eur. Radiother.*, 1982, **3**: 79–89.
20. G. Iliakis, S. Kurtzman. Application of non-hypoxic cell sensitizers in radiobiology and radiotherapy: rationale and future prospects. *Int. J. Radiat. Oncol. Biol. Phys.*, 1989, **16**: 1235–1241.
21. M. M. Kligerman, M. T. Shaw, M. Slavik, J. M. Yuhas. Phase I clinical studies with WR-2721. *Cancer Clin. Trials*, 1980, **3**: 217–221.
22. W. C. Moehler, M. M. Elkind. Radiation response of mammalian cells grown in culture. III. Modification of X-ray survival of chinese hamster cells by 5-bromo-deoxyuridine. *Exp. Cell. Res.*, 1963, **30**: 481–491.
23. L. E. Orr, A. M. N. Syed, A. Puthawala, F. W. George, J. F. McKernan, D. N. Halikis. Radiosentizers in head and neck carcinoma, in: *Front. Radiat. Ther. Onc.*, vol. 13, 215–227, Karger, Basel, 1979.
24. J. Overgaard, H. S. Hansen, K. Jorgensen, M. H. Hansen. Primary radiotherapy of larynx and pharynx carcinoma — an analysis of some factors influencing local control and survival. *Int. J. Radiat. Oncol. Biol. Phys.*, 1986, **12**: 515–521.

25. T.L. Phillips. Effects on lung of combined radiotherapy and chemotherapy. In: *Frontiers in radiation therapy and oncology*, vol. 13 (J.M. Vaeth, ed.), pp.133–135. S. Kärger, New York, 1979.
26. T.L. Phillips. Rationale for initial clinical trials and future development of radioprotectors. pp. 311–329. In: *Radiation sensitizers* (L.W. Brady, ed.). Masson, New York, 1980.
27. L. Revesz, S.B. Balmukhanov. Anaemia as a prognostic factor for the therapeutic effect of radiosensitizers. *Int. J. Radiat. Biol.*, 1987, **51**: 591–595.
28. L. Revesz, M. Edgren. Mechanisms of radiosensitization and protection studied with glutathione deficient human cell lines, in: *Progress in Radio Oncology II* pp. 235–242. (K.H. Kärcher *et al.* eds), Raven Press, New York, 1982.
29. A. Rojas, R.L. Maugham, J. Denekamp. Effects of modifiers on high and low LET responses *in vivo*. *Radioth. Oncol.*, 1984, **2**: 65–73.
30. R. Sealy, J. Korrubel, S. Cridland, G. Blekkenhorst. Interstitial misonidazole. *Cancer*, 1984, **54**: 1535–1540.
31. P.W. Sheldon, J.L. Foster, J.F. Fowler. Radiosensitization of C3 H mouse mammary tumours by a 2-nitroimidazole drug. *Br. J. Cancer*, 1974, **30**: 560–565.
32. P.W. Sheldon, S.A. Hill, J.L. Foster, J.F. Fowler. Radiosensitization of C3 H mouse mammary tumours using fractionated doses of X-rays with the drug Ro-07-0582. *Br. J. Radiol.*, 1976, **49**: 76–80.
33. F.A. Stewart. Modification of normal tissue response to radiotherapy and chemotherapy. *Int. J. Radiat. Oncol. Biol. Phys.*, 1989, **16**: 1195–1200.
34. M. Tubiana. The 1987 Franz Buschke Lecture: The role of radiotherapy in the treatment of chemosensitive tumors. *Int. J. Radiat. Onc. Biol. Phys.*, 1989, **16**: 763–774.
35. R.C. Urtasun, P. Band, J.D. Chapman, M.L. Feldstein, B. Mielke, C. Fryer. Radiation and high dose metronidazole (Flagyl) in supratentorial glioblastomas. *N. Engl. J. Med.*, 1976, **284**: 1364–1367.
36. R. Urtasun, M.L. Feldstein, J. Partington, *et al.* Radiation and nitroimidazoles in supratentorial high grade gliomas. A second clinical trial. *Br. J. Cancer,* 1982, **46**: 101–108.
37. J.M. Vaeth. Combined effects of chemotherapy and radiotherapy in normal tissue tolerance, in: *Frontiers of radiation therapy and oncology*, vol. 13, Karger, Basel, 1979.
38. M. Yuhas, J.M. Stellman, F. Culo. The role of WR 2721 in radiotherapy and/or chemotherapy. In: Radiation sensitizers (L.W. Brady, ed.). pp. 303–308. Masson, New York, 1980.

Bibliography

L.W. Brady. *Radiation sensitizers*. Masson, New York, 1980.
4th Conference on Chemical modifiers of cancer treatment. *Int. J. Radiat. Oncol. Biol. Phys.*, 1984, **10**: 1161–1483 and 1495–1795.
5th Conference on chemical modifiers of cancer treatment, Clearwater 1985. *Int. J. Radiat. Oncol. Biol. Phys.*, 1986, **12**: 1019–1545.
6th Conference on chemical modifiers of cancer treatment, Paris 1988. *Int. J. Radiat. Oncol. Biol. Phys.*, 1989, **16**: 887–1345.

Chapter 11.
Neutrons and other heavy particles

The radiobiological data discussed in the preceding chapters relate for the most part to irradiations with X- or γ-rays. Neutrons and other heavy particles deserve special consideration both because of their increasing importance in radiotherapy and because of the special problems they raise in radiation protection.

Radiotherapy is currently practised with *photons*, mainly high-energy X- or γ-ray beams. During the last 20 years, *beams of high-energy electrons* have gained a place as a valuable technique for well defined applications. Photons and electrons (called low-LET radiation; see Chapter 1) allow irradiation to be delivered with great physical precision. Their therapeutic effectiveness has been proved by long clinical experience. However, these classical techniques are inadequate for certain types of tumour and/or clinical situations, and new approaches are now the subject of clinical trials.

One possible way ahead is the use of radiations whose radiobiological characteristics are different from those produced by conventional radiations. This is the case with *high-LET radiations. Fast neutrons* are an example and are used today in about 20 centres around the world. Another route is research into radiations which enable the *physical selectivity* of the treatment to be further improved (beams of protons, helium ions, heavy ions and negative pi-mesons). Heavy ions and to a lesser extent pi-mesons are high-LET radiations and therefore also have the potential advantage of fast neutron beams.

Application of these radiations requires the use of large and complex equipment, particularly for heavy ions and pi-mesons, which limits the extent of clinical applications.

The advantage to be gained from an improvement in physical selectivity can to a large extent be estimated in advance but it is more difficult to evaluate the benefit to be expected from use of high-LET radiations, although a large amount of radiobiological and clinical data have already been accumulated. Study of the radiobiological properties of high-LET radiations will be the subject of the first part of this chapter. We will then discuss the arguments which form the rationale for therapeutic application of fast neutrons and we will try to evaluate their future in radiotherapy. The other heavy particles which are in use — or might be used — in radiotherapy will be the subject of the third part of the chapter. Finally, we will discuss some specific problems raised by fission neutrons and other high-LET particles in radiation protection.

11.1 Radiobiological properties of high-LET radiations

Linear energy transfer (LET) and relative biological effectiveness (RBE)

Relative biological effectiveness (RBE)

At a given absorbed dose, different types of radiation produce different biological effects; furthermore, the shape of the dose–effect relation may be different. Hence the concept of relative biological effectiveness or RBE.

When comparing two types of radiation, differing in nature and/or energy, the *relative biological effectiveness* (RBE) of the radiation under investigation ('test') compared with a reference radiation ('ref') is the ratio D_{ref}/D_{test}, in which D_{ref} and D_{test} represent the absorbed doses resulting in a given biological effect in a given system. The concept of RBE must therefore refer to a well-defined biological effect at a particular level (Figure 11.1). The RBE depends on several

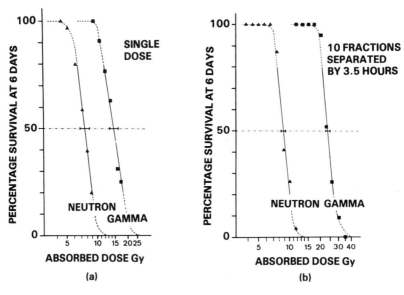

Figure 11.1. Determination of the relative biological effectiveness (RBE) of d(50)+Be neutrons in comparison with ^{60}Co. The test radiation was neutrons produced from a cyclotron by bombarding a thick target of beryllium with 50 MeV deuterons. The reference radiation was γ-rays from ^{60}Co. Randomized groups of similar animals were irradiated and kept under the same environmental conditions. The biological criterion used was the mean lethal dose (LD 50) for a population of female NMRI mice given abdominal irradiation. The proportion of surviving animals was evaluated at 5–6 days after irradiation (gastrointestinal syndrome).
(a) Irradiation given as a single dose. The LD 50 measured at 6 days (LD 50/6) is 14·35±1·45 Gy for ^{60}Co and 7·67±0·60 Gy for d(50)+Be neutrons, giving a neutron RBE of 1·9±0·2.
(b) Irradiation given in 10 equal fractions separated by intervals of 3·5 h. For survival at 5·5 days after irradiation, the LD 50/5·5 is 23·7±1·1 Gy for ^{60}Co and 8·8±0·4 Gy for neutrons, giving a neutron RBE of 2·7±0·2. This value is definitely greater than that measured after a single dose, due to the smaller doses per fraction (2·37 Gy for ^{60}Co and 0·88 Gy for neutrons). The calculation of LD 50 is more straightforward when a system of log-probit coordinates is used; with a normal distribution of radiosensitivity this gives linear relationships between survival and dose (J. Gueulette, personal communication).

factors such as the biological system studied, the absorbed dose, the irradiation parameters (e.g. dose rate) and the environmental conditions (e.g. the level of oxygenation).

Originally it was agreed that the reference radiation should be orthovoltage X-rays (generated at 180–300 kV) [48]; this choice was connected with the large quantity of experimental results which had been gained with this type of radiation. Today there is a tendency to adopt ^{60}Co γ-rays or high energy X-rays (>1MV) as the reference radiation, in agreement with the recommendations of the ICRU [51]. However, an RBE value of a test radiation can be defined with respect to any other type of radiation taken as the reference. This problem arises, for example, in a comparison of the results obtained in different neutron therapy centres with beams of different energy. It is then useful to consider the RBE of the neutrons used in one centre with reference to those used in a different centre.

LET and the shape of cell survival curves

As we have seen in Section 4.3, after irradiation with very high LET radiations survival curves are usually found to be exponential and can be represented by an expression of the form $S=e^{-\alpha D}$. Cell death is due essentially to directly lethal lesions, independent of fractionation and dose rate.

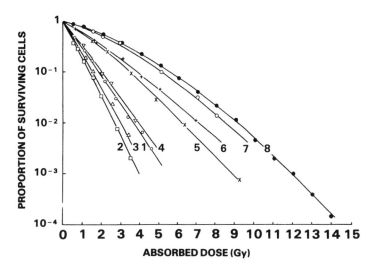

Figure 11.2. Effect of LET on cell survival curves. Survival curves obtained *in vitro* for human kidney cells exposed to radiations of different quality:
1, 2·5 MeV α-particles (LET=166 keV μm^{-1});
2, 4·0 MeV α-particles (LET=110 keV μm^{-1});
3, 5·1 MeV α-particles (LET=88 keV μm^{-1});
4, 8·3 MeV α-particles (LET=61 keV μm^{-1});
5, 26·0 MeV α-particles (LET=25 keV μm^{-1});
6, 3·0 MeV deuterons (LET=20 keV μm^{-1});
7, 14·9 MeV deuterons (LET=5·6 keV μm^{-1});
8, 250 kVp X-rays (mean LET about 1·3 keV μm^{-1}).
As the LET increases the dose needed for a given biological effect (in this case a given level of cell survival) diminishes, except for very high values of LET where it begins to increase once more.
After [1].

Figure 11.2 compares cell survival curves obtained with radiations of increasing LET. As the LET increases there is a progressive increase in the initial slope, a reduction in the shoulder and an increase in the final slope. This corresponds with an increase in the relative importance of lethality by directly lethal lesions in comparison with the accumulation of sublethal lesions. In terms of the linear–quadratic model it represents a progressive increase in the linear component (αD) relative to the quadratic (βD^2).

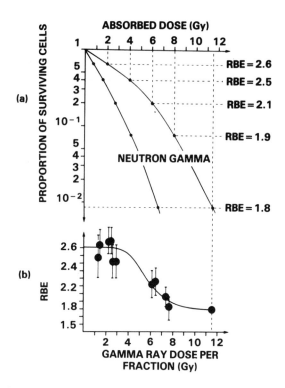

Figure 11.3. The shape of the relation between RBE and absorbed dose.
(a) Survival curves of mouse intestinal crypt cells irradiated with beams of d(50)+Be neutrons and ^{60}Co γ-rays. By means of a comparison of the two curves the values of neutron RBE can be obtained at any survival level (or any dose). Some values of RBE obtained in this way are shown on the right.
(b) The relation between RBE and absorbed dose deduced from a comparison of the neutron and γ-ray curves in part (a) The RBE is 1·8 for the highest doses which could be used (single dose irradiations) and does not vary much in this region of dose where the neutron and γ-ray curves are almost exponential. The RBE increases from 1·8 to 2·6 as the dose is reduced because of the larger shoulder on the γ-ray curve.
The RBE tends towards a plateau at a value of 2·6 which is reached when the γ-ray doses become lower than about 2·5 Gy. This plateau corresponds to the ratio of the initial slopes of the survival curves obtained with neutrons and γ-rays and is reached when the γ-ray curve becomes indistinguishable from its initial tangent. The slope of the relation between RBE and absorbed dose and the point at which the RBE reaches its maximum value (plateau) depend essentially on the shape of the initial part of the γ-ray survival curve.
The black circles are the values of RBE measured directly after fractionated irradiations comparing γ-rays and d(50)+Be neutrons. Up to 20 fractions were used to enable γ-ray doses per fraction to be studied below 2 Gy. The error bars correspond to 95% confidence limits. There is a good agreement between the RBE values obtained directly and those expected from the shapes of the survival curves (J. Gueulette, personal communication).

Relation between RBE and absorbed dose

The differences in the shapes of survival curves with radiations of different LET result in a variation of RBE as a function of the survival level, i.e. as a function of the dose.

Thus, the RBE of fast neutrons relative to γ-rays varies with dose in the following way:

1. For very large doses, the RBE of neutrons shows only a relatively small variation with dose or with the surviving fraction, and as a close approximation the RBE is equal to the ratio of the final slopes of the survival curves.
2. For intermediate doses (in the shoulder region on the curve for γ-rays), the RBE increases as the dose is reduced because of the greater shoulder of the γ-ray curve.
3. Finally, for very low doses (corresponding to the region where the survival curves remain indistinguishable from their initial tangents), the RBE tends towards a limit which is equal to the ratio of the initial slopes of the neutron and γ-ray curves (i.e. the ratio of the α-coefficients or the values of $1/_1D_0$ depending on the symbolism).

Figure 11.3 illustrates, for the stem cells of the intestinal crypts, the different regions of the RBE/absorbed dose relationship. The dose below which the RBE becomes almost constant varies with the cell line, the tissue and the biological effect considered.

Relation between RBE and LET

The variation of RBE with LET can be deduced from survival curves obtained with different types of radiation with different values of LET (Figure 11.2). Figure 11.4 shows RBE as a function of LET for three levels of survival (80, 10 and 1%).

RBE increases with LET, at first slowly and then more rapidly, to reach a maximum value at an LET close to $100 \, \text{keV} \, \mu\text{m}^{-1}$. At higher values of LET the RBE falls again. This observation can be interpreted as follows.

A cell is killed when enough damage has been done to sensitive sites in the nucleus, located on the chromosomes (Section 3.5). With low-LET radiations, much of the damage can be repaired because the energy density within each site is relatively low. As the LET increases, at a given dose (a given amount of energy absorbed in the nucleus) fewer sites are damaged but the sites which happen to be on the tracks of the charged particles receive more energy. A large proportion of the damage is then irreparable and the energy required to kill the cell falls, i.e. the RBE rises. Beyond the maximum, so few sites are damaged that a larger dose of radiation is needed and the RBE falls again. The sites which are damaged receive more energy than is needed and some of the energy is wasted ('overkill effect'). The details of the argument depend on whether one uses a repair model or the theory of dual radiation action but the basic reasons for the rise and fall of RBE are the same.

The 'optimum' LET depends on the biological system (target size and energy needed to inactivate it). At one extreme, certain effects can be obtained with a

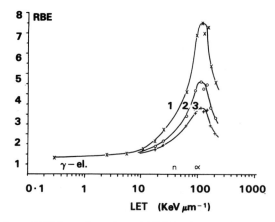

Figure 11.4. Variation of RBE as a function of LET for the survival of human kidney cells T1-g. Curves are given for three levels of survival: 80, 10 and 1%. The difference between the three curves illustrates the fact that the RBE of a given radiation does not have a single value but depends on the surviving fraction considered (that is to say on the dose, see Figure 11.3b). The RBE increases with increasing LET, reaches a maximum at about 100 keV μm^{-1} and then falls again at greater values of LET. Typical LET values of γ-rays, electrons, neutrons and α-particles are shown on the abscissa. After [3].

single ionization and the effectiveness then diminishes steadily with increasing LET. This is the case in radiochemistry ($FeSO_4$ dosemeter and photographic emulsions) and also with certain simple biochemical and biological systems such as viruses (p. 15 in [49]). For the killing of mammalian cells there is little variation in the optimum LET but there is still controversy over certain effects of importance in radiation protection (Section 11.4).

LET and the oxygen effect

With radiations of low-LET (X- and γ-rays and electrons) the doses necessary to produce a given biological effect are 2·5 to 3 times greater if the biological system is irradiated under hypoxic conditions rather than under aerobic conditions (OER=2·5–3) (Section 7.1). Hornsey and Silini [47] compared the survival of Ehrlich ascites cells after irradiation with X-rays and d(16)+ Be neutrons† and found a substantial reduction in OER with neutrons (OER=1·8) in comparison with that of X-rays (OER=3·1). This observation is one of the rationales for the therapeutic use of fast neutrons and other high-LET radiations.

Because of its possible clinical importance, the variation of OER with LET has been studied systematically [44]. As an example, Figure 11.5 shows the survival curves obtained under hypoxic and aerobic conditions with different types of radiation. Figure 11.6 shows the variation of both RBE and OER as a function of LET. The OER which is 2·5–3 for low-LET radiations decreases slowly at first as the LET increases and then more rapidly when the LET reaches 60–100 keV μm^{-1}; for the neutron beams used at present in radiotherapy it is close to 1·6.

---

†d(16)+Be represents the neutrons produced by bombarding a thick beryllium target with 16 MeV deuterons [50].

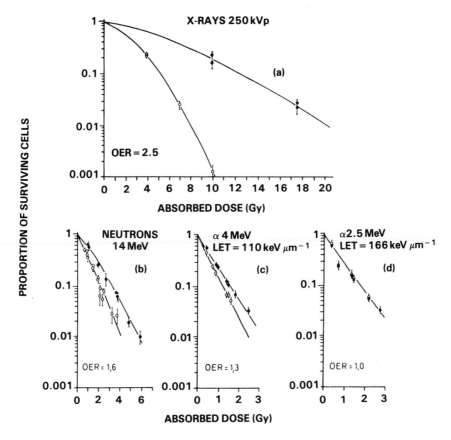

Figure 11.5. Survival curves of human kidney cells T1 irradiated under hypoxic and aerobic conditions with different qualities of radiation.
(a) 250 kV X-rays (LET about 1·3 keV μm^{-1});
(b) 14 MeV neutrons produced by the (d,T) reaction (LET about 12 keV μm^{-1});
(c) 4 MeV α-particles (LET=110 keV μm^{-1});
(d) 2·5 MeV α-particles (LET=166 keV μm^{-1}).
After [1, 10].

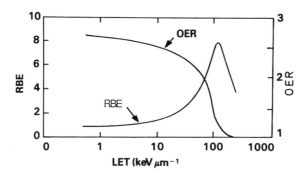

Figure 11.6. Variation of RBE (Figure 11.4) and OER (Figure 11.5) as a function of LET. The curves vary inversely and the most rapid changes occur at about 100 keV μm^{-1}.
After [3].

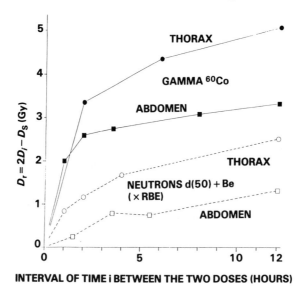

Figure 11.7. **Kinetics of repair of sublethal damage after irradiation with fast neutrons and γ-rays. Acute tolerance of the intestinal mucosa taken as a model of a rapidly renewing tissue is compared with lung tolerance taken as a model of a slowly renewing tissue, both measured in mice. The intestinal tolerance was evaluated from the dose needed for 50% lethality 7 days after abdominal irradiation, and lung tolerance from the 50% lethal dose 180 days after thoracic irradiation. Repair of sublethal injury is shown on the ordinate by the increase in the dose needed to reach the LD 50 when a single dose D_s is replaced by 2 equal doses $2 D_i$ separated by an interval of time i (on the abscissa). After γ-rays, early repair is more important in the lung (D_r=5 Gy) than in the intestine (D_r=3 Gy); it is almost complete after 3–4 h for the intestine but continues for about 12 h in the lung. There is less repair after irradiation by neutrons; it is more marked for the lung (D_r=2·5 Gy) than for the intestine (D_r=0·75 Gy). In order to improve the comparison, the doses of neutrons indicated on the diagram were obtained by multiplying the absorbed doses by the RBE at the LD 50 after a single dose, i.e. RBE=1·8 for the intestine and 1·3 for the lung.**
After [36].

The significance of this reduction in OER for radiotherapy depends on whether hypoxic cells are responsible for local radioresistance in tumours (Section 7.3).

LET and repair phenomena

Repair of sublethal damage

The changing shape of cell survival curves (and of the ratio α/β) seen with increasing LET implies a reduced importance of sublethal damage (Section 4.5). This has been confirmed in many experiments using fractionated irradiation both *in vitro* and *in vivo*. With the fast neutrons used in therapy, when a single dose is replaced by two fractions separated by a few hours, the increase in the dose needed to produce a given effect is smaller than that required with [60]Co γ-rays (Figure 11.7). In the limit, there is no increase with very high-LET radiation (α-particles) for which the survival curves are exponential.

With fractionated irradiation, the isoeffect dose varies less as a function of the dose per fraction for neutrons than for γ-rays (Figures 11.8 and 11.9). There is

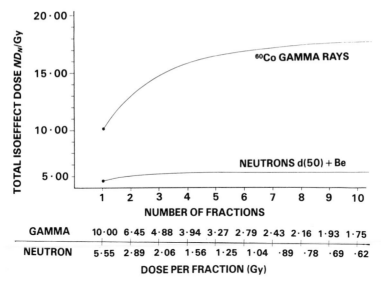

Figure 11.8. Isoeffect dose for acute intestinal tolerance in the mouse. The total dose ($N.d_N$) corresponding to the LD 50 is shown as a function of the number of fractions (N) or of the dose per fraction (d_N) after irradiation with γ-rays or d(50)+Be neutrons. There is little variation in isoeffect dose with neutrons and the increase in RBE when the dose per fraction is reduced (Figure 11.17) is due essentially to an increased tolerance to γ-rays (J. Gueulette, personal communication).

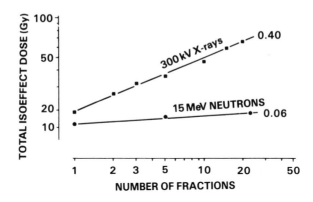

Figure 11.9. Isoeffect dose for late tolerance of the spinal cord in the rat. The total dose corresponding to 50% incidence of myelitis is shown as a function of the number of fractions after irradiation with γ-rays or 15 meV neutrons (A. J. Van der Kogel, personal communication). The exponents in the Elter formula are 0·40 and 0·06.

therefore an increase in RBE when the dose per fraction is reduced (i.e. for a given effect when the number of fractions is increased), as would be expected from the shapes of the cell survival curves.

Repair of potentially lethal damage

Experiments performed both *in vivo* and *in vitro* on the repair of potentially lethal damage after irradiation with high-LET radiations have given contradictory results. For example, after irradiation with d(16)+Be neutrons, Shipley *et al.* [73] found no repair of PLD for Lewis lung carcinoma cells irradiated *in situ* and assayed either *in vivo* or *in vitro*. On the other hand, Guichard *et al.* [42] found similar repair of PLD after irradiation with d(50)+Be neutrons or ^{60}Co γ-rays. These experiments were performed on human melanoma cells (Na-11) transplanted into immune-deprived mice, the tumours being irradiated *in situ* and the cell survival measured *in vitro*.

These contradictions and the lack of information on the role of repair of PLD in conventional radiotherapy (Section 4.5) prevent any firm conclusion on the importance of this factor in neutron therapy.

LET and the cell cycle

The variation in radiosensitivity as a function of the phase in the cell cycle has been studied with neutrons in the same way as with photons (Section 4.4), by irradiation of synchronized populations of cells. Qualitatively there is the same variation of radiosensitivity around the cycle: maximum radiosensitivity during and immediately before mitosis and at the G_1/S junction, and maximum radioresistance at the end of S phase and, when G_1 is long, during the beginning of G_1. However, the amplitude of the variations is reduced with neutrons.

For example, with the intestinal crypt cells of the mouse, Withers *et al.* [95] found after 10 Gy of γ-rays a ratio of 100 between the extreme values of surviving fraction as a function of the cycle and this ratio was reduced to 60 after 6 Gy of d(16)+Be neutrons. As a result there is a variation in RBE as a function of the phase of the cycle. For V79 cells, Gragg *et al.* [31] found that the RBE varied from $1 \cdot 8$ to $5 \cdot 1$, the highest values being obtained when the cells are in the most radioresistant phases. The importance of this effect in radiotherapy will be discussed in the next section.

A systematic study of the variation of radiosensitivity of Chinese hamster cells as a function of LET has been performed by Chapman using different types of ions such as helium, carbon, neon and argon [17]. The large differences in radiosensitivity observed after low-LET irradiation between cells in mitosis, G_1 and in stationary phase diminish with increasing LET and disappear above 100 keV μm^{-1} (Figure 11.10).

11.2 *Radiobiological rationale for the use of fast neutrons in radiotherapy*

Historical reminder

The first trial of fast neutrons in radiotherapy was begun by Stone at Berkeley in 1938 [76]. It was abandoned because of late complications which were considered too severe.

During the 1960s a programme of neutron therapy was set up at Hammersmith Hospital in London. It was stimulated by new radiobiological data, in particular the oxygen effect and the potential importance of hypoxic cells (Section 7.4). In view of the difficulties previously encountered at Berkeley, clinical use of neutrons at Hammersmith was preceded by a long period of radiobiological studies, particularly on the tolerance of normal tissues.

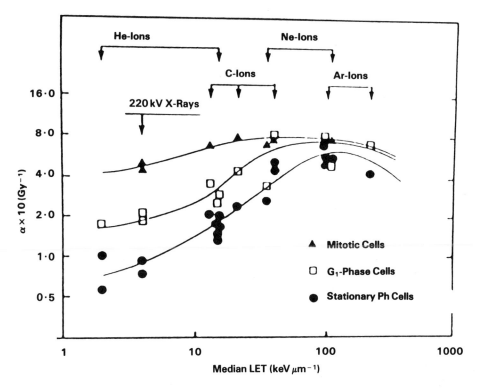

Figure 11.10. Single-hit inactivation coefficients (α) for homogeneous populations of Chinese hamster cells irradiated in mitosis, G_1 phase and stationary phase, with 220 kV X-rays and various beams of charged particles. The α-coefficients are plotted as a function of median LET (in keV μm^{-1}).
After [17].

The first patient was treated in 1966 and the trials of neutron therapy continued until 1985 when the cyclotron was closed [7].

The promising results reported from Hammersmith, which confirmed to a certain extent the radiobiological data on OER, encouraged other groups to consider the use of neutron therapy. This was soon applied in about 20 centres in Europe, the United State and Japan [23, 90]. The neutron generators were mostly cyclotrons of relatively low energy accelerating deuterons to 16 MeV, or (d,T) generators producing 14 MeV neutrons. The dose distributions were rather unsatisfactory and were comparable to those of 250 kV X-rays.

However, the results obtained under technical and physical conditions which were far from optimal were judged sufficiently encouraging for the installation of high energy cyclotrons in hospitals. These facilities are analogous to modern electron linear accelerators, particularly with respect to the depth dose, skin sparing, isocentric mounting and variable collimator. As shown in Table 11.1 this new range of cyclotrons is progressively replacing the old neutron therapy installations. It should be noted in particular that several (d,T) generators are no longer in use; this type of machine does not provide an adequate dose rate and involves some risk of contamination by tritium. Some physical characteristics of fast neutron beams were presented in Chapter 1.

Table 11.1. Neutron therapy facilities in the world.

Centre	Neutron producing reaction	Comments
	EUROPE	
MRC-Clatterbridge, U.K.	p(62)+Be	Rotational gantry Variable collimator
Orléans, France	p(34)+Be	Vertical beam
UCL- Louvain-la-Neuve, Belgium	p(65)+Be	Vertical beam (multileaf collimator and horizontal beam in preparation)
Hamburg, Federal Republic of Germany	(d+T)	Rotational gantry
Heidelberg, Federal Republic of Germany	(d+T)	Rotational gantry
Munster, Federal Republic of Germany	(d+T)	Rotational gantry
Essen, Federal Republic of Germany	d(14)+Be	Rotational gantry
	UNITED STATES	
M D Anderson-Houston, Texas	p(42)+Be	Rotational gantry Variable collimator
Cleveland, Ohio	p(43)+Be	Horizontal beam
UCLA, Los Angeles	p(46)+Be	Rotational gantry Variable collimator
Seattle, Washington	p(50)+Be	Rotational gantry Multileaf collimator
Fermilab	p(66)+Be	Horizontal beam
	ASIA	
National Institute of Radiological Sciences (NIRS), Chiba, Japan	d(30)+Be	Vertical beam Multileaf collimator
Institute for Medical Science (IMS), Tokyo, Japan	d(14)+Be	Horizontal beam
Korea Cancer Center Hospital (KCCH), Seoul, Korea	d(50.5)+Be	Rotational gantry
King Faisal Hospital, Riyadh, Saudi Arabia	p(26)+Be	Rotational gantry
	AFRICA	
National Accelerator Centre (NAC) Faure, Republic of South Africa	p(66)+Be	Rotational gantry Variable collimator

Updated after [55] and [80].

Fast neutrons and the oxygen effect

Historically, the oxygen effect was the rationale for the use of neutrons and other high-LET radiations in radiotherapy. This rationale is based on the following experimental data:

(i)   the presence of hypoxic cells in malignant tumours;
(ii) the great radioresistance (OER=3) of hypoxic cells irradiated with low-LET radiation;
(iii) a reduction in OER with high-LET radiations.

The term *hypoxic gain factor* (HGF) has been used to quantify this advantage. It is defined as the ratio of the OER values for γ-rays and the high-LET radiation (p. 14 in [52]). For fast neutrons it is about $3/1 \cdot 6 = 1 \cdot 9$.

The HGF would represent the therapeutic gain if the hypoxic cells were the determining factor in tumour resistance. In practice, the therapeutic gain is less than the HGF as tumour reoxygenation during fractionated irradiation reduces the population of hypoxic cells. However, there are other factors besides the oxygen effect which may also influence the therapeutic gain and we will discuss them in the following sections.

Fast neutrons and reduction in the differential effect

It is generally accepted that hypoxic cells are a factor in the radioresistance of *some tumours*, but it is not reasonable today to ascribe the radioresistance of *all malignant tumours* to this cause. (Section 6.3)

A wider approach to the rationale of neutron therapy suggests that, with increasing LET, there is a general reduction in differences in radiosensitivity between cell populations [91]. This hypothesis is connected with the microdosimetric characteristics of the neutron beams and with the fact that the recoil protons (and other secondary particles) deposit much more energy per unit path length than do electrons (50–100 times greater). When a cell nucleus is crossed by such particles, there is a much greater probability of lethal damage than

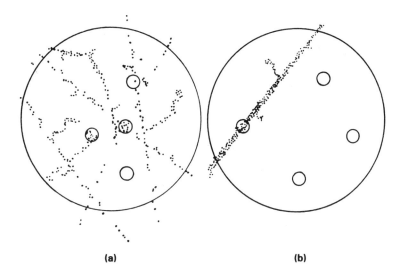

(a)   (b)

Figure 11.11. Distribution of ionizations in a medium irradiated by γ-rays (a) and neutrons (b). The black dots represent the ionizations produced along the tracks of electrons set in motion by γ-rays (a) and of protons, α-particles or heavy ions set in motion by neutrons (b). The distribution of ionizations is very different. After irradiation by neutrons, when a vital sensitive structure (or target, represented by the circles) is crossed by a track, the deposition of energy (or the damage) is so great that there is a high probability of cell death whatever the cell line, the position in the cell cycle, the degree of oxygenation, etc. After irrdiation by γ-rays, the depositions of energy are smaller and more variable. In some cases a single particle deposits enough energy to kill the cell; in others death of the cell requires the accumulation of damage produced by several tracks. After Barendsen, taken from [91].

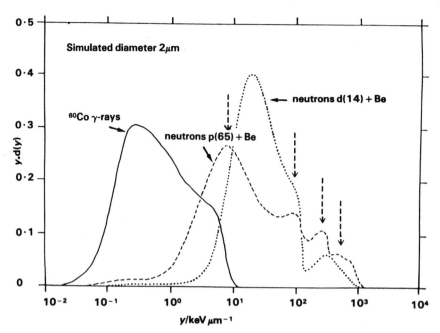

Figure 11.12. Comparison of energy depositions after irradiation with fast neutrons and γ-rays. The curves indicate distributions of individual energy-deposition events in a simulated volume of tissue $2\,\mu m$ in diameter; the parameter y (lineal energy) represents the energy deposited by a single charged particle traversing the sphere, divided by the mean cord length [53]. The maximum with γ-rays is at $0.3\,keV\,\mu m^{-1}$ and with d(14)+Be neutrons at $20\,keV\,\mu m^{-1}$. The spectrum for p(65)+Be neutrons shows 4 peaks: the first is at $8\,keV$ μm^{-1} and corresponds to high energy protons, the second at $100\,keV\,\mu m^{-1}$ corresponds to low energy protons, the third at $300\,keV\,\mu m^{-1}$ is due to α-particles and the last is due to recoil nuclei at $700\,keV\,\mu m^{-1}$.
After [65].

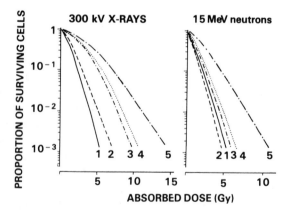

Figure 11.13. Cell survival curves for five lines of mammalian cells irradiated with 300 kV X-rays and 15 MeV neutrons:
1, mouse haemopoietic stem cells;
2, mouse leukaemia cell L5178Y;
3, T-1 g kidney cells of human origin;
4, rat rhabdomysarcoma cells;
5, mouse intestinal crypt cells. When X-rays are replaced by neutrons there is as reduction in the variation of radiosensitivity.
After [2].

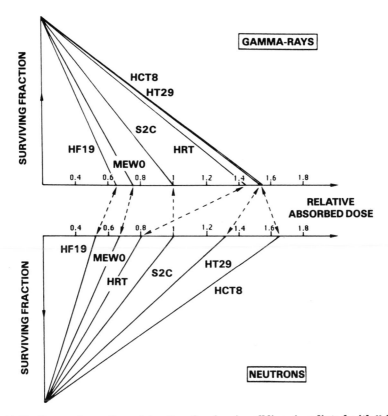

Figure 11.14. Comparison of surviving fraction for six cell lines irradiated with ^{60} Co γ-rays and d(50)+Be neutrons. Survival of the six populations has been calculated for a fractionated irradiation given with fractions of 2 Gy (γ-equivalent). The $_{eff}D_o$ values were deduced from the α- and β-coefficients derived from the survival curves observed *in vitro*. To facilitate the comparison, relative absorbed doses are indicated on the abscissa, the SZC cells being taken as the reference. The variations of radiosensitivity are as important with neutrons as with photons, but the order of radiosensitivities is altered (calculated from the data of Fertil *et al.* [29]).

when the nucleus is crossed by recoil electrons (see Figure 11.11 and 11.12). Some experimental results are presented in order to support this hypothesis.

In 1977, Barendsen and Broerse [2] compared cell survival curves of five cell lines *in vitro* after irradiation with 300 kV X-rays and 15 MeV neutrons. A reduction in the differences of radiosensitivity was observed with neutrons (Figure 11.13). Somewhat different conclusions were reached by Fertil *et al.* [29] who showed that the ranking of radiosensitivity of some cell lines could be altered when X-rays were replaced by fast neutrons (Figure 11.14).

As mentioned above (Figure 11.7–11.9), repair phenomena are less important with neutrons and, consequently, differences in repair capacity are of less significance.

A third differential effect with neutrons is a reduction in the variation of radiosensitivity with the phase of the cell cycle (Section 4.4) and consequently a variation in neutron RBE depending on the phase (Figure 11.10). Based on these findings, Withers and Peters [96] have proposed the idea of a *kinetic gain factor* (KGF) defined as the ratio of RBE values for effects on the tumour and on normal tissues, evaluated by taking account only of the fluctuations in radio-sensitivity with the phase of the cycle. Basing their calculations on data such as those of Gragg *et al.* [31], they obtained gain factors which could, under certain conditions, be as great as 3, i.e. of the same order as the HGF. However, a reduction in OER is always an advantage, because only malignant cells are hypoxic, whereas the KGF may, depending on the situation, represent a gain or a loss.

There may be a gain (KGF >1) for tumours in which cell redistribution is slow, leading to the accumulation of cells in resistant phases of the cell cycle during a fractionated treatment. It may also be effective for tumours whose cells have a long and radioresistant G_1 phase (Section 4.4). These radiobio-logical considerations can be correlated with clinical observations showing that the best results are obtained with slow growing, well-differentiated tumours (see below, and Figure 11.16).

In summary, with photons there are large variations of radiosensitivity between different cell lines or tissues, whether they are normal or malignant. Furthermore, these variations are amplified by fractionation because of differences in repair patterns. With neutrons these variations in radiosen-sitivity are reduced. The reduction in OER with neutrons can then be considered as a particular example of the more general phenomenon of a levelling of radiosensitivity.

Patient selection for neutron therapy and irradiation modalities

Although a reduction in OER is always an advantage, a reduction of differences in radiosensitivity related to cell line, position in the mitotic cycle and repair capacity could be an advantage or a disadvantage, depending on the charac-teristics of the tumour cell population and the relevant normal cell population. This raises the important problem of patient selection.

Patient selection for fast neutron therapy

Schematically, the clinical situations might be divided into three categories (Figure 11.15): (A) Those where the differences in radiosensitivity to photon irradiation between tumour and normal tissue work in favour of the latter. Some typical examples are seminomas, lymphomas, Hodgkin's disease; (B) and (C) those where they work in favour of the tumour.

A change from photons to neutrons involving a levelling of differences between radiosensitivities would be detrimental in (A). By contrast, in situation (B) neutrons bring a benefit by reducing the difference in radiosensitivity which would protect the malignant cell population. A third more favourable situation (C) can be considered where the relative radiosensitivities are reversed. This could be the case when the greater radioresistance of the cancer cell population to X-rays is due to the presence of hypoxic cells. This possibility is also suggested by the data of Fertil *et al.* presented in Figure 11.14. Although this presentation is very schematic, it shows why one cannot hope that neutron therapy (or high-LET therapy) would always have a differential action selec-tively affecting cancer cells and sparing normal tissues.

These considerations also demonstrate the importance of patient selection for

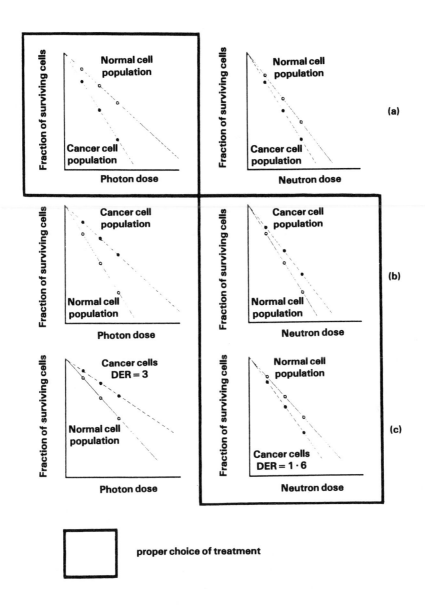

Figure 11.15. Importance of patient selection for fast neutron therapy. Three possible clinical situations are considered.

In the first (a), the cancer cells are more sensitive to X-rays than the critical normal cell population, and there is no argument at all for using neutrons which would reduce a favourable differential effect.

In the second situation (b), neutrons bring a benefit by reducing a difference in radiosensitivity which would selectively protect the cancer cell population.

A third more favourable situation is shown (c) where the relative radiosensitivities are reversed (see text and Figure 11.14). It has been assumed in the figure that the survival curves are exponential after fractionated irradiation, i.e. a constant proportion of the cells is killed at each session. However, the exact shape of the cell survival curve is not essential for the present discussion.

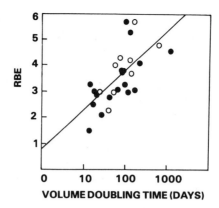

Figure 11.16. Relation between the RBE of neutrons for regression of lung metastases in man and their doubling time. •, Measured values of RBE; ○, values estimated from irradiations with neutrons only. For the 15 MeV neutrons used in this study (produced by a d,T generator) the RBE for tolerance of the most important normal tissues is about 3. Neutrons are therefore a good indication (RBE >3) for tumours having doubling times greater than 100 days. After [5].

neutron therapy and the problems posed by the evaluation of any therapeutic benefit of neutrons in comparative clinical studies. Consider a heterogeneous group of patients, some of whom would be better treated with photons and others by neutrons (respectively the categories A and B (or C) defined above). If the two sub-groups were not identified, the benefits obtained for sub-group B would be masked by the worse results obtained in sub-group A, and altogether there would be no advantage.

Battermann *et al.* [5] have illustrated this interpretation in a study performed on patients with pulmonary metastases. They measured the RBE of neutrons for regression of the volume of the metastases and found a correlation between the RBE and the doubling time (Figure 11.16). The RBE for neutrons produced by a (d,T) generator seemed to be greater than 3 for tumours with a doubling time greater than 100 days while it was about 3 for tolerance of the principal normal tissues. The conclusion is that tumours with long doubling times (>100 days) represent a good indication for neutron therapy, whereas those with doubling times below 100 days should not be treated with neutrons.

Out of more than 200 lung metastases studied, a doubling time greater than 100 days was found in only 30% of the cases. If neutron therapy were evaluated for the whole group of patients it is clear that the verdict would not be positive.

By classifying the tumours according to their degree of histological differentiation, Battermann reached the conclusion that 80–90% of the well-differentiated tumours had a doubling time >100 days and would therefore be likely to benefit from neutrons. Moreover this conclusion is in agreement with the actual clinical results (see later in this section).

Fractionation and overall time

The available radiobiological data suggest that the *dose per fraction* plays a less important role with neutrons than with photons. It is therefore unlikely that changing the dose per fraction will have any significant effect on the clinical results (Figures 11.8 and 11.9). However, we should bear in mind that a treatment regime giving 17·6 Gy (total dose) in 12 fractions over 26 days (i.e. 3 fractions of 1·47 Gy per week) has been used systematically with all the patients at Hammersmith Hospital; it is often put forward as an important factor in the excellent results reported from this centre [15].

As far as *overall time* is concerned there is no specific problem in neutron therapy. Cell proliferation kinetics are not likely to be very different after irradiation with neutrons or photons. The overall time should therefore play a relatively minor role both for slowly growing tumours (which represent a good indication for neutrons, see above) and for slowly renewing normal tissues which are responsible for late complications. However, as the dose per fraction is of minor importance in neutron therapy, it should be possible by using large doses of neutrons per fraction to concentrate the treatment into a short overall time and thus give a more effective treatment to tumours with rapid proliferation [94].

Choice of target volume

Clinical experience in several centres has shown that irradiation of large target volumes with high doses of neutrons often leads to late complications, in particular to severe fibrosis. This can be related to radiobiological data showing that neutrons usually reduce differences in radiosensitivity between tissues and give high RBE values for tolerance of tissues with slow cell renewal (Figure 11.17).

In practice, irradiation of large fields with neutrons can be avoided either by giving a neutron boost to small target volumes or by alternating beams of photons and neutrons (mixed schedule) [43]. Interesting clinical results have

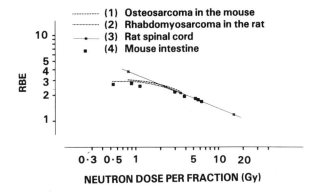

Figure 11.17. Relation between RBE and absorbed dose for fast neutrons relative to γ-rays determined for: two malignant cell lines irradiated *in vitro* by 15 MeV neutrons produced by a d,T generator (A. J. Van der Kogel, personal communication);
late tolerance of the spinal cord in the rat (same neutron energy, same reference);
early tolerance of intestinal mucosa in the mouse (d(50)+Be neutrons produced by a cyclotron).
The shape of the relation between RBE and absorbed dose is similar for effects 1, 2, and 4: the RBE reaches a plateau when the neutron dose per fraction becomes less than about 1 Gy. On the other hand the RBE for late tolerance of the spinal cord continues to rise with lower doses per fraction.
After [91].

been obtained by these methods; however, the best ways of combining neutrons and photons remain to be determined.

Clinical assessment and outlook for the future of fast neutron therapy

A brief clinical assessment of neutron therapy is given here, essentially with the aim of finding a correlation between the clinical results obtained and those which would be expected from the radiobiological data.

Locally extended inoperable tumours of the salivary glands were the type of disease for which the benefit of neutrons was recognized most quickly [38] and is today universally accepted [41, 92]. Historical series give, as an average, local control rates of 67% after neutron irradiation compared with 24% after conventional treatment. These data were confirmed by a randomized trial (although the numbers of patients were small): 9/13 and 2/12 local controls at 2 years respectively [41].

The value of neutrons in the treatment of locally extended prostatic adenocarcinoma was established by a RTOG study which shows a significant benefit of mixed schedule (combination of neutrons and photons) both for local control and survival (Figure 11.18) [69]. This result confirms those found in other centres such as Hamburg [30] and Louvain-la-Neuve [67]. Indeed, prostatic adenocarcinomas are, in general, slowly growing tumours.

Inoperable or recurrent melanomas may also benefit from neutron therapy. Failure of low-LET radiotherapy could be connected with the large shoulder of the cell survival curve found in certain melanomas (Section 8.3). Soft tissue sarcomas, particularly those which are well differentiated and with a slow growth rate, are considered by most neutron-therapy groups as being a good indication [18, 68]. This may be connected with the lower rate of reoxygenation seen in experimental sarcomas.

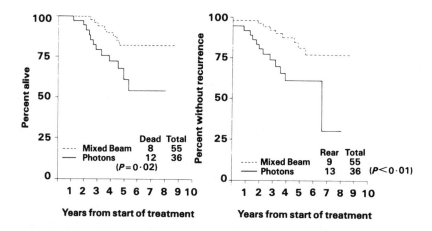

Figure 11.18. RTOG randomized trial comparing a combination of fast neutrons and photons ('mixed schedule') and conventional photon irradiation alone for locally advanced carcinoma of the prostate. Left, actuarial survivals at 8 years are indicated, adjusted by exclusion of intercurrent noncancer death ('determinental' survival rates). Right, local control rates are indicated, combining clinical and biopsy criteria. After [69].

As far as tumours of the head and neck are concerned, contradictory conclusions have been reported [7, 18, 21]. They probably arise from differences in recruitment of the patients, in methods of application of neutron therapy and perhaps also in the way in which the results have been analyzed. It is sufficient to mention here:

(i)   the positive results obtained at Hammersmith Hospital for extended tumours of the maxillary sinus [25];

(ii)   the significant benefit found in a joint study undertaken in several American neutron-therapy centres and initiated by the RTOG, showing the superiority of mixed schedules for the control of metastatic cervical nodes [40];

(iii) the significant benefit found by the same group in a study showing the advantage of neutrons for local control and survival in patients with advanced tumours of the head and neck (Table 11.2) [39].

These results can be correlated with those showing a benefit of hyperbaric oxygen (HBO) for similar patient series: they suggest that hypoxic cells could play a role (Section 7.4). On the other hand, HBO was also shown to bring a benefit for locally extended cervix carcinoma (Table 7.3). Nevertheless, a RTOG randomized trial could not demonstrate any benefit of a mixed schedule (it was stressed, however, that in this study the neutron treatments were given under poor technical conditions.).

Table 11.2. Inoperable squamous carcinoma of the head and neck.
Results of a randomized study undertaken in the USA by the RTOG.

	Photons (66–74 Gy)	Neutrons (20–24 Gy)
Number of patients analyzed	12	23
Local control (primary tumour and nodes)	17%	52% ($p=0 \cdot 035$)
Actuarial survival at 2 years	0%	25%
Severe complications	4	4

After [39].

The value of fast neutrons has also been suggested for other sites: neutron boost for certain lung tumours, Pancoast tumours, osteosarcomas, certain tumours of the rectum, etc. They have been analyzed in several clinical reviews [7, 8, 9, 18, 56, 63].

Finally, two points should be stressed concerning the future of neutron therapy.

First of all, there is a need for improving the technical conditions. High physical selectivity is probably more important with high-LET than with low-LET irradiations as discussed previously.

Until recently, most of the patients who received neutron therapy were treated under conditions which were unsatisfactory from a technical point of view; a large number of complications could have been avoided with better techniques. The potential of neutron therapy cannot be fully appreciated until high-energy cyclotrons are available (giving depth doses at least equal to those of 10 MV photons), with isocentric mounting and variable collimator, located within the hospital. Such machines are now in operation (Table 11.1), allowing the therapist to achieve treatment plans and dose distributions similar to those currently applied with photons [7, 16, 18]. Only under these conditions will it be possible to evaluate the relative merits of high-LET compared with low-LET radiations as a function of the characteristics of the tumours; this is indeed the basic radiobiological question to answer.

Secondly, the major problem which remains is the selection of patients for high-LET therapy. One approach consists of initiating clinical studies and randomized trials in order to define better the categories of patients who might benefit from neutron therapy. Another approach is to develop individual predictive tests and assess their prognostic value; this subject was discussed in Chapter 6.

11.3 Other charged particles used in radiotherapy

Proton beams

Proton beams owe their importance only to the dose distributions which they can provide and to the improved physical selectivity which they make possible (Section 1.3).

To begin with, a proton beam has a well-defined depth of penetration which depends on the energy. Tissues at greater depths are therefore spared. Secondly, high-energy protons have a low density of ionization (they are low-LET radiations), but at the end of the track the LET increases, giving rise to a greater deposition of energy (Bragg peak, Figure 1.3). By modulating the energy of the incident protons, the Bragg peak can be spread out over a greater depth to cover the target volume. When the target volume is thick, the Bragg peak has to be spread out over a large depth, and the ratio between the dose in the spread-out Bragg peak and the dose in the more proximal region is reduced. Nevertheless, there is still usually some skin sparing and some protection of the normal tissues situated in front of the target volume. Finally and thirdly, scattering outside the geometric edge of the beam (penumbra) is smaller with protons than with photons or electrons. The dose distributions obtainable with proton beams are therefore as a rule better than those obtainable with photon beams.

Proton beams are low-LET radiations like photon or electron beams; therefore, no benefit can be expected for radiobiological reasons. The mean LET of a proton beam at its entry into tissue (or in the initial plateau of the depth dose curve) is of the order of $0 \cdot 5 \, \text{keV} \, \mu\text{m}^{-1}$; it increases slowly up to a few micrometres from the end of the range. The RBE of protons in the initial plateau is from $1 \cdot 1$ to $1 \cdot 15$ in comparison with ^{60}Co γ-rays. When the peak is spread over a distance of several centimetres, there is no increase in RBE as energy modulation and range straggling reduce the number of low energy protons.

The radiobiological properties of proton beams with energies of tens or hundreds of MeV are thus completely different from those of the secondary protons produced by fast neutrons (neutron therapy) whose mean LET is 50–100 times greater (Figure 11.12).

Proton beams provide such good physical selectivity that they are the technique of choice for the treatment of radioresistant tumours situated close to radiosensitive and vital normal tissues. Among the first clinical uses of protons was treatment of the hypophysis [57, 78]. Choroidal melanomas are also a good indication for proton beams; this technique which was first used at Harvard has been applied since 1985 at PSI-Villigen, Switzerland (Figure 11.19) [32, 62]. The technique is now under development at other centres such as Clatterbridge and Louvain-la-Neuve. Use of proton beams requires cyclotrons of relatively high energy which are therefore expensive. An energy of 150–200 MeV is needed for treatment of target volumes at 16–26 cm deep. About 60 MeV is enough for treatment of ocular tumours [89].

In addition to use against tumours in particular sites (such as uveal melanomas, chordomas or chondrosarcomas of the base of the skull, paraspinal tumours, hypophysis), there are a number of new projects which aim at treating with protons many other types of tumour and a large proportion of the patients (Table 11.3). One of the most impressive is the Loma Linda programme at Los Angeles, where a variable energy synchrotron (70–250 MeV) and three treatment rooms with isocentric rotating gantries will be the 'core' of a large oncology department. An additional fixed horizontal beam will be reserved for treatment of the eye and brain. When fully operational, the facility is expected to treat 1000 patients per year (cited in [18]). This kind of project really aims at a systematic substitution of proton for photon beams. It raises at least two kinds of problem: the cost versus clinical benefit, and the reliability of the machine and the accuracy in beam delivery and dosimetry.

Beams of other heavy charged particles

Beams of helium ions (^{4}He or He^{2+} or α-particles) have dosimetric characteristics analogous to beams of protons but the energy must be four times greater to obtain the same penetration. The value of helium ions lies in the dose distributions which they provide; they can still be classed among the low-LET

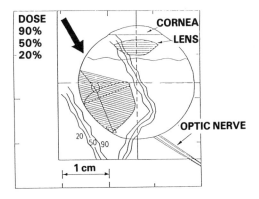

Figure 11.19. Proton therapy for choroidal melanomas. Dose distribution obtained with a beam of 60 MeV protons with a spread out Bragg peak (energy modulated from 14–60 MeV). Transverse section through the centre of the eye. The position of the tumour is indicated by shading. Irradiation with protons gives a homogeneous dose to the tumour with maximum sparing of the normal tissues, but extreme precision is needed when positioning the patient.
After [62].

Table 11.3. Charged-particle biomedical accelerator facilities (excluding pi⁻ mesons).

Location	Ion	Energy (MeV/u)	Accelerator type	Date of first therapy	Current patient total	Date of total
A. Programmes with accrued patients						
184″, LBL, Berkeley (switched to He, 1957)	H	730	Synchrocyclotron	1955	30	1957
184″, LBL (programmes moved to Bevatron, 1/88)	He	231	Synchrocyclotron	1957	1998†	1/88
Bevatron, LBL, Berkeley	He	70–230	Synchrotron	1988	16‡	2/88
GWI, Uppsala, Sweden (see below for upgrade)	H	185	Synchrocyclotron	1957	73	1976
Harvard Cyclotron Laboratory/MGH	H	160	Cyclotron	1961	4300	6/87
ITEP, Moscow, USSR	H	70–200	Synchrotron	1965	1359	10/87
JINR, Dubna, USSR (see below for upgrade)	H	↓80–200	Synchrocyclotron	1967	84	1977
LINPH, Gatchina, USSR	H	1000	Synchrocyclotron	1975	560	10/87
NIRS, Chiba, Japan	H	70,90	Cyclotron	1979	60§	12/88
PARMS, KEK, Tsukuba, Japan	H	↓250	Synchrotron	1983	67	1987
PSI, Villigen, Switzerland	H	100	Cyclotron	1984	429	5/88
BEVALAC LBL, Berkeley (cancer treatment)	Ne,Si	≤670	Synchrotron	1975	296	2/88

Location	Ion	Energy (MeV/u)	Accelerator type	Status		
B. Facilities under construction/development						
Loma Linda, California	H	70–250	Synchrotron	First patient in 1990		
NIRS, Chiba, Japan	He-Ar	800	Synchrotron	First patient in 1993		
NAC, Faure, South AFrica	H	200	Cyclotron	Designing a medical beam line		
GWI, Uppsala, Sweden	H	200	Cyclotron	Upgraded facility ready for therapy		
GWI, Uppsala, Sweden	Ne	20	Cyclotron	For biology experiments only		
JINR, Dubna, USSR	H	200	Synchrocyclotron	Reconstructed and operational in 1987		
IPCR, Tokyo, Japan	H,He	210,135	Cyclotron	To be completed in 1989		
Orsay, France	H	200	Synchrocyclotron	Testing for a medical beam line		
TRIUMF, Vancouver, Canada	H	150	Cyclotron	Developing medical facility		
UCL, Louvain-la-Neuve, Belgium	H	90	Cyclotron	First patient in 1990		
IHP, Beijing, China	H		Cyclotron	First patient in 1989		
MRC, Clatterbridge, UK	H	62	Cyclotron	First patient in 1989		
MEDICYC, Nice, France	H	60	Cyclotron	Plans to develop a medical beam line		

†836 radiation therapy, 292 arterio-venous malformations (AVM), 870 pituitary, etc.
‡6 radiation therapy, 10 AVM
§Including 20 uveal melanomas.
↓ Clinical-energy beams are obtained by degrading higher-energy beams.

radiations. However, the increase in LET at the end of the range is more marked than with protons (an LET of 250 keV μm^{-1} is reached at the end of the range). As a result there is a slight increase in RBE and a small reduction in OER in an extended Bragg peak which can be added to the advantage of the dose distribution (Figure 11.20) [66, 85].

Beams of heavy ions (C^{6+}, Ne^{10+}, Ar^{18+}, etc) give dose distributions comparable with those from protons and helium ions. They suffer even less scattering but produce some long-range particles due to break-up which give a little dosage beyond the theoretical range. The Bragg peaks can be extended for homogeneous irradiation of the tumour volume. The main difference is that heavy ions have a high LET over the whole of an extended Bragg peak. Thus they combine the advantages of protons from the point of view of dose distributions with those of high-LET for the treatment of certain types of tumour. Unfortunately very high energies are necessary (of the order of 300–400 MeV per nucleon, or even more, i.e. 3–4 GeV for carbon ions). The cost and complexity of the installation raises great problems for clinical applications which have until now been undertaken only at a single centre (Berkeley) [15, 66].

A heavy ion therapy programme is planned at the NIRS in Chiba, Japan [18]. Construction of the building started at the beginning of 1989. In Europe, a heavy-ion therapy programme is planned at the GSI-Darmstadt (Federal Republic of Germany).

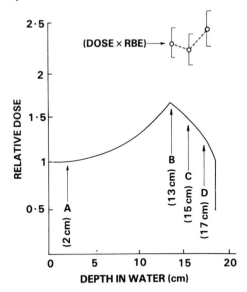

Figure 11.20. Physical and biological depth dose in a beam of helium ions. The continuous line shows the depth dose curve of a 650 MeV beam of helium ions, measured on the synchrotron of CEN at Saclay; the Bragg peak has been extended to cover a target thickness of 5 cm.
The RBE of the beam was measured at the proximal (B), central (C) and distal (D) parts of the extended Bragg peak with reference to the entrance of the beam (A). With growth inhibition in *Vicia faba* as the biological system, the RBE values were found to be 1·4 (B), 1·5 (C) and 2·0±0·2 (D) at an absorbed dose of 0·6 Gy. The dotted line shows the biological depth dose curve calculated by multiplying the physical dose by the RBE at the point considered. The increase in RBE is additional to the advantage of the good dose distribution. After [85].

Negative pi-mesons

Like heavy ions, negative pi-mesons (or pions) have advantages due both to their dose distributions and to their radiobiological properties [66]. They are also very expensive. The depth dose curve of a beam of negative pi-mesons has some similarity to that of a beam of protons or heavy ions. In the initial plateau the dose is given at low-LET, whereas in the extended peak the LET increases due to the contribution of secondary high-LET particles (α-particles, heavy ions, neutrons) set in motion at the end of the range of the pions. The corresponding increase in RBE increases the advantage from the dose distribution. The radio-biological characteristics of negative pi-mesons are intermediate between those of photons and neutrons (OER$\approx 2 \cdot 2$). Figure 11.21 compares the microdosimetric spectra of pi-mesons (static spot or large treatment volume) with those of ^{60}Co γ-rays and d(4)+Be neutrons.

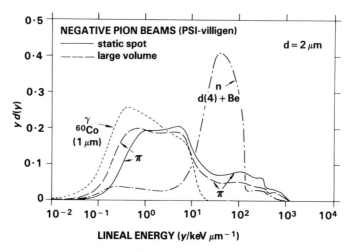

Figure 11.21. Lineal energy *y* spectra for pi-meson beams measured at the therapy facility of the PSI-Villigen. The pi-meson spectra cover a large range in *y* (4 orders of magnitude); they are intermediate between the ^{60}Co and the d(4)+Be neutron spectra shown for comparison. The *y* spectra for pi-mesons are further shifted towards low-LET values when large volumes are irradiated.
Courtesy H. G. Menzel.

A programme of therapy with mesons was set up at Los Alamos in 1973 and continued until 1984 [13]. Another programme has been started at Vancouver (TRIUMF or TRI-University Meson Facility). In Europe, negative pi-mesons are used at the PSI-Villigen (Switzerland). This installation provides 60 small coplanar beams which converge at a point, compensating to some extent for the low dose rate. Each beam is controlled individually and they can be combined to provide the required dose distributions. The small size of the beams limits ir-radiation to a thin slice of tissue and the patient is moved in a direction perpen-dicular to the plane of the beams (Figure 11.22). Individual beams can be adjusted during movement, allowing the optimum dose distribution to be realized in each successive plane ('dynamic treatment') [88].

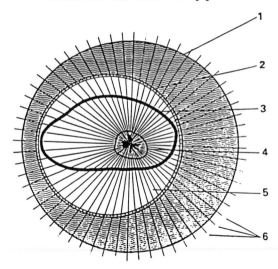

Figure 11.22. Therapy with negative pi-mesons at PSI (Villigen, Switzerland). The diagram shows the plane containing the 60 small convergent beams of pions. The patient lies on a table and is surrounded by a bolus of unit density which is shaped exactly to the patient and has a cylindrical external contour. The combination (patient, table and bolus) is moved within a cylinder of water in such a way as to maintain the target volume at the point of convergence of the 60 beams. The cylinder of water is fixed with respect to the beams: 1, external contour of the cylinder of water; 2, external contour of the bolus surrounding the patient; 3, contour of the patient; 4, target volume; 5, bolus of unit density surrounding the patient; 6, beams of negative pi-mesons. After [88].

Californium-252

Californium-252 (^{252}Cf) is used as a substitute for radium or caesium-137 in interstitial or intracavitary therapy. It makes possible continuous, low dose rate irradiation with neutrons in the geometrical conditions of brachytherapy.

^{252}Cf was identified for the first time at the University of California in Berkeley in 1952. It is produced by the absorption of neutrons by uranium nuclei. More recently it has become possible to make much larger quantities of ^{252}Cf by irradiating ^{239}Pu and its transmutation products with neutrons in a nuclear reactor.

^{252}Cf disintegrates either by a α-emission (97%) or by spontaneous fission (3%) and has a half-life of $2 \cdot 638$ years. The spontaneous fission is accompanied by the emission of $3 \cdot 8$ neutrons on the average. The neutron spectrum shows a maximum at about $1 \cdot 5$ MeV and a mean energy of $2 \cdot 35$ MeV. In addition numerous γ-rays are emitted both at the moment of fission and by the fission products, to which must be added a few γ-rays accompanying the α disintegration. The spectrum of γ-rays has a mean energy of about 1 MeV (p. 219 in [22]).

Miniature sources for medical use have for example the following characteristics: length $4 \cdot 5$ mm, diameter $0 \cdot 7$ mm, content $0 \cdot 3$–$0 \cdot 5$ μg of ^{252}Cf. At 1 cm from a source the contribution of neutrons to the total absorbed dose is about 65% and that of γ-rays about 35%. The RBE of the neutron component depends on the dose, the biological system and the dose rate [86]. As a rule, an RBE of $6 \cdot 5$ is adopted for the doses and dose rates currently used in brachytherapy.

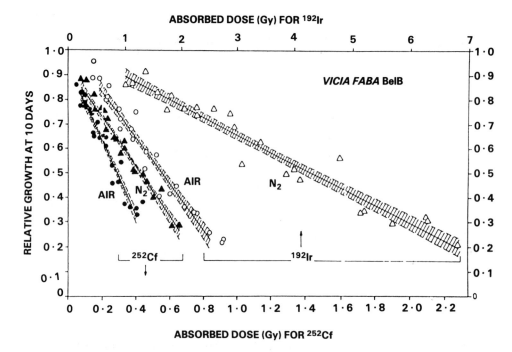

Figure 11.23. OER and hypoxic gain factor (HGF) for ^{252}Cf at low dose rate (conditions analogous to those of brachytherapy). The dose effect curves relate to growth inhibition in *Vicia faba* and were measured with ^{252}Cf and ^{192}Ir, in hypoxic and aerobic conditions. The dose rate of neutrons plus γ-rays from ^{252}Cf was $0\cdot13$ Gy h^{-1}. The dose rate with ^{192}Ir γ-rays was chosen to obtain the same duration of exposure. The OER was found to be $1\cdot4\pm0\cdot1$ for ^{252}Cf and $2\cdot6\pm0\cdot1$ for ^{192}Ir; the HGF is therefore $2\cdot6/1\cdot4=1\cdot8$. After [93].

The potential advantage of ^{252}Cf arises from the combination of irradiation at low dose rate with a reduction in OER. For the dose rates currently used in brachytherapy, the OER of the total emission of ^{252}Cf is about $1\cdot5$ (Figure 11.23) [93]. One of the problems which have limited the clinical use of ^{252}Cf has been the difficulty of producing miniature sources with sufficient activity and free of leakage. In addition there is the high cost of the sources and problems of radiation protection for personnel (barriers against neutrons). The small number of clinical results available do not yet enable a judgement to be made of the therapeutic advantages of this technique in comparison with the difficulties.

Neutron capture therapy

The rationale for this technique is based on the selective uptake of a boron compound by the malignant cells. Irradiation with thermal or epithermal neutrons then leads to the emission of an α-particle by the reaction ^{10}B (n, α)^{7}Li. The α-particle and lithium recoil share an energy of $2\cdot3$ MeV and have ranges of a few micrometres. In this way the cells which have absorbed atoms of boron are irradiated selectively at high-LET.

There are at least three types of clinical situation where a selective uptake of boronated compounds could be expected [28]:

1. The treatment of brain glioblastoma. The blood–brain barrier (BBB) is destroyed at the level of the tumour, but normal CNS cells are protected by the BBB from the boronated compounds present in the blood [37];
2. Some tumours with a specific metabolism through which a boronated compound could be selectively incorporated (e.g. synthesis of melanin in melanoma cells);
3. Tumours against which monoclonal or polyclonal antibodies can be prepared.

So far neutron capture therapy (NCT) has been used only for the treatment of glioblastomas. Two NCT programmes were started in the United States in the 1950s and 1960s. Today NCT is applied only in Japan (Hatanaka [28, 45]). Important progress has been made in developing new boron compounds. Among them, $Na_4 B_{24} H_{22} S_2$, the dimer form of BSH (boron-sulphydrylhydrite or $Na_2 B_{12} H_{11} SH$) seems promising: toxicity tests and pharmacokinetic studies are being performed [28]. As far as the technique of neutron irradiation is concerned, epithermal neutrons appear to be superior to thermal neutrons in providing better penetration and possible skin sparing and so obviating any need for surgery (skin and skull flap). This in turn allows optimization of the beam arrangement and use of fractionated treatments [27].

Besides glioblastomas, extensive animal experiments have been carried out on melanomas: *p*-borono-phenyl-alanine can be selectively incorporated into melanin pigments and thus concentrated in melanoma cells. Promising observations on human tumours have been reported (Mishima [28]).

Monoclonal and polyclonal antibodies can only be used today for diagnosis and tumour localization; unfortunately the achievable concentrations are usually too low for treatment purposes.

NCT will always have definite advantages over simple injections of chemically toxic compounds or of drugs labelled with radionuclides. First, the interval of time between administration of boron and irradiation with neutrons can be selected in order to obtain the optimal boron concentration in the tumour. Second, only the part of the body which contains the target volume will be exposed to neutrons (in general, the boronated compounds themselves are not toxic).

11.4 Specific problems raised in radiation protection by high-LET radiations

Until now we have considered the RBE of fast neutrons for cell killing, i.e. for relatively large doses. In radiation protection other biological effects which occur after much lower doses must be taken into account. The most important high-LET radiations to consider from the point of view of radiation protection are fission neutrons (risks around nuclear reactors, military applications, etc.). Before examining the experimental data it is necessary to consider some methodological aspects.

Methodological approach

RBE at low doses

For the effects of importance in radiation protection (tumour induction, chromosome aberrations, mutations, etc.) the available experimental data are compatible with a dose–effect relation of the linear–quadratic type (Chapter 4) between the effect E and the absorbed dose D:

$$E = \alpha D + \beta D^2 \qquad (1)$$

The relative importance of the linear and quadratic terms depends on the type of radiation, and for high-LET radiations the equation is practically reduced to:

$$E = \alpha D \qquad (2)$$

The variation of RBE with absorbed dose is analogous to that described above (Section 11.1). Thus the RBE of fission neutrons with respect to ^{60}Co γ-rays increases as the dose is reduced (essentially because of the term βD^2 in the equation for γ-rays). In the limit, assuming $E = \alpha D_n$ for neutrons and $E = \beta D^2$ for γ-rays, the RBE would be proportional to $1/\sqrt{D_n}$ and the relation between RBE and dose would be represented on logarithmic coordinates by a straight line with slope $-1/2$. At low doses the RBE tends towards the ratio of the α coefficients for neutrons and γ-rays and reaches a plateau when the dose–effect curves become indistinguishable from their tangents at the origin. This limiting value of RBE will be designated by $\mathrm{RBE_M}$; it is an important factor in radiation protection.

Reference radiation

For experimental determination of RBE, the reference radiation has been either ^{60}Co γ-rays or 200–250 kV X-rays. In radiation protection it has been customary to group together all the low-LET radiations (X-ray, γ-rays, electrons, etc.) and to give them the same value of quality factor ($Q = 1$) (Section 12.5).

The RBE of 200 kV X-rays compared with ^{60}Co γ-rays is close to unity at high doses and high dose rates. In current radiotherapy practice a value of 1·18 (=1/0·85) is usually assumed [51, 74]. However, at low doses and for the effects of importance in radiation protection, much greater values of RBE must be taken into account. Thus for doses below 1 Gy, Underbrink *et al.* [83] found an RBE equal to 2 for the induction of pink mutations in *Tradescantia*. Edwards *et al.* [24] obtained an RBE of 3 for the production of dicentric chromosomes in human lymphocytes. For the same criterion a lower value (RBE=1·5) was found by Fabry *et al.* [26]. From microdosimetric data, an RBE of at least 2 is to be expected [53].

It is also necessary to specify the dose rate and fractionation used for the reference radiation. With low-LET radiations, the effectiveness decreases with reduction in dose rate and with fractionation; data in the literature show that this reduction in effectiveness can reach a factor of 2–10 [61, 84]. Thus, for

example, Grahn and Fritz [34] have studied the influence of dose rate and fractionation on life shortening in the B6CF1 mouse. For irradiation with γ-rays
the life shortening at high dose rate is 43 days per Gy and is reduced to 4 days
per Gy after exposure at low dose rate; after fractionated irradiation (60
fractions) the life shortening is 11–23 days per Gy.

In radiation protection we are concerned usually with small doses received in
many fractions and consequently the most important values of RBE are those
corresponding to highly fractionated irradiation. In practice either X-rays at
high dose rate or γ-rays at low dose rate are used as reference [54]; the latter can
be considered about two times less effective.

Neutron energy

The RBE of neutrons varies with their energy. However, this variation is
relatively small in the energy range 0·1–1 MeV (Figure 11.24). The RBE passes
through a maximum for neutrons of 0·3–0·5 MeV and will therefore be slightly
lower for fission neutrons [44].

The dose rate and fractionation used for irradiation with neutrons can
influence the biological effect, but to a much smaller extent than with low-LET
radiation (Figures 11.8 and 11.9).

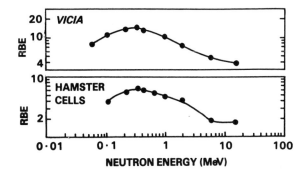

Figure 11.24. RBE of neutrons as a function of energy. Two biological systems are compared:
inhibition of growth in *Vicia faba*;
lethality of Chinese hamster cells. For both systems the RBE shows a maximum at
0·3–0·5 MeV but there is little variation between 0·1 and 1 MeV.
After [44].

Experimental results concerning the RBE of neutrons at low doses

Tumour induction

Several types of tumour have been studied. Shellabarger *et al.* [70–72] have
studied the induction of mammary tumours in the rat (Sprague–Dawley and
ACI) (Figure 11.25). When they compared 0·43 MeV neutrons with X- and γ-
rays, they found that the RBE was proportional to the inverse square root of the
neutron dose ($1/\sqrt{D_n}$). The RBE reached 50 for induction of fibroadenoma in
Sprague–Dawley rats and exceeded 100 at low dose for induction of adenocar-

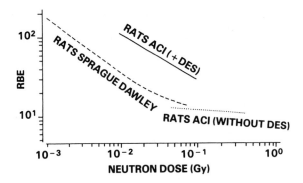

Figure 11.25. RBE of 0·43 MeV neutrons as a function of the neutron dose, for induction of mammary tumours in the rat. For Sprague–Dawley rats, as well as ACI rats after stimulation with oestrogen (diethylstilboestrol, DES), the RBE varies inversely with $\sqrt{D_n}$ over the range of doses explored. At 10 mGy the RBE values are, respectively, about 50 and 100. The RBE is lower (about 10) for ACI rats without hormone stimulation. After [72].

cinoma in ACI rats treated with DES (diethylstilbestrol). The end points were the number of radiation induced tumours and the delay in appearance of the tumours.

Lower RBE values have been obtained at Rijswijk: 15 for induction of adenocarcinoma in the WAG/Rij rat, 13 for induction of fibroadenoma in the same strain of rat and 7 for the induction of fibroadenoma in the Sprague–Dawley rat [10–12].

Grahn *et al.* [35] compared fission neutrons with γ-rays for induction of different types of tumour and obtained RBE values between 8 and 50 depending on the type of tumour: the RBEs for induction of squamous carcinomas were greater than for sarcomas. For induction of lung and mammary tumours in mice, Ullrich [81] found RBE values of 18·5 and 33, respectively at neutron doses of 25 cGy. With another method of analysis and assuming the inverse square root dependence for induction of lung adenocarcinoma, the same authors inferred an RBE of 71 for a neutron dose of 10 mGy.

Other tumours have been studied and large variations in RBE of fission neutrons have been found depending on the type of tumour: from 2 to 3 to more than 200, most RBE values being below 100. A listing is given in Table 11.4.

An important problem is the effect of fractionation or protraction of dose on the effectiveness of neutrons for tumour induction. Fractionation and protraction of low-LET radiation reduce the effectiveness, with only a few exceptions such as the data from Maisin *et al.* [60] on induction of leukaemia, carcinomas and sarcomas. For high-LET radiations, the effects of fractionation and protraction depend on the tumour (Table 11.5). For the induction of ovarian tumours in mice, Ullrich [82] observed that irradiation with fission neutrons was less effective when delivered at low dose rates than at high dose rates. However, for induction of mammary carcinoma, the effect of neutrons was enhanced at low dose rates. Similar observations were made by Vogel and Dickson [87]. In Rijswijk, studies on the induction of mammary carcinoma in WAG/Rij rats with X-rays and 0·5 MeV neutrons indicate that, for equal total absorbed dose, the tumours appeared at approximately the same age after single and fractionated

Table 11.4. **Relative biological effectiveness (RBE) of neutrons for tumour induction (neutron energy 0·43-1 MeV; dose level 10 mGy).**

Tumour	RBE
Lung adenocarcinoma in mice α-neutrons/α photons	18·5
$D_n^{-1/2}$	71
Malignant transformation in hamster embryo cells	10–25
Myeloid leukaemia in mice, daily chronic irradiation	16
Myeloid leukaemia in mice, acute irradiation, square root of α-neutrons/α-photons	13
Myeloid leukaemia in mice	3
Fibroadenoma in Sprague–Dawley rats	
$D_n^{-1/2}$	50
Adenocarcinoma in ACI rats treated with DES,	
$D_n^{-1/2}$	100
Adenocarcinoma in WAG/Rij rats	15
Fibroadenoma in WAG/Rij rats	13
Fibroadenoma in Sprague–Dawley rats	7

After [13].

Table 11.5. **Effect of fractionation or dose rate on tumour induction or life shortening after high-LET irradiation.**

	Change in effectiveness†
Mammary tumours	
Ullrich [82]	+
Vogel and Dickson [87]	+
Broerse *et al.* [11]	=
Ovarian tumours	
Ullrich [82]	−
Pulmonary tumours	
Ullrich [82]	=
Little *et al.* [58]	+ or −
Lundgren *et al.* [59]	+
Life shortening in mice	
Thomson *et al.* [79]	+
Maisin *et al.* [60]	=

†Enhanced (+) reduced (−) or equal (=) with respect to single-dose or high-dose rate.
After [13].

irradiations. As pointed out by Broerse *et al.* [12], experimental studies on mammary carcinogenesis are generally based on whole body irradiation of the animals. The induction of mammary cancer can easily be modified by hormonal factors, and it might well be that specific endocrinological effects caused by the irradiation influence mammary tumour induction to a lesser extent with fractionated or protracted exposures.

As far as induction of pulmonary tumours after exposure to α-particles is concerned, Lundgren *et al.* [59] found in mice that, for a given total dose, a single inhalation of Pu-239 oxide was about four times more effective than repeated exposures. In Syrian hamsters, intratracheal instillation of Po-210 was studied by Little *et al.* [58]. Protraction of the α-irradiation over 120 days was slightly more carcinogenic at lower total lung doses but slightly less carcinogenic at higher doses, in comparison with an exposure limited to a 10-day period.

However, the possible influence of other factors was illustrated by the fact that subsequent weekly instillation of saline alone markedly enhanced the carcinogenic effect of a single intratracheal instillation of Po-210.

Life shortening

Life shortening in the mouse after exposure to low doses is a result exclusively of tumour induction. This criterion is therefore particularly useful for evaluating the totality of tumour induction, complementing the induction of different individual types of tumour. Storer and Mitchell [77] found that the RBE reached a plateau at low doses (RBE=13–22), which may therefore be considered as the RBE_M (see earlier in this section). In these experiments a single dose of fission neutrons was compared with γ-radiation at $0 \cdot 08$ Gy per day.

The influence of fractionation and dose rate have been studied by Grahn and Fritz [34]: fractionated exposure to fission neutrons leads to a life shortening which was greater than or equal to that from a single exposure. With γ-rays on the other hand the effect was reduced as the number of fractions was increased. The RBE of fission neutrons compared with γ-rays lay between 15 and 45 when fractionation was used with both types of radiation. This value represents a plateau which was reached with neutron doses below $0 \cdot 1$ Gy; it may therefore be considered as a value of RBE_M. RBE values of 15 and 12 for life shortening in mice have been reported by Thomson et al. [79] and Covelli et al. [19] respectively for a neutron dose of 10 mGy.

Malignant transformation in vitro

Several teams have studied the RBE of neutrons for the transformation of mammalian cells *in vitro* (Section 12.3). For example Hill et al. [46] have studied the influence of fractionation and dose rate. The RBE of fission neutrons compared with γ-rays was relatively low and close to 3 for a single dose. However, fractionation and reduction in dose rate considerably increased the effectiveness of neutron irradiation (range of doses $0 \cdot 01$–$0 \cdot 1$ Gy). The opposite was found with γ-rays. Consequently high values of RBE were found: $RBE_M=35$ if the neutrons and γ-rays were delivered at low dose rates and $RBE_M=70$ for fractionated irradiation.

Thus the same conclusions are reached as above concerning the role of the time–dose pattern.

Chromosome aberrations

A large number of studies have been made on the RBE of different types of radiation for the production of chromosome aberrations. The principal criterion used is the number of dicentric chromosomes induced in human lymphocytes; the importance of this information in radiation protection is discussed in Sections 3.4 and 12.1.

Table 11.6 summarizes the results of Edwards et al. [24]. At low doses, 250 kV X-rays are about three times more effective than ^{60}Co γ-rays; on the other hand fission neutrons (mean energy $0 \cdot 7$ and $0 \cdot 9$ MeV) are about 50 times more effective than γ-rays. A lower value of RBE of fission neutrons was obtained by

Bauchinger *et al.* [6]: RBE=11 at 0·04 Gy. However, the RBE continued to rise down to the lowest dose studied, implying a greater value of RBE$_M$.

The RBE values of fast neutrons are lower: 16·7 for 14·7 MeV neutrons and 30·3 for 7·6 MeV neutrons [24]. Fabry *et al.* [26] have obtained values of RBE$_M$ relative to ^{60}Co γ-rays of 14, 6·2 and 4·7 for neutrons produced in a cyclotron with deuterons of 16, 33 and 50 MeV, respectively (mean neutron energies 6·5, 14 and 21 MeV) (Table 11.7). These authors found an RBE of 1·5 for 200 kV X-rays compared with ^{60}Co γ-rays.

Table 11.6. Chromosome aberrations in human lymphocytes.

Radiation	α (Gy^{-1})×10	β (Gy^{-2})×10^2	RBE$_M$†
15 MeV electrons	0·55±1·12	5·66±0·55	0·35
15 MeV electrons (pulsed)	0·90±1·92	6·08±0·92	0·57
^{60}Co γ-rays	1·57±0·29	5·00±0·20	1·00
250 kV X-rays	4·76±0·54	6·19±0·31	3·03
14·7 MeV neutrons	26·2±4·0	8·8 ±2·8	16·7
Cyclotron neutrons $\bar{E}$=7·6 MeV	47·8±3·3	6·4 ±2·0	30·3
^{252}Cf neutrons (2·13 MeV)	60·0±1·9	—	38·2
Fission neutrons (0·9 MeV)	72·8±2·4	—	46·4
Fission neutrons (0·7 MeV)	83·5±1·0	—	53·1

†The biological effect (E), or the number of dicentrics per cell, is given by $E=\alpha D+\beta D^2$, D being the absorbed dose. The maximum RBE at low doses, RBE$_M$, is then given by the ratio of the values of α. After [24].

Table 11.7. RBE of fast neutrons and orthovoltage X-rays for the production of dicentric chromosomes in human lymphocytes.

Radiation	RBE at a dose of 2·0 Gy of γ-rays	RBE at a dose of 0·5 Gy of γ-rays	RBE$_M$ αtest/αref
^{60}Co γ-rays	1	1	1
250 kV X-rays	1·2	1·3	1·5
Neutrons d(50)+Be	1·8	3·0	4·7
Neutrons d(33)+Be	2·3	3·8	6·2
Neutrons d(16)+Be	4·0	8·2	14·0

After [26].

Genetic effects

The RBE of neutrons for genetic effects has been studied in a variety of biological systems. The mechanisms of production of mutations are to a certain extent similar, allowing the results to be extrapolated cautiously to man.

High values of RBE have been found in plant systems. For example, for pink mutations in *Tradescantia*, Underbrink *et al.* [83] found an RBE of 100 for fission neutrons compared with ^{60}Co γ-rays and of 50 when compared with 200 kV X-rays. For fast neutrons, Pihet *et al.* [64] found lower values: in comparison with γ-rays, the RBE of neutrons produced with 65 MeV protons (p(65)+Be) was found to be 12±4 at a neutron dose of 4 mGy.

Grahn *et al.* [33] studied various effects in mice (dominant lethal mutations, chromosomal translocations and other abnormalities in spermatogonia). They found values of RBE$_M$ of 10–45 for fission neutrons compared with X-rays, depending on the biological criterion. Higher values of RBE have been seen for chromosomal translocations in spermatogonia and for neutrons given once per week compared with γ-rays at low dose rate.

Cataracts

For production of cataracts, high values of RBE have been obtained by Bateman *et al.* [4] who compared fission neutrons (0·43 MeV) with 200 kV X-rays. RBE values greater than 100 were seen at 1 mGy of neutrons and, in addition, the RBE was found to increase in proportion to $1/\sqrt{D_n}$ for doses at least as low as 1 mGy. These studies have been repeated by Di Paola *et al.* [20] who found values of RBE from 25–40 at 10 mGy of neutrons.

Conclusions

The available data concerning the RBE of fission neutrons are summarized in Table 11.8. There are very large variations of RBE (from 3 to 200) depending on the criterion and, for a given criterion, from one study to another. However, there are a number of values in the range 15–70 [75]. A large proportion of the recent results provide justification for a reevaluation of the quality factor Q [54]. The RBE of fast neutrons used in therapy is lower than that of neutrons with energies of 0·43–1 MeV such as those produced by fission.

Finally allowance must be made for the reference radiation since there is evidence that the RBE of 200 kV X-rays could be as high as 2 compared with ^{60}Co γ-rays at low doses and low dose rates.

Table 11.8.   RBE$_M$ of fission neutrons (with respect to γ-rays in fractionated exposures).

Effect	RBE$_M$
Tumour induction	$\approx$ 3 to $\approx$ 200
Life shortening	15–45
Cell transformation	35–70
Chromosome aberrations	40–50
Genetic effects in mammals	10–45
Cataracts	25–200
Micronuclei	6–60
Loss of weight of the testis	5–20

After [75].

References

1. G. W. Barendsen, Responses of cultured cells, tumours and normal tissues to radiations of different linear energy transfer. *Curr. Top. Radiat. Res. Quarterly*, North-Holland, Amsterdam, 1968, 4: 293–356.
2. G. W. Barendsen, J. J. Broerse. Differences in radiosensitivity of cells from various types of experimental tumors in relation to the RBE of 15 MeV neutrons. *Int. J. Radiat. Oncol. Biol. Phys.*, 1977, 3: 211–214.
3. G. W. Barendsen, C. J. Koot, G. R. van Kersen, D. K. Bewley, S. B. Field, C. J. Parnell. The effect of oxygen on impairment of the proliferative capacity of human cells in culture by ionizing radiations of different LET. *Int. J. Rad. Biol.*, 1966, 10: 317–327.
4. J. L. Bateman, H. H. Rossi, A. M. Kellerer, C. V. Robinson, V. P. Bond. Dose-dependence of fast neutron RBE for lens opacification in mice. *Radiat. Res.*, 1972, 51: 381–390.

5. J.J. Battermann., K. Breur, G.A.M. Hart, H.A. van Pepenzeel. Observations on pulmonary metastases in patients after single doses and multiple fractions of neutrons and cobalt-60 gamma rays. *Eur. J. Cancer* 1981, **17**: 539–548.
6. M. Bauchinger, L. Koester, E. Schmid, J. Dresp, S. Streng. Chromosome aberrations in human lymphocytes induced by fission neutrons. *Int. J. Radiat. Biol.*, 1984, **45**: 449–457.
7. D.K. Bewley. The physics and radiobiology of fast neutron beams. Adam Hilger, Bristol and New York, 1989.
8. A. Breit, G. Burger, E. Scherer, A. Wambersie (eds). Advances in radiation therapy with heavy particles. *Strahlentherapie*, 1985, vol. 161, No. 12.
9. N. Breteau, J.P. Le Bourgeois, J.J. Battermann, A. Wambersie (eds). High LET particles in radiation therapy. *J. Eur. Radiothérapie*, 1984, **5**, No. 3. 115–264.
10. J.J. Broerse, G.W. Barendsen, G.R. van Kersen. Survival of cultured human cells after irradiation with fast neutrons of different energies in hypoxic and oxygenated conditions. *Int. J. Radiat. Biol.*, 1967, **13**: 559–572.
11. J.J. Broerse, L.A. Hennen, M.J. van Zwieten. Radiation carcinogenesis in experimental animals and its implications for radiation protection. *Int. J. Radiat. Biol.*, 1985, **48**: 167–187.
12. J.J. Broerse, L.A. Hennen, M.J. van Zwieten, C.F. Hollander. Mammary carcinogenesis in different rat strains after single and fractionated irradiations, in: *Neutron carcinogenesis* (J.J. Broerse, G.B. Gerber, eds), Report EUR 8084 (Commission of the European Communities, Brussels). 1982. 155–168.
13. J.J. Broerse, D.W. Van Bekkum, C. Zurcher. Radiation carcinogenesis in experimental animals. *Experientia*, 1989, **45**: 60–69.
14. S.E. Bush, A.R. Smith, S. Zink. Pion radiotherapy at LAMPF. *Int. J. Radiat. Oncol. Biol. Phys.*, 1982, **8**: 2181–2186.
15. J.R. Castro, W.M. Saunders, C.A. Tobias, G.T. Y.-Chen, S. Curtis, J.T. Lyman, J.M. Collier, S. Pitluck, K.A. Woodruff, E.A. Blakely, T. Tenforde, D. Char. T.L. Phillips, E.L. Alpen. Treatment of cancer with heavy charged particles. *Int. J. Radiat. Oncol. Biol. Phys.*, 1982, **8**: 2191–2198.
16. M. Catterall, R.D. Errington, D.K. Bewley, F. Paice, S. Blake. Observations on thirteen years fast neutron therapy. *J. Eur. Radiother.*, 1984, **3**: 132–137.
17. J.D. Chapman. Biophysical models of mammalian cell inactivation by radiation, in: *Radiation biology in cancer research* (R.E. Meyn, H.R. Withers, eds), pp. 21–32. Raven Press, New York, 1988.
18. P. Chauvel, A. Wambersie (eds). EULIMA Workshop on the potential value of light ion beam therapy. Publication EUR 12165 EN of the Commission of the European Communities, c ECSC-EEC-EAEC, Brussels-Luxembourg, 1989.
19. V. Covelli, M. Coppola, V. Di Majo, S. Rebessi, B. Bassani. Tumor induction and life shortening in $BC3F_1$ female mice at low doses of fast neutrons and X-rays. *Radiat. Res.*, 1988, **113**: 362–374.
20. M. Di Paola, M. Coppola, J. Baarli, M. Bianchi, A.H. Sullivan. Biological responses to various neutron energies from 1 to 600 MeV. II. Lens opacification in mice, *Radiat. Res.*, 1980, **84**: 453–461.
21. W. Duncan, S.J. Arnott, J.J. Battermann, J.A. Orr, G. Schmitt, G.K. Kerr. Fast neutrons in the treatment of head and neck cancers: the results of a multi-centre randomly controlled trial. *Radiother. Oncol.*, 1984, **2**: 293–300.
22. A. Dutreix, G. Marinello, A. Wambersie. *Dosimétrie en curiethérapie*. Masson, Paris, 1982.
23. J. Dutreix, Neutrons pour la radiothérapie. *J. Biophys. Méd. Nucl.*, 1981, **5**: 3–11.
24. A.A. Edwards, D.C. Lloyd, R.J. Purrott, J.S. Prosser. The dependence of chromosome aberration yields on dose rate and radiation quality, in: *Research and development report*, 1979–1981, RAD 4, pp. 83–85. National Radiological Protection Board, Chilton, Oxon, U.K., 1982.
25. R.D. Errington. Advanced carcinoma of the paranasal sinuses treated with 7.5 MeV fast neutrons. *Bull.Cancer (Paris)*, 1986, **73**: 569–576.
26. L. Fabry, A. Leonard, A. Wambersie. Induction of chromosome aberrations in Go human lymphocytes by low doses of ionizing radiations of different quality. *Radiat. Res.*, 1985, **103**: 122–134.
27. R.G. Fairchild, V.P. Bond. Current status of ^{10}B-neutron capture therapy: enhancement of tumor dose via beam filtration and dose rate, and the effects of these parameters on minimum boron content: a theoretical evaluation. *Int. J. Radiat. Oncol. Biol. Phys.*, 1985, **11**: 831–840.
28. R.G. Fairchild, V.P. Bond, A.D. Woodhead (eds), *Clinical aspects of neutron capture therapy*. Plenum Press, New York and London, 1989.
29. B. Fertil, P.J. Deschavanne, J. Gueulette, A. Possoz, A. Wambersie, E.P. Malaise. *In vitro* radiosensitivity of six human cell lines. II. Relation to the RBE of 50- MeV neutrons. *Radiat. Res.*, 1982, **90**: 526–537.
30. H.D. Franke, G. Langendorff, A. Hess, Die Strahlenbehandlung des Prostata-Carcinoms in Stadium C mit schnellen Neutronen. *Verhandlungsbericht der Deutschen Gesellschaft für Urologie*, 32 Tagung 1980, pp. 175–180. Springer-Verlag, Berlin, Heidelberg, New York, 1981.

31. R. L. Gragg, R. M. Humphrey, H. D. Thames, R. E. Meyn. The response of Chinese hamster ovary cells to fast neutron radiotherapy beams. III. Variation in relative biological effectiveness with position in the cell cycle. *Radiat. Res.,* 1978, **76**: 283–291.

32. E. S. Gragoudas, M. Goitein, L. Verhey, J. Munzenreider, H. D. Suit, A. Koehler. Proton beam irradiation. An alternative to enucleation for intraocular melanomas. *Ophtalmology,* 1980, **87**: 571–581.

33. D. Grahn, B. A. Carnes, B. H. Farrington, C. H. Lee. Genetic injury in hybrid male mice exposed to low doses of ^{60}Co γ rays or fission neutrons. I. Response to single doses, *Mutat. Res.,* 1984, **129**: 215–229.

34. D. Grahn, T. Fritz. Studies on chronic radiation injury with mice and dogs exposed to external whole-body irradiation at ANL, in: *Proceedings of the 22nd Symposium on Life Sciences,* Battelle Pacific Northwest Laboratory, Hanford, 27–30 September, 1983, U.S. DOE CONF-830951, 1984.

35. D. Grahn, J. F. Thomson, F. S. Williamson, L. S. Lombard. Somatic and genetic effects of low doses of fission neutrons and ^{60}Co gamma rays, in: *Proceedings of the Seventh Intl. Congress of Radiation Research,* Amsterdam, 3–10 July 1983, Abstract Book C, C2-05, Martinus Nijhof, 1983.

36. V. Grégoire, J. Gueulette, M. Octave-Prignot, B. M. de Coster, A. Wambersie. Réparation cellulaire précoce, du poumon et de l'intestin, chez la souris, après irradiation par neutrons rapides et rayons gamma. *C. R. Soc. Biol.,* 1986, **180**: 372–378.

37. V. Gregoire, A. Keyeux, A. Wambersie. Blood–brain-barrier impairment after irradiation: implication in boron neutron capture therapy, in: (R. G. Fairchild, V. P. Bond, A. D. Woodhead, eds), *Clinical aspects of neutron capture therapy,* pp. 299–309. Plenum Press, New York and London, 1989.

38. T. Griffin, J. Blasko, G. Laramore. Results of fast neutron beam radiotherapy. Pilot studies at the University of Washington, in: *High-LET radiations in clinical radiotherapy,* (G. W. Barendsen, J. J. Broerse, K. Breur, eds), pp. 23–29. *Eur. J. Cancer.,* Suppl. 1979.

39. T. W. Griffin, R. Davis, F. R. Hendrickson, M. H. Maor, G. E. Laramore. Fast neutron radiation therapy for unresectable squamous cell carcinomas of the head and neck: the results of a randomized RTOG study. *Int. J. Radiat. Oncol. Biol. Phys.,* 1984, **10**: 2217–2221.

40. T. W. Griffin, R. Davis, G. E. Laramore, D. H. Hussey, F. R. Hendrickson, A. Rodriguez-Antunez. Fast neutron irradiation of metastatic cervical adenopathy. The results of a randomized RTOG study. *Int. J. Radiat. Oncol. Biol. Phys.,* 1983, **9**: 1267–1270.

41. T. W. Griffin, T. F. Pajak, G. E. Laramore, W. Duncan, M. P. Richter, F. R. Hendrickson, M. H. Maor. Neutron vs photon irradiation of inoperable salivary gland tumors: results of an RTOG-MRC cooperative randomized study. *Int. J. Radiat. Oncol. Biol. Phys.,* 1988, **15**: 1085–1090.

42. M. Guichard, J. Gueulette, M. Octave-Prignot, A. Wambersie, E. P. Malaise. Effect of combined misonidazole and d(50)+Be neutrons on a human melanoma transplanted into nude mice. *Radiology,* 1980, **136**: 479–484.

43. E. J. Hall, R. G. Graves, T. L. Phillips, H. D. Suit (eds), *Particle accelerators in radiation therapy.* Pergamon, Oxford, 1982.

44. E. J. Hall, J. K. Novak, A. M. Kellerer, H. H. Rossi, S. Marino, L. J. Goodman. RBE as a Function of Neutron Energy. I. Experimental observations, *Radiat. Res.,* 1975, **64**: 245–255.

45. H. Hatanaka. Clinical experience of boron neutron capture therapy for malignant brain tumors. *Proc. of First International Symposium on Neutron Capture Therapy,* 12–14 Oct. 1983, Brookhaven National Laboratory Report No. 51730, 1983, pp. 384–393.

46. C. K. Hill, B. A. Carnes, A. Han, M. M. Elkind. Neoplastic transformation is enhanced by multiple low doses of fission-spectrum neutrons, *Radiat. Res.,* 1985, **102**: 404–410.

47. S. Hornsey, G. Silini. Comparisons of the effects of X-rays and cyclotron neutrons on mouse ascites tumours, mouse testis and chick embryos. *Br. J. Radiol.,* 1963, **36**: 92–97.

48. International Commission on Radiation Protection. Report of the RBE Subcommittee to the International Commission on Radiation Protection and the International Commission on Radiation Units and Measurements. *Health Physics,* 1963, **9**: 357–386.

49. International Commission on Radiation Units and Measurements. *Linear Energy Transfer.* ICRU Report 16, 1970.

50. International Commission on Radiation Units and Measurements. *Neutron dosimetry for biology and medicine.* ICRU Report 26, 1977.

51. International Commission on Radiation Units and Measurements. *Dose specification for reporting external beam therapy with photons and electrons.* ICRU Report 29, 1978.

52. International Commission on Radiation Units and Measurements. *Quantitative concepts and dosimetry in radiobiology.* ICRU Report 30, 1979.

53. International Commission on Radiation Units and Measurements. *Microdosimetry,* ICRU Report 36, 1983.

54. International Commission on Radiation Units and Measurements. *The quality factor in radiation protection.* ICRU Report 40, 1986.

55. International Commission on Radiation Units and Measurements. *Clinical neutron dosimetry, Part I: Determination of absorbed dose in a patient treated by external beams of fast neutrons.* ICRU Report 45, 1989.

56. C.M. Lalanne, G. Mathieu, D.K. Bewley, A. Wambersie (eds), Fast neutrons in radiation therapy, *Bull. Cancer*, 1986, **73**: 546–561.

57. B. Larsson. Use of medium energy particles in radiobiology and radiotherapy. *J. Eur. Radiother.*, 1984, **5**: 223–234.

58. J.B. Little, A.R. Kennedy. R.B. McGandy. Effect of dose rate on the induction of experimental lung cancer in hamsters by α radiation. *Radiat. Res.* 1985, **103**: 293–299.

59. D.L. Lundgren, N.A. Gillett, F.F. Hahn, W.C. Griffith, R.O. McClellan. Effects of protraction of the α dose to the lungs of mice by repeated inhalation exposure to aerosols of $^{239}PuO_2$ *Radiat. Res.*, 1987, **111**: 201–224.

60. J.R. Maisin, A. Wambersie, G.B. Gerber, G. Mattelin, M. Lambiet-Collier, B de Coster, J. Gueulette. Life-shortening and disease incidence in C57Bl mice after single and fractionated gamma and high-energy neutron exposure. *Radiat. Res.*, 1988, **113**: 300–317.

61. National Council on Radiation Protection and Measurements. *The influence of dose and its distribution in time on dose-response relationships for low-LET radiations.* NCRP Report 64, 1980.

62. Ch. Perret. L. Zographos, C. Gailloud, R. Greiner. Die behandlung Intraokularer Melanome mit Protonen am Schweizerischen Institut für Nuklearforschung (SIN) in: *Neue Aspekte radiologischer Diagnostik und Therapie, Jahrbuch der Schweizerischen Gesellschaft für Radiologie und Nuklearmedizin*, pp. 307–318. Hans Huber, Bern, 1985.

63. L.J. Peters, M.H. Maor, G.E. Laramore, T.W. Griffin, F.R. Hendrickson. Review of clinical results of fast neutron therapy in the USA. *Strahlentherapie*, 1985, **161**, 731–738.

64. P. Pihet, H.G. Menzel, H. Haut, G. Garot, A. Wambersie. Shape of the RBE-dose relationship for fast neutrons at low doses for somatic mutations in *Tradescantia*, in: *Fifth Symposium on Neutron Dosimetry*, vol. 1, Radiation protection aspects. (H. Schraube, G. Burger, J. Booz eds), pp. 45–55. Commission of the European Communities: EUR. 9762en, Brussels, Luxembourg, 1985.

65. P. Pihet, C. Norman, J. Gueulette, H.G. Menzel, A. Wambersie. Microdosimétrie des faisceaux de neutronthérapie d(50)+Be et p(65)+Be à Cyclone, Louvain-la-Neuve pp. 269–277, in: *Radiophysique*, XXIV Congrès de la Société Française des Physiciens d'Hôpital, Tours, 1985.

66. M.R. Raju. *Heavy particle radiotherapy*, Academic Press. New York, 1980.

67. F. Richard, L. Renard, A. Wambersie. Current results of neutron therapy at the UCL, for soft tissue sarcomas and prostatic adenocarcinomas. *Bull. Cancer*, 1986, **73**: 562–568.

68. F. Richard, L. Renard, A. Wambersie. Neutron therapy of soft tissue sarcoma at Louvain-la-Neuve (interim results 1987) *Strahlenther. Onkol.* 1989, **165**: 306–308.

69. K.J. Russell, G.E. Laramore, J.M. Krall, F.J. Thomas, M.H. Maor, F.R. Hendrickson, J.N. Krieger, T.W. Griffin. Eight years experience with neutron radiotherapy in the treatment of stages C and D prostate cancer: Updated results of the RTOG 7704 randomized clinical trial. *The Prostate*, 1987, **11**: 183–193.

70. C.J. Shellabarger, R.D. Brown, A.R. Rao, J.P. Shanley, V.P. Bond, A.M. Kellerer, H.H. Rossi, L.J. Goodman, R.E. Mills. Rat mammary carcinogenesis following neutron or x radiation, in: *Symposium on the effects of neutron irradiation upon cell function*, Munich 1973 pp. 391–401. International Atomic Energy Agency. Vienna, 1974.

71. C.J. Shellabarger, D. Chmelevsky, A.M. Kellerer. Induction of mammary neoplasms in the Sprague-Dawley rat by 430-keV neutrons and X-rays. *J. Natl. Cancer Inst.*, 1980, **64**: 821–833.

72. C.J. Shellabarger, D. Chmelevsky, A.M. Kellerer, J.P. Stone, S. Holtzman. Induction of mammary neoplasms in the ACI rat by 430-keV neutrons, X-rays, and diethylstilbestrol. *J. Nat. Cancer Inst.*, 1982, **69**: 1135–1146.

73. W.U. Shipley, J.A. Stanley, V D. Courtenay, S.B. Field. Repair of radiation damage in Lewis lung carcinoma cells following in situ treatment with fast neutrons and γ-rays. *Cancer Res.*, 1975, **35**: 932–938.

74. W.K. Sinclair. The relative biological effectiveness of 22 Mevp X-rays, Cobalt-60 gamma rays and 200 Kvcp X-rays. VII. Summary of studies for five criteria of effect. *Radiat. Res.*, 1962, **16**: 394–398.

75. W.K. Sinclair. Experimental RBE values of high-LET radiations at low doses and the implications for quality factor assignment. *Radiation Protection Dosimetry*, 1985, **13**: 319–326, Nuclear Technology Publ.

76. R.S. Stone, Neutron therapy and specific ionization. *Am. J. Roentgenol.*, 1948, **59**: 771–785.

77. J.B. Storer, T.J. Mitchell. Limiting values for the RBE of fission neutrons at low doses for life shortening in mice. *Radiat. Res.*, 1984, **97**: 396–406.

78. H. Suit, M. Goitein, J. Munzenrider, L. Verhey, P. Blitzer, E. Gragoudas, A.M. Koehler, M. Urie, R. Gentry, W. Shipley, M. Urano, J. Duttenhaver, M. Wagner. Evaluation of the clinical applicability of proton beams in definitive fractionated radiation therapy. *Int. J. Radiat. Oncol. Biol. Phys.*, 1982, **8**: 2199–2205.

79. J. F. Thomson, F. S. Williamson, D. Grahn. Life shortening in mice exposed to fission neutrons and gamma-rays. *Radiat. Res.,* 1985, **104**: 420–428.
80. H. Tsunemoto, S. Morita, S. Satho, Y. Iino, S. Yul Yoo. Present status of fast neutron therapy in Asian countries. *Strahlenther. Onkol.,* 1989, **165**: 330–336.
81. R. L. Ullrich. Tumor induction in BALB/c female mice after fission neutron or γ-irradiation. *Radiat. Res.,* 1983, **93**: 506–515.
82. R. L. Ullrich. Tumor induction in Balb/c mice after fractionated or protracted exposures to fission-spectrum neutrons. Radiat. Res, 1984, **97**: 587–597.
83. A. G. Underbrink, A. M. Kellerer, R. E. Mills, A. H. Sparrow. Comparison of X-ray and gamma-ray–dose response curves for pink somatic mutations in Tradescantia clones 02, *Radiat. Environ. Biophys.,* 1976, **13**: 295–303.
84. United Nations Scientific Committee on the Effects of Atomic Radiation (UNSCEAR). *Sources effects and risk of ionizing radiation.* Report to the General Assembly with annexes, United Nations, New York, 1988.
85. J. Van Dam, G. Billiet, A. Wambersie, A. Bridier, A. Dutreix, C. Bouhnik. RBE of d(50)+Be neutrons and of 650-MeV helium ions at different depths for growth reduction in Vicia faba. *Radiat. Res.,* 1980, **81**: 31–47.
86. J. Van Dam, J. Bronte, A. Dutreix, H. Bouhnik, A. Wambersie. RBE of californium-252 at low dose rate for growth inhibition in Vicia faba. *J. Eur. Radiother.,* 1982, **3**: 109–120.
87. H. H. Vogel, H. W. Dickson. Mammary neoplasia in Sprague-Dawley rats following acute and protracted irradiation, in: *Neutron Carcinogenesis. EUR 8084* (J. J. Broerse, G. B. Gerber, eds), pp. 135–154. Commission of the European Communities, 1982.
88. C. F. Von Essen, G. Bodendörfer, J. E. Mizoe, H. Tsujii, A. J. Wijnmaalen, A. Zimmermann. Recent clinical results of the SIN pion therapy program. *J. Eur. Radiother.,* 1984, **5**: 167–169.
89. S. Vynckier, J. P. Meulders, P. Robert, A. Wambersie. The protontherapy program at the cyclotron 'Cyclone' of Louvain-la-Neuve (first dosimetric results). *J. Eur. Radiother.,* 1984, **5**: 245–247.
90. A. Wambersie. The European experience in neutron-therapy at the end of 1981. *Int. J. Radiat. Oncol. Biol. Phys.,* 1982, **8**: 2145–2152.
91. A. Wambersie, G. W. Barendsen, N. Breteau. Overview and prospects of the application of fast neutrons in cancer therapy. *J. Eur. Radiothér.,* 1984, **5**: 248–264.
92. A. Wambersie, J. J. Battermann. Review and evolution of clinical results in the EORTC heavy-particle therapy group. *Strahlentherapie,* 1985, **161**: 746–755.
93. A. Wambersie, A. Dutreix, H. Bouhnik, J. Van Dam, J. Bonte, OER of californium-252 at low dose rate for growth inhibition in Vicia faba. *J. Eur. Radiother.,* 1984, **5**: 3–9.
94. H. R. Withers. Neutron radiobiology and clinical consequences, *Strahlentherapie,* 1985, **161**: 739–745.
95. H. R. Withers, K. Mason, B. O. Reid, N. Dubravsky, H. T. Barkley, B. W. Brown. J. B. Smathers. Response of mouse intestine to neutrons and gamma rays in relation to dose fractionation and division cycle. *Cancer,* 1974, **34**: 39–47.
96. H. R. Withers, L. J. Peters. The application of RBE values to clinical trials of high-LET radiations, in: *High LET radiations in clinical radiotherapy* (G. W. Barendsen, J. J. Broerse, K. Breur eds), pp. 257–261. Pergamon Press, Oxford, 1979.

Chapter 12.

Effects of irradiation on the human body: radiopathology

There has been concern with the risks of ionizing radiation since the beginning of the 20th century. Research on the subject has increased in parallel with the rapid development of the medical uses of ionizing radiation. Also the first victims of radiation were the physicists and doctors involved in research in radiology. This helps to explain why for nearly a century the effects of ionizing radiation on man have been studied more intensely than those of other noxious agents, physical or chemical. The feelings of guilt which Hiroshima and Nagasaki produced in the scientific community explains why the study of radiopathology became even more extensive after 1945.

It may seem paradoxical that the extent of these researches has given rise to some misgivings. It may be thought that the scale of the research is not commensurate with the gravity of the danger. Moreover, as the risks of radiation were the first to be quantified they have received special attention, particularly as ionizing radiation can be detected more easily than any of the other noxious physical and chemical agents, thanks to the extraordinary sensitivity of the measuring equipment. Thus a Geiger counter can measure doses several tens of thousands of times lower than the minimum dose which can produce any observable biological effect.

In Europe and the USA several hundred thousand people in hospitals and clinics work with ionizing radiation (diagnostic radiology, nuclear medicine, radiotherapy). A million patients are treated each year by radiotherapy and many millions are examined by diagnostic radiology. In Europe about a hundred thousand people work in nuclear establishments. In the United States more than a million workers are exposed to ionizing radiation in the course of their work.

In spite of the large number of people exposed, accidental irradiations are rare in hospitals and very exceptional in nuclear establishments where working practices can be much stricter. Accidents are a little more frequent in other industrial applications: industrial radiography and crystallography make up two thirds of the 40 accidents which have occurred in France during the last 25 years, none of which has been fatal. In the whole world the number of deaths due to accidental irradiation was less than 30 during the 40 years up to the date of the accident at Chernobyl. These remarkable results are due to a rigorous organization of radiation protection, which specialists in hygiene consider as a model for protection against noxious agents.

Since 1928 groups of specialists, doctors and physicists, have met to discuss the risks and the necessary precautions and have founded the International Commission for Radiological Protection (ICRP) whose first recommendations were published in that very year. Knowledge of the biological effects of ionizing radiation in man is based on the study of several hundred thousand patients treated with X-rays or radioactive isotopes, several groups of workers — painters of luminous dials, radiologists, etc. — and the survivors at Hiroshima and Nagasaki [7, 63–66].

In addition to early somatic effects caused by exposure above the threshold of tolerance, two types of late effect must be distinguished. One is caused by the death of a large number of cells in a tissue (somatic effect) or an embryo (teratogenic effect). The other type, referred to as stochastic, originates from a defect occurring in a single cell: carcinogenesis and genetic effects. We will examine each of these in turn.

12.1 Somatic effects

These lesions occur in all subjects who have received radiation above a threshold and their severity increases with the dose. No effect can be detected below the threshold. The threshold varies between a few Gy and a few tens of Gy depending on the effect considered; it is always greater than several tens of cGy per year.

The effects depend on three factors: dose, fractionation and volume irradiated. For example, a single acute dose of 5 Gy to the whole body results in death of about half the irradiated subjects, whereas the same dose has no effect if it is delivered over a sufficiently long time and causes only a slight erythema when given as a single dose to a small area. We will examine first irradiation of the whole body, followed by that of more localized areas.

Total body irradiation

This occurs in three circumstances: preparation for organ transplantation, treatment of certain types of lymphoma, and accidental irradiation. In the first two the irradiation is homogeneous, but it is usually heterogeneous in the third.

In animals, particularly in the mouse, it is conventional to distinguish three ranges of dose:

1. With very large doses (100–150 Gy) death occurs in a few hours or 1 or 2 days, caused by neurological complications (disorientation, loss of co-ordination, respiratory distress, convulsions, coma), probably caused by vascular damage and cerebral oedema. In man only 2 accidents of this type have been reported; in both cases death occurred in less than 48 h.
2. With doses of 12–20 Gy, death is due to intestinal damage and occurs at the time when this damage is expressed, 4–7 days later (see Chapter 5). The clinical picture is dominated by diarrhoea and wasting followed by septicaemia, haemorrhage and intestinal perforations.

3. With doses of about 10 Gy the intestinal symptoms are less intense and death is caused by aplasia of haemopoietic tissues leading to infection and haemorrhage about 15 days after irradiation. With doses below 12 Gy mice can be rescued by a bone marrow transplant from histocompatible animals.

In man the symptomatology may be different as treatment profoundly modifies the development of the lesions [9, 61]. Beginning in 1958, use was made for organ transplantation of the immunosuppression occurring after irradiation. Kidney grafts after total-body irradiation were performed simultaneously at Boston and Paris in 1958. It was seen that doses of 3·5–4 Gy induced immunotolerance of the grafted kidney and were well tolerated if the patients were protected against infection during the period of bone marrow aplasia. Later it was found with patients suffering from leukaemia that it was necessary to give a dose of 8–10 Gy to induce tolerance to a bone marrow transplant, but the first patients treated in this way died from graft-versus-host disease. With progress in the understanding of tissue typing (HLA), it has been possible to reduce the frequency and severity of these reactions and so to use total body irradiation for the treatment of leukaemia. In chronic lymphatic leukaemia and non-Hodgkin's lymphoma much lower doses are given and the radiation is divided into fractions of 5–15 cGy, up to a total dose of a few gray at most. These patients are sometimes very radiosensitive, probably because of the reduction in the pool of haemopoietic stem cells.

The experience gained from these medical irradiations has led to a better understanding of the development of effects after accidental irradiation.

(1) In the absence of a bone marrow graft the mean lethal dose (LD 50) for man is about 4·5 Gy. One can arrive at this figure both from accidental irradiation [42] and therapeutic treatment [61]. In 1969 Lusbaugh [39] estimated it to be 3 Gy based on data from Hiroshima and various accidents. However, it is definitely greater for therapeutic irradiations, reaching 4 Gy after conventional treatment and 5 Gy if the subject is isolated under germ-free conditions with transfusion of platelets and intensive medical treatment. Without a bone marrow graft the probability of survival is small after doses above 6–7 Gy [9]. Thus man is more radiosensitive than the mouse or the rat in which the LD 50 is about 9 Gy, but his radiosensitivity is close to that of the dog and other large mammals (Table 12.1).

(2) At these doses, in man as in animals, death is the result of aplasia of haemopoietic tissue, leading to haemorrhage and infection. After the

Table 12.1 50% lethal dose (LD 50) in mammals.

Species	LD 50 (Gy)
Sheep	1·55
Pig	1·95
Goat	2·30
Dog	2·65
Rabbit	8·40
Mouse	9·00
Rat	9·00
Hamster	9·00
Guinea-pig	2·55
Monkey (according to the species)	3·5–5
Man	4·5–5

immediate symptoms caused by the radiation (nausea), the subject is asymptomatic until the appearance of an intense asthenia, shivering, fever and buccal ulceration. With lower doses the aplasia is less marked, develops later and is repaired more slowly. A fall in lymphocyte count is the earliest symptom and changes in the number of platelets, polynuclear cells and reticulocytes run in parallel. When regeneration begins, it takes place simultaneously and very rapidly in all three cell lines (Section 5.3).

(3) After a histocompatible bone marrow graft and in subjects less than 40 years old, there is a very high survival rate with doses of 10–12 Gy. At this dose given in a single session the critical tissue is the lung and the number of deaths due to pneumonopathy during the 6 months following irradiation is greater than that due to haemopoietic aplasia. Consequently the lung should be protected during irradiation before grafting. Subjects more than 50 years old are more sensitive and a large proportion do not survive this dose.

(4) During the first few hours the most important symptoms are nausea and vomiting. At 1 Gy these occur in more than half the patients and in nearly all beyond 5 Gy; they develop earlier and are more severe as the dose is increased.

(5) The frequency of attacks of nausea and the severity of the post-irradiation syndrome is markedly reduced when the dose rate is lower than $0 \cdot 3 \, \text{cGy min}^{-1}$.

(6) The other symptoms develop later or are more variable and they do not have much prognostic value (Table 12.2).

Table 12.2 Immediate and early clinical symptoms connected directly with the irradiation for a dose of 10 Gy given at low dose rate ($2 \, \text{Gy h}^{-1}$).

	Frequency	Time of onset	Duration
Nausea, vomiting	++	1 h	3–6 h
Fever, tachycardia	++	2 h	—
Headache	+	3 h	—
Diarrhoea			
Immediate	rare	2 h	6–12 h
Early	+	3 days	1–2 weeks
Parotiditis	++	1 day	2–3 days
Erythema	++	1 day	2–3 days
Dryness of mouth	++	1 day	1–2 days
Oesophagitis	+	1 week	1–3 weeks
Pneumonopathy	+	2–10 months	

Accidental irradiations

Accidental irradiations [1, 17, 19, 30, 33] differ from medical irradiations in several ways.

1. The dose is usually non-uniform when the irradiation is at high dose rate; it is more uniform at low dose rate as the subject changes position. Protection of part of the body (e.g. a limb) markedly reduces the haemopoietic effect of irradiation.

2. The dose level is not known. Usually one tries to reconstruct the circumstances of the accident in order to estimate the dose. In the case of irradiation by neutrons or very high energy X-rays (more than 10 MeV) the induced radioactivity gives some information on the dose received. The radioactivity is usually very small and presents no problem of radiation

protection for the teams of rescue workers and doctors unless there has been extensive contamination by radioactive isotopes.

To estimate the importance of the irradiation several factors must be taken into account.

CLINICAL DATA

Nausea and vomiting are, as we have seen, the most trustworthy symptoms. They develop earlier and are more severe as the dose is increased. Diarrhoea is a later symptom with less prognostic value as it appears only after several days and is more variable. Nevertheless, if it is severe and continues for several days it indicates a serious degree of irradiation. A neurological syndrome with headache, depression, early state of shock and pyrexia occurs only with very high doses beyond any possibility of therapeutic action. Early erythema is also seen with high doses but if it is localized it is compatible with survival.

Three types of biological data give useful information.

Lymphopenia: the number of circulating lymphocytes falls quickly after irradiation and the rate of fall is a function of dose for an acute irradiation at high dose rate. This is why the first lymphocyte count must be performed as quickly as possible; given the variability in the number of lymphocytes in normal subjects, changes in lymphocyte count are more useful than absolute numbers. Doses as low as 30 cGy are enough to induce a detectable reduction. The minimum is reached towards the third day but by 48 h the reduction in count gives a useful dosimetric indication (Figure 5.12).

Changes in the number of granulocytes: as we have seen in Chapter 5, the fall in the number of granulocytes is preceded by an early rise which is due to mobilization of reserves of granulocytes and is also seen in animals. This peak in granulocyte count may take place during the first few hours and lasts for 1 or 2 days; its height is variable but it is usually seen when the mean dose is greater than 1·5 Gy. Later the number of granulocytes falls rapidly; then with doses lower than 6 Gy it stabilizes from the 10th day until the beginning of the third week when it falls further (Figure 5.14). The initial slope of the curve gives little information; on the other hand the shape of the later part of the curve and the minimum number reached between the second and fifth week, depending on the dose, are of fundamental importance as they are an expression of the severity of the damage suffered by the haemopoietic tissue.

After whole body irradiation, a critical level of neutrophils ($<300\,\mu l^{-1}$) is reached in 7–10 days after a dose greater than 6 Gy, in 15–20 days after 4–6 Gy and later than 20 days after doses below 4 Gy.

Chromosome aberrations: karyotype analysis and counting of chromosome aberrations (dicentrics) for biological dosimetry has been discussed in Chapter 3. Experience gained at Chernobyl has shown the value of this technique. It is reliable for doses above 1 Gy but is still difficult for various reasons:

1. The standardization curve varies from one laboratory to another depending on the experimental conditions. Counting is reliable only in specialized laboratories. In the future, automation of karyotype analysis should reduce this cause of uncertainty.
2. After irradiation by X- or γ-rays the number of aberrations is influenced by the dose rate, e.g. it is reduced by a factor of 3 when the dose rate falls from 1

to $0.3\,Gy\,min^{-1}$. For very low dose rates the standardization curve loses its reliability.

3. The standard curve is less useful for non-uniform irradiation as the distribution of lymphocytes varies from one region of the organism to another. In addition, the irradiated lymphocytes do not react in the same way to mitogens as unirradiated lymphocytes, which leads to errors in estimation of the proportion of lymphocytes carrying an aberration. Study of fibroblasts from the irradiated region can also supply information in the case of localized irradiation but the technique is more difficult.

4. Even under the best technical conditions it is impossible to detect any effect after a dose below 20 cGy. Chromosome aberrations exist in all subjects, particularly in the aged; if the karyotype has not been studied before irradiation it is difficult to interpret a small number of aberrations, particularly since a large number of physical and chemical agents (tobacco, various mutagens, heavy metals, high frequency electromagnetic radiation) also produce aberrations.

In spite of these limitations, counting of chromosome aberrations is the best method of biological dosimetry in subjects irradiated at high dose rate, but unfortunately a delay of several days is needed to obtain the result.

Steps to be taken after accidental irradiation

If the dose is known it is simple to adapt the treatment to the expected symptoms [30]. As soon as possible after irradiation, blood should be taken for karyotype analysis, counting of lymphocytes and HLA-typing.

After doses below 1·5 Gy no treatment is needed; it is enough to adopt a watching policy and to take blood counts and to be ready to take the subject into hospital if the number of granulocytes falls below 1000 or the number of platelets below $50\,000\,\mu l^{-1}$, which should not normally occur.

Between 2 and 5 Gy, after a symptom-free period, bone marrow aplasia with granulopenia and thrombopenia is to be expected between the 15th and 30th day after irradiation. It is therefore necessary to protect the patient against the risk of infection, by isolation in a relatively sterile laminar air-flow environment, with oral antibiotics to modify the endogenous flora of the gastrointestinal tract. It is not necessary to give systemic antibiotics before the temperature rises above 38·5 °C, usually coinciding with the beginning of aplasia. During the phase of agranulocytosis, intensive supporting care is necessary: correction of dehydration and electrolyte imbalance, administration of antimicrobial, antifungal and antiviral drugs, extensive transfusion of red blood cells and platelets irradiated to 30 Gy before infusion in order to inactivate immunocompetent cells originating from the donor, parenteral nutrition in patients suffering from enteritis and/or severe mucositis of the upper digestive tract.

If the dose is unknown or uncertain, treatment must be based on the functional symptomatology (nausea, vomiting) and particularly on biological dosimetry (karyotype) [1, 9]. If there is neither nausea nor skin erythema and if lymphopenia is moderate (minimum number greater than $500\,\mu l^{-1}$), a simple policy of watching is adequate.

The experience gained after the nuclear accident at Chernobyl (April 1986) showed that the role of bone marrow transplantation following accidental irradiation is complex [1, 9, 19]. First, let us recall that transplantation of histocompatible haemopoietic stem cells can reconstitute haemopoiesis and rescue both animals and humans from otherwise lethal doses of radiation. However, after transplantation of mismatched bone marrow the graft may be rejected or graft-versus-host disease (GVHD) may kill a high proportion of recipients. The cells responsible for graft rejection are the T lymphocytes of the host, those responsible for GVHD are the T cells of the graft. The use of T cell depleted bone marrow transplants markedly reduces the risk of GVHD but increases that of rejection.

The potential efficacy of bone marrow transplants also depends on the dose of radiation. Following low doses the graft is rejected, following high doses an engraftment is observed. Mice that received doses of radiation in the range 2–4 Gy followed by transplantation of incompatible bone marrow have decreased survival compared with controls, probably because conflict with donor bone marrow somehow decreases endogenous haemopoietic recovery [14]. However, this effect is not observed in dogs or monkeys and it is not known whether or not it exists in man.

Finally, experimental data show that following high doses of radiation and transplantation of incompatible T-cell depleted bone marrow, a temporarily functioning transplant can permit the animal to survive sufficiently long for recovery of its own haemopoietic system. In this experimental model, survival is improved only if the T cells are removed from the graft; failure to do so results in sustained donor rather than host haemopoiesis.

In man, bone marrow transplantation for accidental irradiation had been attempted twice before the accident at Chernobyl. In a reactor accident at Vinca (Yugoslavia) in 1958, five workers who received doses ranging from 3–6 Gy were treated at the Curie Institute in Paris with allogenic bone marrow grafting. All but one survived. In most of these patients a transitory take was demonstrated and the data suggested that it might have had a beneficial effect. In another accident (USA), a patient who had been exposed to a total body dose of more than 6 Gy received marrow from an identical twin brother on the eighth day post-irradiation; by day 21 marrow competence was restored. This confirms that in normal individuals, as in experimental animals, transplantation of identical bone marrow is well tolerated and effective. In patients with leukaemia or aplastic anaemia, bone marrow transplantation is usually carried out only when there is a related donor with histocompatible bone marrow; the recipients are conditioned for transplantation with a high dose of total body radiation (~ 10 Gy) with or without high dose chemotherapy. Sustained engraftment has also been reported following transplants of partially HLA-mismatched bone marrow but then the risks of rejection and GVHD are much higher.

During the Chernobyl accident more than 200 individuals received doses above 1 Gy and 35 above 5 Gy; 13 of them received bone marrow transplants and 6 received infusion of foetal liver cells [1, 9]. Foetal liver was used in severely burned patients in whom adequate HLA-typing was impossible because of severe lymphopenia; all died within a few weeks. A total of 113 potential donors, close family members in most cases, were evaluated to select the 13 bone marrow transplantations. Seven of the marrow recipients died between the 9th and 19th days after transplant (15–25 days after irradiation) from acute skin and gastrointestinal damage. In the remaining recipients who received T cell depleted marrow, a temporary take was observed in four. Two of them died from mixed viral and bacterial infection and complications which might be related to the immunosuppression induced by the bone marrow transplant (doses 5·2 and 6·4 Gy); for them the transplant probably had a deleterious effect. Conversely, in two of them (doses 5·6 and 8·7 Gy), an initial donor engraftment probably had a beneficial effect and allowed reconstitution of recipient haemopoiesis; both had haplo-identical female donors (sisters) and rejected the functioning transplant one month later. In two recipients an early rejection was observed but during this time their own myelopoiesis was restored; they nevertheless died.

These data show that marrow transplantation should play only a limited but still non-negligible role in overall management. In each patient the potential benefits and risks of a marrow transplant should be carefully evaluated.

The first risk is GVHD; its probability depends on the histocompatibility between donor and recipient and on the efficacy of measures designed to prevent or modify GVHD (such as T-cell depletion, cyclosporine and monoclonal antibodies against T cells). The age and sex of the recipient and donor are also important since these are determinants of the likelihood and severity of GVHD. This emphasizes the necessity of early HLA-typing of the patient and potential donors in the family as well as in the pool of volunteer donors.

The second risk is rejection. Rejection of HLA-mismatched bone marrow is likely to occur following a dose of radiation such as 8–10 Gy which is associated with a high risk of death from bone marrow suppression but which is insufficient to permit sustained engraftment. In this instance additional immune suppression (cyclophosphamide or anti-T cell antibodies before the transplant) might facilitate engraftment. In this setting, temporary engraftment (slow rejection) is an optimal outcome when it does not interfere with recovery of the recipient's haemopoiesis.

A third risk is related to the existence of other lesions. For example, in the rat a whole body dose of 2 Gy results in 100% survival. Likewise a 1 cm skin burn causes no immediate mortality. If, however, these injuries are combined the mortality rises to 50%. In patients it has been observed that the healing of wounds stops at the beginning of the phase of agranulocytosis. Thus bone marrow transplantation can potentially save lives since these other lesions will not compromise the outcome of the transplant. The existence of associated lesions, abdominal wounds or extensive burns, therefore increases the indications for bone marrow grafting.

In summary, the physician has a range of therapeutic options. Intensive supportive care is associated with a high rate of survival in individuals receiving less than 6 Gy total body irradiation. For doses below 8 Gy to the whole body it may be possible to expedite bone marrow recovery by administration of haemopoietic growth factors (CSF). Beyond 8 Gy, bone marrow transplantation may be envisaged if a compatible bone marrow is available. The risk of GVHD should be carefully weighed, in particular in patients over 40 years old. The use of T-cell depleted, partially compatible bone marrow should be envisaged only for doses in the range 9–14 Gy. However, each situation must be considered individually. In patients without associated lesions, transplantation is not urgent. As aplastic subjects can be kept alive in a sterile environment, one can wait for a week or more before deciding upon a graft unless there are burns or wounds, as agranulocytosis prevents healing and encourages infection. In this case surgery must be performed quickly and a decision must be made about grafting taking account of all the factors involved [61].

Chronic irradiation

Accidental irradiation at low dose rate

Several fatal accidents have occurred due to handling radioactive sources which had been stolen or lost (Morocco, Algeria, Mexico, Brazil). Exposures were spread over times from a few days to several months [33]. In these cases death was due to irreversible bone marrow failure. In the Mexican accident a survivor received between 10 and 17 Gy in 100 days. In the Algerian accident four survivors received doses between 12 and 14 Gy in 40 days. Extended observation of sheep receiving chronic irradiation at constant dose rate shows that the accumulated dose required to kill from haemopoietic damage increases at a rate of 0·12 Gy per day when the daily dose is decreased and exposure is consequently prolonged. The operational equivalent dose (OED) is OED=total accumulated dose−150−10t where t is in days and dose in cGy [40]. The expected mortality of individuals for a given value of OED is that expected to follow a single brief exposure of the same magnitude. This formula is consistent with the limited human data.

Critical organs

In radiation protection there are four critical organs which must be distinguished because of the frequency with which they are damaged after many small doses or irradiation at low dose rate [64].

Skin

For a long time the skin was considered to be the critical organ. When low energy X-rays were the only radiation in use, the skin received greater doses than the deeper tissues; moreover it was easy to see the damage. Historically it was damage to the skin which led to the development of ideas of a tolerance dose and a threshold. An acute dose of a few gray produces an erythema, as we have seen in Chapter 5; however, if the dose is fractionated the effect is reduced and the skin can be completely restored between two irradiations. Low but repeated doses give rise to subacute lesions; nevertheless smaller doses still, even if repeated indefinitely, do not lead to any detectable change in its structure. The threshold of tolerance was evaluated in 1925 at about $0 \cdot 2 \, \text{cGy day}^{-1}$ and this was for a long time the basis of all the recommendations in radiation protection.

The existence of chronic cutaneous damage, particularly in the hands where it is easily recognizable, indicates that the subject has received at least several tens of gray at a rate greater than $0 \cdot 5 \, \text{cGy day}^{-1}$, as there is no obvious damage with lower doses and dose rates.

Severe skin damage, such as late necrosis or ulceration which heals poorly and is liable to breakdown, often appears after minimal trauma in skin that has already been altered. The skin is either dry and atrophied, giving the impression of premature ageing, or thick and oedematous. Fissures round the nails, hyperkeratoses, telangiectases and pigmentation which may be uniform or streaked are also seen in the hands and constitute a warning, as it is likely that the tolerance dose has been exceeded. Loss of finger prints is an early sign of skin damage, particularly in radiologists practising fluoroscopy.

Eyes

Cataracts leading to total blindness have occurred in patients irradiated for disease situated close to the eye. Their frequency increases with dose. They are very rare after doses of 2 Gy of X- or γ-rays given in a few weeks. With doses below 5 Gy they usually have no clinical significance. They occur in all subjects when the dose exceeds 11–12 Gy in fractionated irradiation. After irradiation of children for retinoblastoma, cataracts are seen only beyond 13 Gy. These cataracts are due to damage to the germinal zones of the epithelium of the lens. The long latent period is connected with the slow rate of cellular renewal.

The RBE of neutrons relative to X-rays for this effect may be 10 or more. Cataracts have been seen in physicists working with cyclotrons and exposed to neutron radiation. They can be treated by surgery.

Gonads

The importance of the testes and ovaries as critical organs is connected with the action of radiation on the germinal cell lines with the double risk of mutation and sterility. Because of the great radioresistance of the interstitial tissues, irradiation of the testes even with high doses does not lead to impotence (see Chapter 5).

A dose of 5 cGy day^{-1} in mice and 1 cGy day^{-1} in dogs delivered over a long period of time causes total sterility in males; 0·1 cGy day^{-1} for several months is enough to reduce the number of spermatozoa.

The doses received by professional workers do not lead to any detectable reduction in fertility in men or amenorrhoea in women. From this point of view the maximum permissible doses (Table 12.11) give a large factor of safety. No reduction in fertility has been detected in the survivors of the atomic bomb.

Haemopoietic tissues

Changes in blood cell counts are one of the most sensitive symptoms of irradiation. An acute dose of 25 cGy is enough to cause lymphopenia and 5 cGy produces a reduction in erythropoiesis in animals which can be demonstrated by means of radioactive iron. Doses of the order of 2 cGy day^{-1} given over a period of many months lead to haemorrhage, thrombopenia and fatal anaemia. Both in animals and man doses of 0·1 cGy week^{-1} cause changes in the numbers of blood cells. This is the reason why blood counts have been taken routinely on workers exposed to ionizing radiation. However, data collected during several decades have shown that detailed haematological examinations do not give information specific to the radiation received.

The numbers of different blood cells or the differential blood count is not a reliable index of the effect on the organism. Leukaemia not preceded by any change in the differential blood count has been seen in irradiated subjects. On the other hand many common conditions, such as influenza, angina and viral diseases may disturb the blood count. Moreover, in the absence of any disease, the blood count may vary markedly from one examination to another and between ethnic groups. Finally the magnitude of the changes in blood count do not always match the severity of the damage.

However, surveillance of the blood count still has considerable value:

(a) Variations in the differential blood count represent the only biological test available to evaluate the changes caused by chronic irradiation in man: continuous irradiation at about 0·1 cGy week^{-1} may be enough to lead to slight leucopenia.

(b) A change in the differential blood count is seen after local or whole body irradiation and is a marker of the total effect of irradiation on the organism.

However, the fall in the number of leucocytes and the change in the differential count often appears only many weeks or more after the time of irradiation. Repeated examinations are useful as the time course of changes is more instructive than a single isolated result. But this type of surveillance is of practical value only if the technical conditions are sufficiently rigorous to allow comparison of examinations performed with an interval of many months or years.

After chronic irradiation, the occurrence of any of the following indices must be taken as a sign of alarm: permanent reduction in leucocyte count below 4000 or an increase above 15 000 μl^{-1} with absolute lymphocytosis; relative lymphocytosis (inversion of the normal distribution) with a normal number of leucocytes, particularly if the lymphocytosis disappears when the subject is no longer irradiated; an increase in mean volume or diameter of the red cells; reticulocytosis greater than 2%; a red cell count above 5 800 000 μl^{-1}; macrocytic anaemia.

Some authors emphasize the importance of pathologically abnormal lymphocytes, changes in their colour, the presence of bilobed lymphocytes or segmented polynuclear cells. The development of leukaemia may be preceded by an increase in the number of basophils and a reduction in the alkaline phosphatase of the leucocytes. Biochemical changes may therefore precede the morphological alterations. Also there is a slow and progressive appearance of abnormal immature cells in the blood.

The need for a comparison with an analysis of blood taken before irradiation is the reason for the value of this examination at the beginning of employment. If this initial examination is abnormal some employers will refuse to take on the person concerned. This policy removes subjects who may be beginning to develop a haematological disease which might otherwise have been attributed to the effects of radiation, but it raises several problems:

    (i) there is no absolute separation between a normal and an abnormal count;

    (ii) some changes arising from common diseases are temporary and may cause a subject who is perfectly suitable to be refused employment because, for example, he has just been suffering from influenza;

    (iii) there is no evidence that subjects with idiopathic leucopenia are more likely than others to develop radiation induced leukaemia. Any fixed criterion is therefore to some extent arbitrary.

12.2 Effects on the embryo and fetus: teratogenesis

Diagnostic and therapeutic radiologists are often confronted by the question of the danger of irradiating a pregnant woman, a problem which has been the subject of many studies [32, 45, 64–66].

The value of human observations is limited by dosimetric uncertainties. In addition, often the age of the embryo at the time of irradiation is not known exactly. The effects of irradiation depend on the moment at which it is given. Consequently animal studies are indispensable despite the difficulties of extrapolating to man.

Radiation effects as a function of the chronology of embryonal development

Comparisons between animal species must take into account the chronology of embryonal development. This takes place in the same order in all mammals, making possible the construction of tables of equivalence. Three periods can be distinguished. The first finishes at the time of implantation; its duration is similar in all mammals (Table 12.3). The second is that of organogenesis. The third, that of fetal development, varies greatly from one species to another.

Before implantation (until the ninth day in women), the effects of irradiation are of an all or nothing character and may lead to death of the embryo; this is often unnoticed as the woman is not aware that she is pregnant. Otherwise development and postnatal survival are normal. In animals, malformations induced during this period are very rare and there is no delay in growth. At this stage the cells are not yet differentiated and the death of a cell is not serious; a single surviving cell may be enough.

During organogenesis, irradiation may cause serious malformations whose nature depends on the moment of irradiation. An embryo is a mosaic of many clones of cells undergoing proliferation and differentiation which gives rise to tissues and organs; this mosaic changes from day to day. Thus each tissue passes through periods of maximum radiosensitivity corresponding to the stages of differentiation and organization of the tissue. Death of one cell at a moment when there are still very few differentiated cells may lead to an arrest of development of the organ or of one of its parts and therefore to a major anomaly. When allowance is made for the chronology of embryonal development, the periods of maximum risk are the same in all mammalian species. At the moment of maximum radiosensitivity, doses as low as 5 cGy can lead to significant malformations; before and after this critical period the probability and severity of the malformations is much lower.

In man embryonal development is much slower than in small mammals and there is a lower rate of cell division. In addition the duration of each stage of

Table 12.3 Principal periods of embryonal development (days).

	Pre-implantation	Organogenesis	Fetal period
Mouse	0–5	6–12	13–16·5
Rat	0–7	8–15	13–21·5
Man	0–8	9–60	60–270 (proliferation of neuroblasts from the 60th to the 110th day)
Effects of irradiation	Intra-uterine death	Intra-uterine death (beginning of organogenesis)	Malformations of the CNS and mental retardation (from 60th to 110th day)
	Growth and postnatal survival normal	Malformations Neonatal and postnatal death	Growth defects Postnatal weakness Childhood cancers

organogenesis is longer, allowing more time for processes of repair and regeneration. There is another factor contributing to the reduced sensitivity of the human embryo: in animals heterozygotes have a much greater resistance than homozygotes of in-bred lines to the teratogenic and lethal effects; most experimental work has been done on in-bred lines of mice.

During the fetal period, which begins at the end of the second month in women, the frequency and severity of malformations are smaller and the morphological effects of irradiation become progressively less important since the number of cells in each tissue is so great that there is little probability of damage to enough cells to cause a serious malformation. Nevertheless, in this stage irradiation may cause a delay in growth or some functional deficiency, particularly of the human brain.

Mortality

The radiosensitivity of the embryo and fetus varies considerably. In mice, radiosensitivity before implantation is high and the 50% lethal dose (LD 50) for intra-uterine mortality is of the order of 0·5 Gy. Beyond 0·2 Gy the relation between dose and effect seems to be linear with an increase in the frequency of death of about 1% cGy^{-1}. After implantation, radiosensitivity remains high and in certain species may even show a maximum during the first stages of organogenesis. Later the LD 50 increases during the embryonal period. In addition there is some neonatal and postnatal mortality. A dose of 1 Gy given during the embryonal phase produces a slight increase in postnatal mortality. With doses above 2 Gy there is in addition some shortening of life. During the fetal period the LD 50 at 30 days increases steadily with the age of the fetus and at birth becomes equal to the LD 50 of adult mice.

Human data on the lethal effect of irradiation *in utero* are uncertain. A dose of the order of $3 \cdot 5$–4 Gy seems great enough to cause a miscarriage in most cases. Out of 30 pregnant women who suffered radiation sickness at Hiroshima and Nagasaki immediately after the explosion, indicating relatively large doses, intra-uterine or neonatal death was of the order of 40%. This has not been seen with lower doses. In the 1300 children who were irradiated *in utero*, mortality was greater than normal during the first year and has been correlated with the dose received.

Malformations and developmental defects

In addition to malformation due to lesions occurring during the embryonal phase there are also *developmental deficiencies*, without observable morpho-logical defects, which are connected with a lack of cells in the tissue [43, 66]. The most important are microcephaly and mental retardation caused by a deficit of brain cells.

Brain

Malformations of the brain are caused by a defect in the development of certain structures, due to the death of cells or a defect in migration during the critical period of growth of these structures [18, 47]. The frequency and types of malformation therefore depend strictly on the time at which the irradiation takes place, the sensitive structures being those which are in the process of development at the time of irradiation.

In mice various lesions are produced by irradiation. Exencephalus, anencephaly, hydrocephalus, microcephaly and lesions of the cerebral cortex can be seen with doses above $2 \cdot 5$ Gy but their frequency is very low with doses below 1 Gy and reaches about 15% at $1 \cdot 5$ Gy. The frequency of a particular type of lesion depends on the age of the embryo and changes markedly over a period as short as 24 h.

In man the primitive brain begins to develop during the first 6 weeks. The hemispheres then continue to grow and differentiate during the whole fetal life and in the infant. The period between the 8th and 16th weeks corresponds to the proliferation of neuroblasts which are very radiosensitive and have a limited capacity for proliferation; thus only a small depletion of cells can be compensated by an increase in the number of divisions. Moreover irradiation may interfere with the migration of the cells destined to become neurones. The period from the 8th to the 15th week is also the time in the human embryo when the cortical neurones migrate to the cortex from the region situated close to the ventricles. Accordingly to Otake and Schull [47] this explains why this period is critical.

This conclusion is based on observations made on subjects irradiated *in utero* at Hiroshima and Nagasaki. In the two towns together there were 49 cases in which a reduction in the perimeter of the head was seen in embryos irradiated between the 3rd and 17th week, which is a frequency of 20% compared with 4% in non-irradiated subjects. A correlation was found between the reduction in perimeter and the dose above $0 \cdot 2$ Gy. With doses greater than $0 \cdot 5$ Gy mental retardation also occurred in some subjects. Mental retardation without reduction in head perimeter has also been reported after irradiation between the 8th and the 15th week and with doses greater than 0·5 Gy. No cases were seen when the irradiation occurred before the 3rd week; however, one cannot conclude with certainty that irradiation at this time is innocuous. The risk diminishes between the 15th and the 25th week. After 25 weeks and with doses below 1 Gy no case of severe mental retardation has been reported. It is not impossible that malnutrition and epidemics of disease which occurred in these cities may also have played a role.

This is the reason why the study of pregnant women receiving radiotherapy is of particular interest. Microcephaly or mental retardation was seen in 26 cases out of 200 in which the embryo received a dose greater than 2·5 Gy. The mental retardation was more significant when the irradiation was given before rather than after the 11th week. No anomalies have been reported when the irradiation occurred after the 19th week. In spite of their lack of precision, these data are consistent with those from Hiroshima and Nagasaki [66].

Some authors argue that there may be no threshold and that the dose–effect relation remains linear at low doses; this would imply that death of a single neuroblast would be enough to induce some intellectual deficit. This appears doubtful and it must be noted that at the present time no mental retardation has been found after doses below 0·5 Gy. It seems increasingly likely that there is a practical threshold below which there is no detectable effect. The 1986 UNSCEAR report [65] used the hypothesis of a linear dose–effect relationship and estimated the probability of induction of mental retardation to be 0·4% cGy^{-1} at the time of peak sensitivity and 0·1% between 16 and 25 weeks from conception. However, the 1988 UNSCEAR report [66] stated that information becoming available suggests that these risk estimates may need substantial revision downward, particularly in the low dose range.

Eye

Malformations are seen in mice and rats with doses above 0·25 Gy given during the stage of embryogenesis corresponding to differentiation of the eye. At 0·5 Gy the frequency is 7% during the most critical stage. The dose–effect relationship seems to be curvilinear.

Skeleton

This is very suitable for studies of teratology as the defects are easy to quantify in animals as in man. In animals, irradiation produces various malformations, particularly when given during the embryonic phase, and for each there is a critical period when radiosensitivity is at a maximum.

The frequency of malformations increases with dose above 0·20 Gy. The shape of the dose–effect curve varies with the type of malformation. In man, a number of studies have shown that the incidence of bony anomalies is not changed by doses of the order of a few cGy, excluding the hypothesis of a high radiosensitivity of the human embryo. In animals the probability of malformations varies between 0·2 and 0·5% cGy^{-1}, depending on the age of the embryo, over a range of doses from 0·25 to 1·5 Gy. In 1986 the UNSCEAR report [65] estimated that a dose to the conceptus of 1 cGy delivered over the whole pregnancy would add a probability of less than 2 per 1000 of adverse health effects in the live born, including mortality and risk of induction of mental retardation, malformations and malignancy (the normal risk to a non-irradiated live born is about 6%). In 1988 UNSCEAR [66] felt that this risk estimate also needed substantial revision downward.

Epidemiological data do not make it possible to demonstrate or exclude the presence of a threshold because at low doses the incidence becomes so small that statistical significance cannot be achieved. Nevertheless the existence of a practical threshold is likely.

Growth retardation

In rodents, doses of about 10 cGy during embryogenesis or the fetal period cause retardation of development *in utero*, demonstrated by a reduction in birth weight and retardation of postnatal growth.

In infants irradiated *in utero* at Hiroshima and Nagasaki who received at least 0·5 Gy of γ-rays, by the age of 17 there was a mean reduction in height of 2·3 cm together with a loss of weight of 3 kg and a reduction in head perimeter of 1 cm. Also there was a delay in the age of menarche and a retardation of ossification which does not seem to be correlated with dose. On the other hand there has been no alteration in fertility: the number of marriages, births and the interval between marriage and the first birth have been identical to those in the controls. No abnormalities have been found in the descendants.

Study of children irradiated *in utero* for medical reasons confirms the existence of a growth delay but there is some disagreement between the findings after medical and non-medical irradiations. This suggests that the children whose mothers were irradiated for medical reasons were not altogether normal and indicates that some caution is needed in the interpretation of studies made on these children.

As with other biological effects, the teratogenic action of radiation is reduced at low dose rate and with fractionated exposures.

Carcinogenesis after irradiation *in utero*

There have been two types of survey. At Hiroshima and Nagasaki no increase in the incidence of leukaemia has been seen in children born to mothers who were pregnant at the time of the explosions [66]. The other studies relate to children whose mothers received therapeutic or diagnostic irradiation during pregnancy [3, 60]. The work of Stewart and her colleagues [3] showed a small increase in the incidence of leukaemia and cancers (malignant lymphomas, nephroblastoma, tumours of the CNS, neuroblastoma, etc.) in the irradiated children. However, this result raises an objection: were the irradiated children comparable to the non-irradiated controls? It has been suggested that the women whose children have an increased likelihood of developing malignant disease might themselves be more likely to be irradiated during pregnancy for the diagnosis of already existing disease. In reply to this criticism Mole [25, 41] analyzed the results in twins. Whereas pelvimetry was performed in 10% of the single births the figure for twins was 50%. Although the incidence of leukaemia in the twins and the single births was different in the absence of irradiation *in utero*, the excess of cancers and leukaemias found in the children irradiated *in utero* was the same in twins as in the single births. This suggests the reality of the carcinogenic effect but does not provide a definite proof.

Other studies have also shown an increase in the incidence of leukaemia but have not demonstrated any excess of other types of cancer. However, the radiogenic cause cannot be proven in view of the conflicting Japanese and experimental data. It is surprising that the leukaemogenic effect *in utero* should be three to four times greater than in adolescents and adults. Furthermore, animal experiments have failed to show any particular sensitivity of the embryo or foetus to radiation induced cancer. Altogether, the 1986 UNSCEAR report [65] concludes that the carcinogenic effect remains doubtful. On the assumption that the effect is real, the number of additional leukaemias and cancers would not be large, about 0·05% for a dose of 2 cGy. At such low doses no increase has been seen in animals. In dogs, irradiation with doses from 20 to 80 cGy causes an increase in the incidence of malignant haematological disease and of cancers of the breast, lungs and thyroid. The age of the foetus at the moment of irradiation may be an important factor. Some findings suggest that the risk is greater during the first trimester.

Practical measures

What should one do when there has been an accidental irradiation [30]? Even if we assume that there is no threshold and that any dose, however small, has a certain probability of causing damage, the risk with very small doses is negligible. In practice no damage has been observed in man with doses lower than 20 cGy. All authors are in agreement that no special action is needed when the dose received by the embryo or fetus is less than 10 cGy. Some authors suggest therapeutic abortion when the dose is greater than 10 cGy. However, as a rule no arbitrary decision should be made; between 10 and 20 cGy account should be taken of family circumstances before recommending termination of the pregnancy. Above 20 cGy abortion can be recommended. It is only in exceptional family circumstances that one should accept the risk when the dose received by the uterus was greater than 25 cGy.

Although a relaxed attitude can be taken to accidental irradiation, it is imperative to avoid any unnecessary irradiation greater than 1 cGy. When radiology is indicated, the cost and benefit must be compared and the risks should be accepted only when the radiological investigation is beneficial for the health of the mother.

It used to be recommended that irradiation of the pelvis should be avoided during the last 2 weeks of the cycle (the 10-day rule); in fact there is a risk only after the ninth day post-conception and one should avoid pelvic irradiation only during the last 5 days of the cycle. Most importantly, any delay in the cycle, even slight, should be a contra-indication for radiology until pregnancy is excluded by a biological test.

12.3 Carcinogenesis

The carcinogenic effect of ionizing radiation has been known since 1902, the date of the first case of radiogenic cancer of the skin. Subsequently many other pioneers of X-rays and radioactivity have died of skin cancer or leukaemia.

In 1910 P. Marie succeeded in obtaining radiogenic cancers in animals and in 1966 Borek and Sachs [6] showed that it was possible, by irradiation *in vitro*, to 'transform' a normal cell into a cell having malignant characteristics. In order to evaluate the risk of induction of cancer, there are therefore three sources of information: (i) studies *in vitro* of isolated cells, (ii) animal experiments and (iii) epidemiological studies in man. The last source of information is the most important as it is always difficult to extrapolate from cells or animals to man, and epidemiology is the only way of obtaining a quantitative estimate of the risk. However, the other methods are useful for comparing risks in different tissues and establishing the shape of the dose–effect relation.

Epidemiological studies

The principal sources of human data are: (1) patients irradiated for medical reasons; (2) survivors at Hiroshima and Nagasaki; and (3) occupationally exposed workers [7, 36, 50, 66, 67].

Irradiated patients

A number of studies have been made on patients treated by radiotherapy. Two of them are particularly important.

The first is concerned with 14 000 patients suffering from ankylosing spondylitis treated between 1933 and 1954 with regular follow-up thereafter (Figure 12.1). The bone marrow dose varied between 2 and 6 Gy. The overall incidence of leukaemia was increased by a factor of 3 and was at a maximum 3–5 years after irradiation; it was about 2 per 1000 for a dose of 3 Gy to the whole spine, i.e. half the bone marrow. In lightly irradiated tissues the ratio of the observed over expected incidence of tumours was about 1·2 and was not significantly different from 1; any increase in the incidence of cancer is therefore small or zero. In heavily irradiated tissues the ratio of observed to expected (based on a control population) for solid tumours was definitely increased and equal to about 1·5. The proportional increase reached a maximum of 70% between 10 and 12 years after irradiation and then declined. There was a 7% increase in mortality from the excess of malignant tumours more than 25 years after irradiation and the relative risk was significantly raised in this period only for cancer of the oesophagus.

Another study is concerned with 82 000 women irradiated by external beam therapy and/or intracavitary radioactive sources for cancer of the uterine cervix, who were followed for 5–20 years [4, 5]. The number of excess cancers was calculated from the number of second cancers observed (3324) less the incidence of cancers in untreated women of the same age (3063), a difference of 261. A similar study was made on women treated by surgery alone. In both groups there was a considerable excess of cancers of the lung, no doubt due to the increased use of tobacco by women suffering from cervical cancer than by the rest of the population. After excluding cancers due to tobacco (lung, buccal cavity, etc.) the excess of other cancers was relatively small despite the large doses given to the whole body during intracavitary therapy. This confirms that the carcinogenic effect of radiation is limited and the total number of cancers which could be attributed to irradiation has been estimated at about 125, which

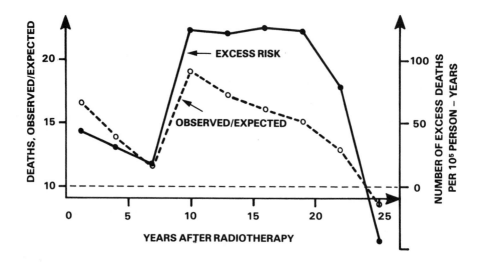

Figure 12.1. Excess deaths due to malignant disease as a function of time after irradiation in patients treated for ankylosing spondylitis. Both the ratio observed/expected and the absolute number of excess deaths have been calculated. The number of leukaemias reached a maximum 3–5 years after irradiation and then diminished. The number of solid tumours in the irradiated region was at a maximum 9–11 years after irradiation and diminished after 20 years, but this reduction was not statistically significant. After [12].

Table 12.4 Comparison of predicted and observed excess second cancers in women irradiated to treat cervical cancer.

Second primary cancers	Risk coefficient (cases per 10^4 PYGy)	Organ dose (Gy)	Predicted excess cancers	Observed excess cancers†
Stomach	1·68	2·0 (0·5–3·5)	60	+3
Colon	1·12	5·0	100	+15
Liver	0·70	1·5 (0·5–2·5)	20	0
Pancreas	0·99	1·5 (0·3–3·0)	25	+9
Lung	3·94	0·3 (0·1–0·6)	25	+77
Breast	5·82	0·3 (0·1–0·6)	37	−101
Kidney	0·88	2·0 (0·6–3·5)	30	−6
Bladder	0·88	30	475	+82
Thyroid	5·80	0·1 (0·0–0·3)	15	+4
Lymphoma	0·27	~10 (3·0–13)	50	+15
Acute and NL	2·70	7·5 (3·0–13)‡	1000	+13
leukaemia		2·5 (0·8–3·3)§	350	+13
		0·3 (0·1–0·4)¶	45	+13

†In women, except those with leukaemia, living more than 10 years; for women with leukaemia, values are for 1–20 years after irradiation.
‡Averaged over entire bone marrow.
§Excluding pelvis contribution.
¶Excluding pelvis, lumbar spine, and upper femur contributions.
From [51], p. 515.

is lower than the expected number based on published coefficients of risk (Table 12.4). From 10 years after irradiation the incidence of cancers was slightly but significantly increased in the regions which had received doses greater than 1Gy, in particular the bladder and rectum. It is also possible that the incidence of cancers of the bone and intestine were increased although the differences are not significant. There was only a small increase in the incidence of leukaemia, much lower than that expected. There was no increase in the incidence of cancer of the colon, kidney, pancreas or stomach. The incidence of breast cancer was markedly reduced (about 60%), probably a result of castration due to radiotherapy. This survey is consistent with earlier studies of women irradiated for cancer of the uterine cervix, in which an increase in the incidence of cancer of the bladder and rectum was also found.

Some other studies have also produced significant results. Patients suffering from Hodgkin's disease have been followed after treatment by radiotherapy alone (40 Gy to very large volumes) or combined with various forms of chemotherapy. Ten years after treatment the cumulative incidence of leukaemia after radiotherapy alone was small, about 1%. On the other hand it reached 8–10% in patients treated by a combination of radiotherapy and chemotherapy with a number of drugs or chemotherapy alone, particularly when alkylating agents were used (nitrogen mustards). After a long delay there was also a significant increase in solid tumours, particularly in patients treated by a combination of radiotherapy and chemotherapy [27, 66, 67].

After other types of radiotherapy the percentage of second radiogenic cancers varies between 0·5 and 2%; they are mostly bone tumours and soft tissue sarcomas. The carcinogenic effect seems larger in children, of the order of 4%, but with large variations depending on the original cancer, as children suffering from cancers in which genetic factors play a role (retinoblastoma, nephroblastoma, Ewing's sarcoma) also show an increased susceptibility to the induction of a second cancer, particularly bone sarcomas. In children the tissues in which radiogenic cancers are commonest are the thyroid, bone, haemopoietic tissue and breast.

Two studies (one in New England and the other in Canada) have been made on women suffering from pulmonary tuberculosis whose pneumothorax was followed regularly by fluoroscopy. An increase in the incidence of breast cancer was noted [37] but there was no increase in leukaemia or cancer of the skin. Similarly an increased incidence of thyroid cancer has been seen in children irradiated in the cervical region, the thymus, or the scalp for tinea capitis [7, 29, 66, 67].

No increase in the incidence of leukaemia or thyroid cancer has been found in subjects treated by radioactive iodine for hyperthyroidism or in those receiving radioactive iodine for scintigraphy [29].

A number of studies have been made to determine whether normal radiological examinations lead to an increase in the incidence of cancer and particularly of leukaemia. After critical analysis of these studies is has been concluded that no increase in incidence has been seen either in adults or in children [53]. On the other hand it is not impossible that irradiation of the fetus *in utero* in the course of prenatal radiography may increase the incidence of leukaemia, although as discussed above the results of different studies have not all been in agreement.

Survivors at Hiroshima and Nagasaki [10, 56, 57, 66, 70]

The 285 000 survivors at Hiroshima and Nagasaki have been followed for more than 40 years; 80 000 died of natural causes between 1950 and 1978; 400–500 of these deaths appear to be due to radiogenic cancer, among which there was an excess of about 90 leukaemias and 80 skin cancers. The carcinogenic effect is therefore certain but in quantitative terms it is relatively small (of the order of 1%) and hardly alters the overall number of survivors. In the two cities the carcinogenic effect showed itself first by an increase in the number of leukaemias at the end of the 1940s. After passing through a peak between 1952 and 1965, the number of leukaemias declined and returned towards normal, while the number of radiogenic solid tumours increased (Figure 12.2), mostly in the thyroid, breast, lungs, stomach, oesophagus, ovary, bladder, multiple myeloma and CNS. The number of cancers of the colon, bones, larynx and pharynx may have increased slightly but none of these sites showed a significant dose–response relationship. No increase in cancers of the gall bladder, uterus, salivary glands, pancreas, or lymphomas has been detected. In children the number of excess cancers has diminished with time, but no such reduction has been seen in adults, which is at variance with the results of surveys carried out on patients treated by radiotherapy.

A complete re-evaluation of the A-bomb dosimetry was carried out in 1986. Under the new dosimetric system (DS86) the difference between the radiation effects in the two cities is smaller than under the old, nevertheless a small inter-city difference in dose–response is still present. The contribution of neutrons to the radiation at Hiroshima appears to be smaller than formerly estimated, but is still not negligible. The revision of the dosimetric system had little influence on the cancer risk coefficients when the absorbed doses received by the organs were used and the new risk coefficients are slightly smaller for all organs except breast and ovary. The risk coefficients calculated with the shielded kerma (inside the dwellings) are occasionally quoted; they are

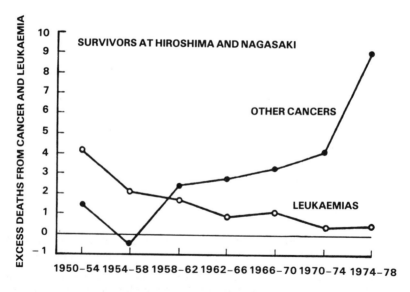

Figure 12.2. Number of additional deaths (per million persons and per centigray) due to leukaemia and solid tumours in the survivors at Hiroshima and Nagasaki as a function of time after the explosion.
After [34].

35–60% higher but meaningless from a medical point of view. Nevertheless, the cancer risk recently assessed is higher than had been estimated previously because 40 years after exposure the incidence of several types of cancer remains greater than in the control population. This justifies the use of projection models in order to assess the lifetime risk, as discussed later. Over the dose range from 0 to 6 Gy a linear-quadratic model fits the dose–response curve for all cancers; however, linear or quadratic relationships cannot be excluded for several types of cancer.

With the exception of cataracts and a slight retardation of growth in children who were exposed when very young, studies of the survivors have shown no evidence of any other effects due to irradiation: no increase in morbidity, acceleration of ageing, life shortening, nor reduction in the number of children.

Occupational exposure

A few studies have produced quantitative information [7, 66, 67]. During the 1920s, for example, 1700 people painted luminous dials with luminescent paint containing radium. In the course of their work they were contaminated quite heavily and the mean dose received by the skeleton was evaluated at 17 Gy, mostly due to α-rays; 48 of them died of osteosarcoma [52]. In these subjects, as in those who received therapeutic intravenous injections of radium, no cases of bone cancer were seen with low doses and the shape of the dose–effect curve suggests the existence of a practical threshold [8] (Figure 12.3). In particular no one who began work after 1927, when the working conditions were improved, has presented with osteosarcoma. People treated for various diseases with short-lived α-emitters (Ra 224) experienced an increase in osteosarcomas from 3·5 to 25 years after the initial injection.

Several extensive analyses of lung cancers in underground miners who inhaled radon have been published in Czechoslovakia, Canada (Ontario), France, Sweden and the USA (Colorado) [8, 66]. Radon and thoron are α-

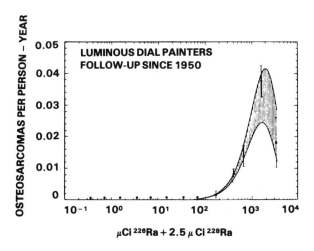

Figure 12.3. Dose–effect relation for osteosarcomas in luminous dial painters caused by internal irradiation by radium 226+228 (α-emitter with half-life 1600 years). No increase in incidence of cancer was seen with low doses. Above an activity corresponding to a dose of a few gray, the incidence (expressed as the number of cases per year per person exposed) increases at first very slowly, then more rapidly and passes through a maximum for several tens of gray and then decreases. A function which fits this dose–effect relation is $I=(c+\beta D^2)\,e^{-\gamma D}$ where D is the quantity of radium fixed. The hatched area shows the band covered by the function. Error bars correspond to standard errors. After [52].

emitting gases which cause long-term, low-level exposure to the lung. There have been large differences in the exposure levels in the various mining cohorts and in risk coefficients derived from the epidemiological data. However, in all cohorts an excess of lung cancer and a dose–effect relationship were found. Large differences were reported between smoking and non-smoking miners. The BEIR IV [8] modelled the effect of smoking as interacting multiplicatively with radiation but other models are also consistent with the data. Excess lung cancers appeared about 5 years after the onset of exposure, peaked at 15–20 years and were no longer significant after 25–30 years.

Exposure of the lung to α-particles from radon is customarily expressed in terms of working levels (WL). The WL is any combination of radon and its daughter products in a litre of air that will result in the emission of $1\cdot3\times10^5$ MeV of potential α-energy. The working level month (WLM) is the exposure resulting from the inhalation of air with a concentration of 1 WL of radon for 170 (working) h. A reference conversion is 6 mGy mean bronchial dose per WLM with the usual conditions in the mine. Recent data from the various surveys suggest an average lifetime risk of about 3×10^{-4} per WLM for uranium miners, with a range $1\cdot5$–$4\cdot5\times10^{-4}$ per WLM. BEIR IV [8] estimated that occupational exposure to 4 WLM per year from age 20 to 40 would increase the male lung cancer deaths by a factor of $1\cdot6$, most of the cases being in smokers. Extrapolation of the risk coefficient to the effect of indoor radon will be discussed later and is inconclusive.

Among radiologists working in the USA between 1920 and 1939, the incidence of leukaemia and the number of fatal skin cancers was 10 times greater than in doctors of the same age practising general medicine, while it was three times greater in radiologists working between 1940 and 1959. There was no excess in radiologists starting practice after 1959. In England, out of 3339 radiologists who began work between 1897 and 1921, there were 62 deaths from cancer instead of 35 expected from comparison with controls. In those who began work after 1921, there were 72 cancer deaths instead of $68\cdot6$ expected and the difference is not significant; the dose received by the latter group during their professional life has been estimated at a few gray (<5). Efforts have been made to determine whether radiology technicians and individuals employed in the nuclear industry do or do not have increased risks of cancer. A number of surveys of workers exposed to ionizing radiation have been reviewed recently; some were carried out on cohorts of 6000–46000 individuals [2, 11, 15]. They failed to disclose any statistically significant increase in cancer incidence, even in the groups exposed to relatively high doses. In some studies, a deficit or an excess of mortality was reported for various sites, but when the findings were combined the excesses seen in one of the studies were no longer significant. This suggests that the individual findings could be due to chance. A much larger study is currently in progress at IARC which will combine data from a large number of countries.

Conclusions

In summary, several generalizations can be made for radiation effects in man [7, 10, 38, 66, 67]. (a) If the dose is large enough, either a single or chronic exposure can be carcinogenic. However, at equal doses acute exposures are more effective than chronic. (b) There is no cell type uniquely susceptible to radiogenic cancer. (c) Some malignancies (such as leukaemias, sarcomas) appear after a short latent period, peak rapidly thereafter and then decline, but some small excess risk may persist for several decades. The latent period for leukaemia is at least 2 years and has a mean value of 8 years, for solid tumours a minimum of 10 years and for osteosarcomas a mean value of 20 years, and it may be even longer for certain solid tumours. (d) Radiogenic tumours may appear at a much later time after exposure than the growth period of the tumour. Many solid tumours have an age-onset pattern similar to that of non-radiogenic tumours at the same site, after a latency of about 10 years. This is, for example, the case with breast cancer and squamous carcinomas of the digestive tract, where the incidence is increased but the mean age of appearance is not changed. Thus the latency may be very long, particularly in young subjects in whom radiogenic cancers may not appear until an advanced age. The latent period for many sites is a function of age at exposure, but in some types of cancer it is shorter after high doses (Figure 12.4). (e) Age at exposure is the most general host susceptibility factor, with higher risks associated with exposure at younger ages.

Compared with cytotoxic drugs, natural carcinogenic chemicals (such as aflatoxin) and products of the combustion of fossil fuels, ionizing radiation appears to be a rather weak carcinogenic agent.

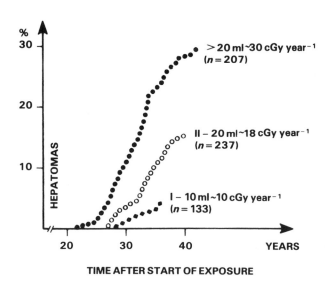

Figure 12.4. Hepatomas in man caused by injection of thorium dioxide or thorotrast, a contrast medium once used in vascular radiology. The dose rate due to this α-emitter is very heterogeneous owing to its fixation by the parenchyma of the liver. Out of 1689 deaths in 2135 subjects there were 256 cases of liver cancer 16–40 years after injection of thorotrast, the total dose being between 2 and 15 Gy. The figure shows that the incidence of hepatomas is greater with larger doses. Also there seems to be a slightly shorter latent period with high doses.
After [69].

Risk factors

Several epidemiological studies can be used to estimate the risk of doses equal to or greater than 1 Gy. For total body irradiation several methodological approaches are possible. The risks in each tissue or organ can be added together. One can also compare the incidence of all solid tumours with that of leukaemia; this ratio is about 5. Knowing that the risk of leukaemia is in the region of $0\cdot2$ or $0\cdot3\%\,Gy^{-1}$ the total risk of fatal cancer would then be of the order of $1\cdot2\%\,Gy^{-1}$ (Table 12.5). This is the value which was used by the ICRP in 1977 [31]. More recently other groups, particularly BEIR and UNSCEAR, have evaluated the risk coefficients for cancer deaths following a dose of 1 Gy. The most recent is that of UNSCEAR [66] which relies mainly on the survivors at Hiroshima and Nagasaki. From these data it concludes that, after a high dose of low-LET radiation delivered at a high dose rate, the lifetime risk coefficient for death due to cancer for the whole population is between 4 and $11\times10^{-2}\,Gy^{-1}$. The wide range is partly due to the lack of sufficient data for children; in the adult population the range is between 5 and $6\times10^{-2}\,Gy^{-1}$. The marked increase in the risk coefficient is only to a small extent related to the revised A-bomb dosimetry and the longer follow-up. The main reason for the increase in risk and uncertainty is related to the use of projection models in BEIR III [7] and UNSCEAR 1988 [66]. This question deserves some explanation.

Table 12.5 Risk from dose of 1 Sv† (1 Gy of X- or γ-rays)

Organ or tissue	Pathological effect	Risk coefficient‡	W_T‖
1 Gonads	Genetic effects in the first two generations	$0\cdot40\times10^{-2}$	$0\cdot25$
2 Breast§	Death due to cancer	$0\cdot25\times10^{-2}$	$0\cdot15$
3 Red bone marrow	Death due to leukaemia	$0\cdot20\times10^{-2}$	$0\cdot12$
4 Lung	Death due to cancer	$0\cdot20\times10^{-2}$	$0\cdot12$
5 Thyroid gland	Death due to cancer	$0\cdot05\times10^{-2}$	$0\cdot03$
6 Bone	Death due to cancer	$0\cdot05\times10^{-2}$	$0\cdot03$
7 Other tissues¶	Death due to cancer	$0\cdot50\times10^{-2}$	$0\cdot30$
Total		$1\cdot65\times10^{-2}$	$1\cdot00$

†The total risk of fatal cancer is 125 cases for a population of 10 000 persons receiving 1 Sv. The risk involved by the irradiation of each tissue or organ enables risk factors to be calculated; this is used to calculate the effective dose equivalent.
‡The risk factor is expressed per Sv and over the whole life of the irradiated subject.
§The value of the risk factor corresponds to a mean for both sexes.
¶Other tissues must be understood in the following way: (i) hands, lower arm, feet, ankles, skin and lens of the eye are excluded; (ii) a risk factor of $0\cdot1\times10^{-2}$ is allowed for each of the remaining five organs or tissues in which the dose equivalents are greatest. The risks in the other tissues can be neglected.

‖ $W_T = \dfrac{\text{relative detriment in tissue T}}{\text{relative detriment for the whole body.}}$

After [31] p. 515.

In some studies, in particular that of the A-bomb survivors, the increase in the incidence of cancer has persisted for more than 40 years after irradiation. Complete data on many sites over a lifetime are not yet available. Thus, in order to estimate the impact of a given radiation exposure on the lifetime cancer incidence of an exposed cohort, it is necessary to project the lifetime risk from data based on only a portion of the life of exposed individuals. Several models have been used to this end. When the risk in the exposed individuals exceeds the spontaneous, non-exposed, risk level by the same amount at all ages, the effect of exposure is termed absolute or additive. When the risk to the exposed is some constant fraction greater than the spontaneous risk, with the relative risk constant at all ages, this is termed a multiplicative effect. Both additive and multiplicative models assume that a cancer excess will persist till death.

The value of the risk coefficient varies widely with the model chosen, with the multiplicative one leading to a higher risk. In view of the uncertainties which are associated with the choice of model, the UNSCEAR report [66] has defined upper and lower limits of the risk. However, Muirhead and Darby [44] have shown that neither of these two projection models fit well with the actual data. Hence the validity of both models remains debatable. Other models should be explored [38], in particular models in which the cancer risk declines or fades away at a given time after exposure (25–30 years). This has been observed with leukaemia and osteosarcoma (Figure 12.1) and in the young age cohort (<19 years) of the A-bomb survivors. Another example illustrates the limits of the relative risk concept. For breast cancer the absolute number of cancers induced per unit dose at a given age is almost the same in the survivors from Hiroshima and Nagasaki, the patients suffering from tuberculosis irradiated during fluoroscopy for pneumothorax (100 irradiations every 15 days with a dose of about 1·5 cGy per exposure), and in women treated for mastitis (1–8 exposures to irradiation). The spontaneous incidence is much greater in North America than in Japan. In this case the excess observed corresponds therefore to an absolute risk and not to a relative risk [31, 67].

In conclusion, a projection is necessary to assess the lifetime risk, but current data cannot yet provide a model by which to project accurately or even to bracket the range of likely risks [38]. This underlines the need for more sophistication in risk assessment when all types of cancer are considered together. Another problem is the discrepancy between the various data, the risks evaluated from A-bomb survivors appearing to be 2–5 fold greater than those based on irradiated patients (Table 12.6).

To evaluate the carcinogenic risk of occupational exposure or radiodiagnosis, i.e. from doses of a few cGy or less, there are no reliable data. Some studies of subjects who had received doses of this order have reported an increase in the incidence of certain types of cancer, but methodological errors have subsequently been recognized and often these studies have been mutually contradictory. For this reason the risks attached to low doses cannot be based on such studies [7, 64]. Nevertheless these surveys can provide some information regarding the upper limit of the risk coefficient. It has been suggested that the data from those surveys which have been carried out with an adequate methodology should be pooled because it is necessary to obtain information on hundreds of thousands of individuals receiving annual doses of 10–100 mGy to the whole body in order to obtain a reliable estimate of effect. Studies of this kind are in progress. Meanwhile the only way to estimate the risk of low doses is to make an extrapolation from the risks observed after doses of the order of 1 Gy. For this purpose (Figure 12.5) it is necessary to know the shape of the dose–effect relationship in the region of low doses, in addition to the influence of dose rate and radiation quality on this relation [38]. As epidemiology cannot by itself deal with these questions it is necessary to consider the results of experimental research before discussing this problem later in this chapter.

Table 12.6 Summary of the estimated risk of cancer per gray of organ absorbed dose obtained from the atomic bomb, ankylosing spondylitis and cervical cancer series.

Organ or tissue	Atomic bomb survivors	Spondylitis series	Cervical cancer series
	Excess relative risk		
Leukaemia	5·21 (3·83–7·12)†	3·5‡	0·88
All cancers except leukaemia	0·41 (0·32–0·51)	0·14§	¶
Bladder	1·27 (0·53–2·37)	0·19	0·07 (0·02–0·17)
Breast	1·19 (0·56–2·09)	–	0·03 (0·00–1·29)
Kidney	0·58 (−0·09–1·94)‖	0·12	0·71 (0·03–2·24)
Large intestine	0·85 (0·39–1·45)	–	0·00 (0·00–0·02)
Larynx	0·51 (−0·05–1·68)‖	0·15	
Lung	0·63 (0·35–0·97)	0·13	
Multiple myeloma	2·29 (0·67–5·31)	–	
Oesophagus	0·58 (0·13–1·24)	0·29	
Ovary	1·33 (0·37–2·86)	0·00	0·01 (0·00–0·14)
Rectum	0·00 ‖	0·03	0·02 (0·00–0·04)
Stomach	0·27 (0·14–0·43)	0·004	0·69 (0·01–2·25)
	Absolute risk (excess deaths per 10^4 PYGy)		
Leukaemia	2·94 (2·43–3·49)	2·02	0·61
All cancers except leukaemia	10·13 (7·96–12·44)	4·67	¶

†Values in parentheses are 90% confidence intervals. They are those given by the authors.
‡This figure was derived by the Committee using data from individuals receiving a mean marrow dose of 3 Gy or less.
§All cancers except leukaemia and colon cancer.
¶An estimate of the risk of all cancers except leukaemia cannot be made for this series. An estimate of the whole body dose does not exist, and probably cannot be estimated given the nature of the exposures.
‖Shielded kerma.
After [66], p. 523.

Mechanisms of carcinogenesis: studies *in vitro* [6, 20–23, 35, 64, 66]

At the cellular level, cancer is a clonal molecular-genetic disease. Carcinogenesis is a multi-stage process. This means that for a cell to be affected a series of events must occur in its lineage, the last event rendering it malignant and causing it to become the progenitor of the tumour and its metastases. Study of chemically induced cancers shows that at least two stages of carcinogenesis can be distinguished: initiation and promotion.

Initiation is an irreversible process in which a normal cell acquires pre-neoplastic characteristics following modification of its genetic material (DNA). The 'initiated' or 'transformed' cell may remain indefinitely in a quiescent state without proliferating. Promotion is the result of events whereby a transformed cell gives rise to malignant cells capable of multiplying and invading neighbouring tissues. Promoters are physical or chemical agents with the property of stimulating cell proliferation. They probably also act on DNA. Ionizing radiations are both initiators and promoters.

Much research has been performed on initiation by ionizing radiation. An important methodological step was taken when it became possible to study this phenomenon *in vitro* [6]. It was noted in 1966 that irradiation of cells in culture transformed some of them, giving rise to new features:

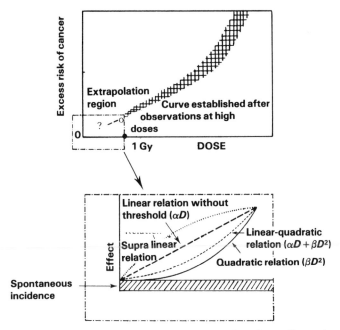

Figure 12.5. Extrapolation of the dose–effect relation to low doses. Several studies have established a dose–effect relation with doses greater than 1 Gy, but none have provided reliable data below 1 Gy. The effect of these low doses is the relevant factor in radiation protection. For this purpose it is necessary to know the shape of the dose–effect relation in order to extrapolate between the spontaneous incidence and that found after irradiation to 1 Gy. The figure shows that the evaluation of risk depends on the function chosen. The linear relation gives the greatest risk which, at 0·5 Gy, is about double that given by the linear–quadratic relation which is scientifically much more plausible.

1. Immortalization: whereas fibroblasts can divide only a limited number of times, usually about 60, transformed cells are capable of an unlimited number of mitoses. However, although all transformed cells are immortal there are also immortal cells which are not transformed.
2. Morphological changes, particularly in the cellular membrane, so that the cell no longer needs to be anchored on a solid medium in order to divide.
3. Loss of contact inhibition: on a petri dish normal cells remain in a monocellular layer whereas the transformed cells infiltrate among their normal neighbours and give rise to a small heap composed of several superimposed layers. It is therefore easy to count them (see Figure 12.6).
4. Often, but not always, when colonies of transformed cells are injected into an isologous animal, they give rise to a malignant tumour. However, some of these regress spontaneously.

These four properties are not acquired simultaneously, as transformation, although it represents only certain stages in carcinogenesis, is itself the result of several distinct events.

The study of transformation *in vitro* makes possible two types of research: (i) analysis of the factors affecting the frequency of transformation; (ii) research on the mechanism of carcinogenesis [20–24].

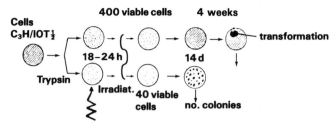

Figure 12.6. Scheme of an experiment on neoplastic transformation *in vitro*. C₃H/10 T½ cells are cultivated in Petri dishes, harvested and trypsinized to obtain a cell suspension which is then irradiated. About 400 viable cells are seeded 18–24 h later in a Petri dish; after 4 weeks the number of clones of transformed cells is counted. These clones are easily identified as the colonies of transformed cells are composed of several cell layers (whereas normal cells lie in a single layer) and form heaps which are immediately visible. The lower line of the figure shows how the percentage of viable cells is measured: 18–24 h after irradiation about 40 viable cells are seeded per Petri dish; 14 days later the number of colonies is counted (this includes both normal and transformed cells).

Analysis of the factors influencing the frequency of transformation

The proportion of surviving cells which are transformed can be determined by the use of *in vitro* techniques.

DOSE–EFFECT RELATION

The proportion of transformed cells rises with increasing dose. Figure 12.7 shows this relationship for the number of transformed cells per survivor; the relation is linear at low doses but this is difficult to appreciate in the figure as the ordinate is logarithmic. Fractionation with γ-rays reduces the proportion of transformed cells, but with neutrons the proportion is increased.

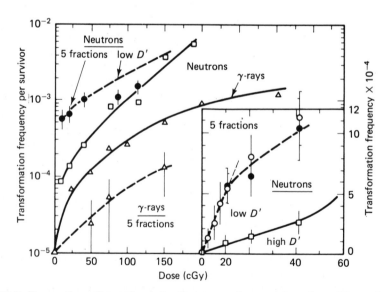

Figure 12.7. Proportion of transformed cells per survivor as a function of dose of γ-rays and neutrons, single doses and 5 fractions. Fractionation decreases the frequency with γ-rays but increases it with neutrons.
After [28].

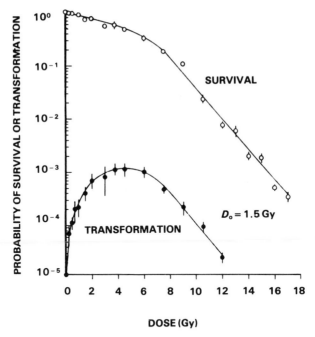

Figure 12.8. The upper curve shows the probability of survival of 10T ½ cells irradiated *in vitro* by cobalt γ-rays at 1 Gy min⁻¹. The lower curve shows the probability of transformation of a cell of the same line irradiated under the same conditions; the reduction seen above 4 Gy is due to the death of cells potentially transformed. The radiosensitivity of transformed and untransformed cells is the same ($D_0=1.5$ Gy). After [20].

The number of transformants as a proportion of the number irradiated (rather than per survivor) rises to a maximum near 4 Gy and then diminishes (Figure 12.8). This decrease is due to the fact that the transformed cells can be killed in the same way and with the same radiosensitivity as the normal cells [23, 24, 67]. This is also the reason why the number of transformed cells, expressed as a proportion of the surviving cells, remains small, of the order of 0.1%.

When doses greater than 1 Gy are given in 2 fractions with an interval of 5 h, enough for full repair of radiation damage, the frequency of transformation is reduced. With shorter intervals of time there is incomplete repair of subtransformations, in analogy with that of sublethal damage. This repair is also shown by varying the dose rate: the frequency of transformation is reduced by a factor of 3 when the dose rate is reduced from 1 Gy min⁻¹ to 1 mGy min⁻¹. However, as the reduction in dose rate is even more effective in reducing cell lethality, the number of transformed cells at doses above 10 Gy is greater at low dose rate than at high dose rate (Figure 12.9).

With neutrons, fractionation or a reduction in dose rate increases the effectiveness for transformation (perhaps because of misrepair) particularly with low doses; the data suggest that even with neutrons transformation is caused by several distinct events. However, with neutrons reduction in dose rate does not alter cell mortality.

The RBE of neutrons for transformation therefore varies as a function of the dose and of the dose rate. It is very high for doses below 0.1 Gy and for low dose

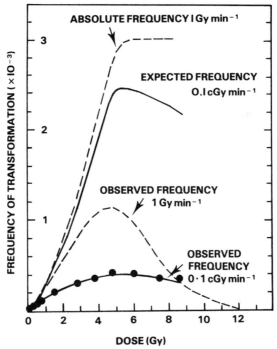

Figure 12.9. Frequency of transformation as a function of the conditions of irradiation. The curve for a dose rate of 1 Gy min^{-1} is that of Figure 12.8. The upper curve of absolute frequency is deduced from it by taking account of cell mortality at each dose; it indicates the total number of cells which have been transformed. The expected frequency at 0·1 Gy min^{-1} is that which would have been obtained if the frequency of transformation had been the same as at 1 Gy min^{-1}, greater than the observed frequency at 1 Gy min^{-1} because of the lower cell mortality at the lower dose rate. The observed frequency at 0·1 Gy min^{-1} is much lower than the expected frequency, demonstrating the role of repair of subtransformations (see text).
After [20]

rates and is of the order of 10 for higher doses and dose rates [24] (see Section 11.4).

Mechanisms of carcinogenesis

The study of transformation *in vitro* has contributed towards a better under-standing of the carcinogenic action of radiation.

After irradiation, if the cells are maintained in a quiescent state without dividing, the number of transformed cells gradually falls over a period of 24 h, showing the existence of repair processes analogous to the repair of sublethal or potentially lethal damage (Figure 12.10). Therefore, even though the DNA has been damaged, its repair within a few hours or days of initiation can prevent the development of a tumour. The time between DNA damage and the next mitosis is critical: proliferation after exposure results in a higher number of transformed cells. This may be due to the shorter time available for repair before the lesion is fixed during mitosis. Also transformation is not expressed unless the cells divide a sufficient number of times after irradiation; between

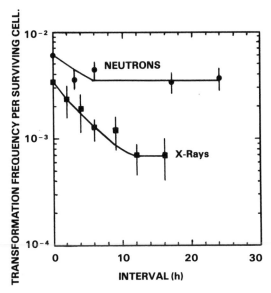

Figure 12.10. Effect of fractionation on the proportion of transformed cells per surviving cell (line 10 T½). Lower curve, 2 fractions of 2·5 Gy of X-rays as a function of the interval between fractions. Upper curve, 2 fractions of 1·89 Gy of neutrons. Repair of subtransformation damage is greater after irradiation with X-rays than after neutrons. After [23].

four and six mitoses must occur after irradiation to produce a fixed transformation and the first mitosis must take place within the first day. If it does not, the potentially carcinogenic character of the initiated cell may be lost. This suggests that expression requires a second event which occurs at random but infrequently (of the order of 10^{-6}) during mitosis; the greater the number of cell divisions the greater is the number of transformed cells.

This dissociation between the stages of initiation and expression of transformation has been shown in many experiments. The most important are those of Kennedy and Little [35]. These authors irradiated the cells to a dose of 4–6 Gy and then seeded a variable number into petri dishes and allowed them to grow to confluence; they then counted the number of clones of transformed cells. One might expect that the number of transformed cells would be proportional to the number of irradiated cells seeded. In fact, whatever the number of cells seeded the number of clones was the same. This suggests that in this cell line initiation is a very frequent phenomenon (affecting one cell in two after a dose of 5 Gy). On the other hand expression of transformation is a very rare event whose frequency is proportional to the number of divisions during the week following irradiation.

A similar result was obtained by Gould [21] who grafted thyroid cells into the fat pads of rats which were fed a diet deficient in iodine. These cells gave rise to colonies of thyroid cells. If they had been irradiated, about one colony in six was found to contain a thyroid tumour. Whether the cells had received 1 Gy or 5 Gy, there was very little increase in the proportion of colonies containing tumours although the number of irradiated cells which were grafted was increased at the higher dose.

These two experiments therefore suggest that expression is a much rarer phenomenon than initiation and that the probability that an initiated cell should be transformed depends much more on the number of mitoses after irradiation than on the dose. Also, by culturing the cells at different times after irradiation, it has been shown that the initiated lesion can express itself for about a week but that later the probability of expression diminishes. Expression can also be inhibited if cell division is blocked by the mechanism of contact inhibition when the cell density becomes very large. In addition, promoters are often agents which disturb intercellular communication.

These studies give no information on the nature of the lesions responsible for transformation. However, some progress is being made [48, 66]. Initiation can be due to a point mutation or a chromosomal rearrangement. In some experiments carcinogenesis appears to be related to symmetrical chromosome translocations (reciprocal translocations without loss of chromosome material). The similarity in the rate of induction and repair of transformation *in vitro* and of sister chromatid exchanges suggests that the latter may play a role.

Experiments with particles of different LET enable the cross-section of the target to be determined from the probability of induction of an irreversible lesion after passage of a particle across the cell. For cell death the cross-section for the most effective particles is only a little less than the area of the nucleus, showing that the passage of a single particle at high LET through the nucleus has a high probability of killing the cell. For gene mutations the cross-section is about 10 000 times smaller, of the order of $0 \cdot 005 \, \mu m^2$, which is, however, larger than the size of a gene. For transformations the target is 10–100 times greater, suggesting either that there are many sensitive sites in which damage leads to transformation, or that the targets are larger than those responsible for point mutations [20]. Lesions leading to chromosome breaks and the translocation of certain chromosomal regions may be one of the main mechanisms through which a normal cell becomes malignant.

Malignant cells contain oncogenes. These are also present in normal cells but they are not activated (proto-oncogenes). Activation can be caused by gene mutation (transformation of a proto-oncogene into an oncogene), or by a disturbance in the mechanism whereby the gene is regulated. This may be due to insertion, next to the proto-oncogene, of an activator gene perhaps of viral origin, or to the translocation of a normal regulator gene to the neighbourhood of the proto-oncogene by a chromosomal rearrangement.

About 30 oncogenes have been identified. Study of carcinogenesis by chemical or physical agents has shown that in many cases an oncogene of the family *Ras* has been activated, but this is only one of the events which lead to transformation. Mouse cells may be transformed by chemical carcinogens which activate *Ras* oncogenes by substitution of adenine for guanine. The same point mutation of guanine to adenine in a *Ras* oncogene was observed in the induction by radiation of a thymoma in mice. These findings suggest that, at the molecular level, the carcinogenic effects of radiation are similar to those of other carcinogens.

An isolated somatic mutation is insufficient, but irradiation can also cause transpositions of genes, recombinations and deletions. It is not surprising that these lesions, or errors occurring during repair, can activate one or several proto-oncogenes (Chapter 3).

Besides the incorrect activation of a normal gene or the activation of a mutant version of a normal gene, some tumours such as retinoblastoma are caused by a gene deletion which inactivates an 'antioncogene' (suppressor) or a gene repressor region. With regard to these antioncogenes, there is evidence that after a first mutation at one of the two loci, a somatic recombination event may occur which replaces the normal gene on the unmutated chromosome by the mutated gene, leading to cell transformation. Another possibility is a second somatic mutation at the suppressor gene located on the intact homologous chromosome or its deletion.

Thus, studies *in vitro* have extended our understanding. However, most initiated cells never result in a tumour. *In vivo*, several mechanisms ensure that most potentially carcinogenic cells do not cause a cancer. This can be illustrated by the induction of leukaemia by radiation which occurs in about 1% of irradiated subjects after a dose of 3 Gy. Allowing for the number of haemopoietic cells in each subject, less than one cell in 10^{14} gives rise to leukaemia. Even if it is only the pluri-potential stem cells which can give rise to leukaemia, there are still 10^{11} of these and there remains an enormous disproportion between the large frequency of effects seen *in vitro* and the extreme rarity *in vivo*. It is therefore likely that transformation *in vitro* is only one out of many stages of carcinogenesis.

In the past it was tempting to assume that the relation between dose and carcinogenic effect would be linear, at least at low doses, on the assumption that transformation of a cell was a very unlikely event caused by a lesion in a particular region of the genome which could be produced by a single particle. However, this idea must be abandoned as the initial event appears to be frequent and its expression depends on a series of later stages whose probability is influenced by external factors, particularly the administration after irradiation of promoters (16) or anti-promoters [36, 66]. Certainly current knowledge does not exclude the existence of a linear relationship but it shows that there is no theoretical argument in its favour, in contrast with past thinking [68].

Finally, it should be emphasized that most *in vitro* experiments have been conducted with rodent cells which are easily immortalized, whereas this is rare and difficult to achieve with human cells. Extrapolation to the situation *in vivo*, particularly in man, must therefore be made with caution, particularly as far as the dose–effect relationship is concerned.

Animal experiments

Many experiments have been made with different species of animal [16, 63–66]. We will only discuss certain points.

In animals, as in man, the incidence of tumours arising after a given dose varies markedly from one tissue to another and, for a given tissue, from one species to another. In mice there are large variations between strains, emphasizing the role of genetic factors. Radiation-induced cancers are much commoner in mice than in man and the difference becomes even greater if one relates it to the number of cells at risk. It is likely that these differences are due, at least in part, to the fact that a potentially malignant cell has a different probability of giving rise to a tumour, depending on the species; these differences must be due to the characteristics of the host.

Extrapolation from one species to another is not possible in the current state of knowledge. It seems, however, to a first approximation, that the number of radiation induced cancers in a given tissue and species is greater when the number of spontaneous tumours is large [16].

Dose–effect relationship

The shape of the dose–effect relation has been the subject of many experiments and depends on the type of tumour (Figure 12.11). With X-rays the incidence is usually very small with doses below 1 Gy. It then increases slowly, passes through a maximum and thereafter decreases. The initial part of the curve can often be well fitted to a second degree polynomial, the linear–quadratic relation. The final part of the curve decreases exponentially; as we have seen, this is due to the death of transformed cells. However, other shapes sometimes occur: a curve with threshold, a quadratic relation, a linear relation and even a reduction in incidence with dose, suggesting the killing by radiation of potentially malignant cells already present in the animal.

This variability from one tissue to another shows that the mechanisms of induction may be different. Radiation can act both as an initiator and a promoter and may be particularly effective during cell proliferation which takes place after doses great enough to cause the death of a large proportion of cells, thereby inducing a compensatory proliferation of the tissue.

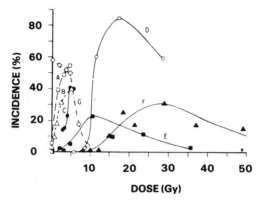

Figure 12.11. Dose–effect relations for the induction of different types of tumours in animals given external irradiation.
A, Myeloid leukaemia in the mouse, irradiation with X-rays;
B, mammary tumours in rats after irradiation with cobalt γ-rays;
C, thymomas in mice irradiated with X-rays;
D, tumours of the kidney in rats irradiated with X-rays;
E, skin tumours after irradiation with α-rays (incidence × 10);
F, skin cancer after irradiation with electrons (incidence × 10);
G, reticulosarcomas in mice irradiated with X-rays.
After [63].

The influence of the promoter on the development of radiation induced tumours has been shown in many experiments. For example, the incidence of mammary or ovarian tumours in the mouse is considerably increased by administration of oestrogen, that of tumours of the kidney by unilateral nephrectomy (which causes hypertrophy of the remaining kidney), that of leukaemia in the rat by bleeding, etc. Remote effects (abscopal) of radiation occur with certain types of tumour, e.g. tumours of the hypophysis induced by irradiation of the thyroid leading to hypersecretion of TSH.

The importance of events occurring after irradiation is illustrated by several data. For example, carbon tetrachloride which has a toxic effect on the liver, increases the incidence of hepatoma after irradiation. In man the incidence of skin cancer after irradiation with X-rays is greater in white than in coloured people, no doubt because of the effects on the former of ultraviolet rays in sunlight as an associated factor.

Also the shape of the curve may be very different depending on the conditions of irradiation (Figure 12.12). A promoter such as phorbol ester has a considerable effect in modifying the shape of the dose–effect relation [16]. This shows that the probability of induction of a tumour is the product of at least two probabilities: the induction of a single potentially malignant cell and the

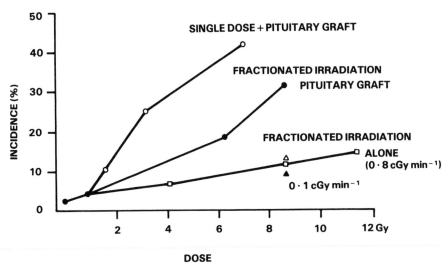

Figure 12.12. Incidence of Harderian gland tumours after irradiation with γ-rays. A pituitary graft maintaining a high level of prolactin increases considerably the incidence of the tumours, particularly after fractionated irradiation. This suggests that fractionation reduces the effectiveness of radiation carcinogenesis both by reducing the number of lesions causing initiation and by reducing the expression of these lesions due to the reduced cell mortality.
After [16].

proliferation of this cell. For example, irradiation of BALB/c mice with a dose of 1 Gy of γ-rays produces mammary cancers in 14% of the mice. Now, if the mammary tissue is excised after irradiation and the cells are dissociated and grafted into fat pads, nodules of malignant cells can be found in all the grafted animals. Thus inhibition of proliferation in a normal tissue, caused by homeostatic mechanisms, prevents the development of potentially malignant cells.

To set these results in the context of our understanding of carcinogenesis in man, we must recall that the clinical emergence of a tumour is the result of a series of successive stages. This is shown particularly by studies on cancer of the uterine cervix: the first pre-cancerous lesions appear at about 25 years of age, followed by more malignant lesions around 40 and invasive cancer at about 50. Thus the process extends over more than 20 years. Moreover there are 10 times as many pre-cancerous lesions as there are invasive tumours. Every pre-cancerous lesion does not give rise to a frank tumour.

Similarly, in all countries about 10% of elderly men examined post-mortem are found to have occult tumours of the prostate, whereas the actual incidence of clinically detectable prostate tumours is much lower and very variable from one country to another. This suggests that the transition from latent cancer to definite tumour requires an additional factor, variable from one country to another and probably connected with diet.

Thus it seems likely that the dose–effect relation for clinical carcinogenesis is different from that obtained for cell transformation. Moreover, after low doses which produce no tissue reactions and therefore no compensating cell proliferation, the effect per cGy is probably much lower than that forecast on the basis of observed effects after doses of a few gray [16, 46, 66, 67].

Influence of dose rate [46, 66]

In all the experimental systems studied, the carcinogenic effect of X-rays and γ-rays is reduced at low dose rate. The reduction factor at low doses lies between 2 and 10. However, the value of this factor is not the same at all doses and even the shape of the dose–effect curve may be altered. A reduction in dose rate affects both the probability of initiation (Figures 12.13 and 12.14) and that of promotion, since in the absence of tissue damage there is no effect on promotion due to cell multiplication. High doses of radiation or moderate doses at high dose rate can reduce the effectiveness of DNA repair mechanisms (Section 4.5). This may in part explain the influence of dose rate.

Effects in different tissues

There are large differences in the rate of induction of tumours in different tissues. In animals, as in man, radiogenic cancers are relatively frequent in the thyroid, the breast and the bone marrow and very rare in the prostate and testis. After irradiation no excess of cancer of the uterine cervix, chronic lymphocytic leukaemia or Hodgkin's disease has been reported. Factors such as

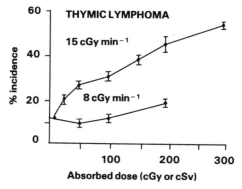

Figure 12.13. Effect of dose and dose rate on the incidence of thymic lymphomas in mice. After [62].

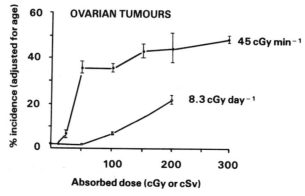

Figure 12.14. Effect of dose and dose rate on the incidence of ovarian tumours in mice. After [62].

the importance of promotion may contribute to explaining these differences. Also, the frequency of transformed cells *in vitro* varies widely from one type of tissue to another. *In vivo*, only relatively poorly differentiated cells become malignant, essentially the stem cells; their number varies between different tissues. Within a given tissue, important differences are seen as a function of age. For example, susceptibility to radiation induced cancer of the breast is relatively high in women between 5 and 20 years of age and then declines in adults and elderly women. Two factors explain this influence of age: changes in the number of stem cells susceptible to carcinogenesis, and a longer interval between irradiation and the menopause during which partially transformed cells can proliferate and hence be vulnerable to a final transforming event.

The relationship between age at irradiation and delay between exposure and emergence of cancer is complex. There are several possibilities. (i) If the first of the sequence of transforming events is induced by the exposure, the proportion of individuals in whom there are already partially transformed cells is increased. For a long time after exposure these individuals will remain at excess risk, their cells having to await only a smaller number of events in subsequent years before becoming fully malignant. However, the age at cancer emergence might be the same as that in an unexposed cohort because a significant number of other events will still be required for full malignancy. (ii) Conversely, if a late stage of cell transformation is affected by irradiation, those cells that have already experienced some events will quickly become malignant; however, after a relatively short delay there will be no further excess risk in the exposed cohort relative to the unexposed one. In this case late age of exposure should manifest more excess cancers than in younger individuals, because elderly individuals possess a higher proportion of cells which have already experienced several transforming events. (iii) If an intermediate event is affected by the exposure, some time later individuals in a non-exposed cohort will also have cells which have accumulated these stages and the excess risk in the exposed cohort will diminish. These considerations illustrate the fallacy of the use of a single, additive or multiplicative, projection model for all cancer types and all ages at exposure [38, 66].

Radiation quality

At a given dose, carcinogenic effectiveness varies considerably with the type of radiation. High-LET radiations (neutrons, α-rays, etc.) have a high RBE and the dose–effect relation is different and often linear. Changes in dose rate have a smaller effect than with radiation of low LET (X-, β- and γ-rays). Consequently the RBE may reach very high values for low doses and low dose rates, as under these conditions the effect of X-rays is very small or zero.

In summary, animal experiments have made possible a study of the influence of dose, dose rate and radiation quality and have demonstrated the role of the conditions of life and promoting factors. Thanks to animal experiments we are beginning to understand the differences in frequency of radiation induced cancers depending on tissue, species, sex and age. This valuable information is of a qualitative nature. Quantitative extrapolation to human beings remains hazardous.

Evaluation of the carcinogenic risk at low doses in man [7, 13, 31, 48–50, 66]

As we have seen, with doses of the order of 1 Gy or more of low LET radiation given as a single dose (dose rate >1 cGy min^{-1}), a fairly reliable estimate of the short- and medium-term risks can be obtained from epidemiological data.

Below 0·4 Gy most investigations have not detected any effect. When there was an effect, uncertainties in evaluation of the dose have made the risk estimate unreliable or have provided only an upper limit to the risk. With doses below 0·2 Gy no increase in incidence of tumours has been observed; given the small effect which would be possible, enormous surveys would be necessary to obtain direct information. Risk assessment following irradiation at low doses delivered at low dose rates therefore requires an extrapolation from the risk coefficient computed for high doses. Experimental analysis (see earlier in this section) does not enable one to exclude the possibility that there is an effect with doses of 10 cGy. It cannot be evaluated from a linear extrapolation of the effect at high doses as the form of the dose–effect relationship is usually linear–quadratic or quadratic and so may have a practical threshold.

A linear extrapolation leads to an overestimation of the risk. In neither animals nor man is there any argument suggesting that the risk is greater than the value estimated by linear extrapolation, whatever may be the radiobiological effect studied. This would only be conceivable if there were a sub-group of individuals much more sensitive to radiation induced carcinogenesis than the rest of the population. The proportion of radiosensitive individuals (heterozygotes with ataxia telangiectasia) seems too small to modify significantly the dose–effect relation [48]. Table 12.5 indicates the risk estimates at 1 Sr given in the report of the US Academy of Sciences [7] which are slightly greater than those of the ICRP [31] and less than those of the 1988 UNSCEAR report [66].

In animals, the shape of the dose–effect relation depends on the tissue and the dose rate and is influenced by exogenous factors. With X- and γ-rays it is usually quadratic or linear–quadratic at low doses. There is no reason to think that the shape would be different in man.

When there are adequate epidemiological data they are usually in favour of a linear–quadratic relationship. For the survivors of the atomic bombs, the linear–quadratic relation represents the best fit to the totality of the data.

It has been claimed that the dose response is linear for a few types of cancer. The first is *leukaemia*. However, several sets of data challenge the concept of a linear dose–effect relationship for leukaemogenesis. Among the A-bomb survivors the data suggest a curvilinear relationship with a smaller relative risk for individuals exposed to doses below 0·5 Gy and no detectable effect below 0·3 Gy. In the study of cervical cancer the incidence of leukaemia was much lower than expected on the basis of current estimates. This relative deficit of excess cases was partly attributed to local cell killing of pelvic bone marrow cells. Nevertheless, peripheral marrow received doses of about 1 Gy at a low dose rate from radium sources; the data suggest a leukaemia induction per gray about 5-fold smaller than in the A-bomb survivors. This strong influence of dose rate is consistent with a non-linear dose response. *Breast*: Three out of the four studies are consistent with a linear dose–response pattern but cannot exclude a linear–quadratic relationship. The fourth, on breast cancer secondary to chest fluoroscopy in which the irradiation was fractionated, is consistent with a quadratic or a linear–quadratic dose–effect relationship. There was a definite excess of tumours even after doses of 0·2 Gy, but retrospective evaluation of doses delivered during fluoroscopy is uncertain [37, 66, 67]. *Thyroid*: The thyroid gland is particularly susceptible to radiation induced cancer especially when exposure occurs in the first two decades of life. In the A-bomb survivors the incidence fitted a linear model. An increase in the incidence of thyroid tumours was seen in children treated by radiotherapy for tinea capitis [7, 66]. The dose to the thyroid in the children who later developed thyroid cancer has been estimated at $0 \cdot 1$ Gy, but in this case also estimation of the doses is subject to uncertainty as it was performed many years after irradiation and a small change in the position of the head and neck would have caused the thyroid gland to receive a much greater dose. Also other surveys of children who had received radiotherapy for tinea capitis failed to find any increase in the incidence of thyroid cancer [67].

No excess incidence of thyroid cancer has been found in the population of Nevada exposed to iodine-131 from fall-out from atomic explosions. The same is true for 35 000 individuals investigated by scintigraphy with ^{131}I and studied by Holm *et al.* (29). Holm's data lead to a reduction factor greater than or equal to 4 between the effects of a given dose on the thyroid gland by external irradiation at high dose rate or by internal irradiation with ^{131}I. In the Marshall Island cohort a group of 250 individuals has now been followed for 30 years. The dose was 7–14 Gy in young children, delivered by ^{131}I and short-lived radioiodines. There has been a large number of cases of benign thyroid nodules, but it is uncertain whether an excess of malignant thyroid cancer has occurred. The data suggest a linear dose–response relationship for thyroid nodules and show that internal irradiation at high dose rate delivered by short-lived isotopes is more effective than low dose rate irradiation from ^{131}I.

No increase in incidence of *bone sarcomas* has been detected after contamination with less than 30 μg of radium and doses below 7 Gy (Figure 12.3). Similarly, as we have seen in women treated for cancer of the uterine cervix, the incidence of tumours in tissues which had received low doses was not increased and even when part of the bone marrow received greater doses (at a low dose rate) there was only a small excess of leukaemia.

In summary, the shape of the dose–effect relationship is still uncertain. Furthermore, as stated in the BEIR IV report [8] for bone sarcomas, 'the appearance time increases with decreasing dose and dose rate and characterizes a practical threshold of about $0 \cdot 8$ Gy average skeletal dose, below which the chance of developing bone cancer from Ra 226 and Ra 228 during the normal lifetime is extremely small and possibly zero'. This remark may be valid for several other types of cancer and is consistent with animal experiments performed with bone-seeking radioisotopes.

Risk coefficients at low doses received at low dose rate

The UNSCEAR report [66] proposes the use of a linear relationship associated with a reduction factor for low doses and low dose rates. It estimates its value to be between 2 and 10, in keeping with the NCRP report [7]. Use of a reduction factor applied to the risk coefficients that were determined for high doses leads to risk coefficients at low doses and low dose rates between 0·4 and $5 \cdot 5 \times 10^{-2}$ Gy^{-1}. This range includes the value $1 \cdot 25 \times 10^{-2}$ Gy^{-1} formerly adopted by ICRP [31].

It should be emphasized that in the UNSCEAR report [66] the risk estimates are based only on A-bomb survivors. This survey is subject to several pitfalls, in particular the immunosuppression induced by high doses of total body irradiation, a dose rate far higher than that of exposures in civilian life, and the presence of some neutron irradiation which was small but not negligible. Epidemiological studies carried out on patients lead to risk coefficients which are 2- to 5-fold smaller [33, 66]. It has been argued that susceptibility to carcinogenesis might be different in patients and normal individuals. This statement has no scientific basis. It might be true for some types of cancer (such as retinoblastoma, nephroblastoma) in which the genetic constitution of the host plays a crucial role, but these tumours are very rare; moreover, even in these subjects the risk is increased and not decreased. The hypothesis that in some patients the risk might be reduced is contradicted by all that we know about carcinogenesis [38]. Furthermore, surveys on patients avoid some of the biases encountered in the study of the A-bomb survivors.

In conclusion, the 1988 UNSCEAR report [66] proposes to re-evaluate by a factor of $1\cdot6$–$4\cdot4$ its 1977 [63] estimates of the risk coefficient applicable for high doses and introduces a reduction factor between 2 and 10 for low doses and low dose rates. These figures do not exclude the possibility that the risk at low doses and low dose rate may be lower than has so far been estimated. Moreover they are based only on A-bomb survivors whereas risk coefficients derived from surveys on patients are smaller (Table 12.6). On-going studies should provide more precise assessments of risk coefficients.

12.4 Genetic risk

Radiation is the longest known and best understood of the mutagenic agents present in the environment [7, 55, 59, 66], but there are many others, particularly the molecules produced during combustion of coal, oil and tobacco. The mutations caused by radiation are no different from the others. In comparison with chemical agents, radiation is a mutagen of low efficiency.

In Chapter 3 we examined the different lesions caused by radiation in the genetic material of cells. Here we are concerned only with hereditary effects, i.e. the result of lesions in the germinal cells. In the male, the dividing stem-cell spermatogonia constitute a permanent stem-cell population which continues to multiply throughout the reproductive lifespan of the individual. In the female, the relevant cells are the oocytes. Female mammals are born with a finite number of oocytes which are arrested in meiosis from prenatal life. Shortly before ovulation they have to complete meiotic divisions before pronuclear fusion. The mutability of the germinal cells of the male is much greater than that of the female, by a factor of about 5. In the female there are two periods which are sensitive to mutagenesis; (i) a short period during foetal life before the seventh month, and (ii) the period of reproductive life after puberty. In men spermatogonia appear to have low sensitivity before puberty. Because of the importance of repair processes, the genetic risk falls off with time after irradiation, which is the reason why people are advised to wait at least 6 months after irradiation before procreation.

Many research studies have measured the frequency per unit dose of various types of genetic mutation in mice and *Drosophila*. Experiments with cells in culture suggest that the dose—effect relation is of the linear—quadratic type in all species and in particular in man. The influence of dose rate is important: in males the number of mutations is reduced by a factor of about 4 when the dose rate is lower than $0 \cdot 1$ mGy min^{-1}. In the female the influence of dose rate and fractionation is even more pronounced.

There is little information whereby the genetic risk in man can be directly estimated. One important fact is that studies of the descendants of subjects irradiated at Hiroshima and Nagasaki have shown no genetic or cytogenetic effects: the frequency of congenital defects, the electrophoretic characteristics of blood proteins, morphology, fecundity and life expectancy have been no different in descendants of the survivors in comparison with children of non-irradiated parents [55, 66]. The follow-up is now so long that this conclusion appears to be definite. This absence of any detectable effect can only be explained on the assumption that the mutagenic effect is at least four times lower in man than in the mouse [55]. Similarly, surveys of descendants of patients treated by radiotherapy have revealed no increase in the frequency of congenital defects. However, epidemiological surveys are of limited precision and human studies are made difficult by lack of understanding of the genetics of pathology; for this reason experts continue to extrapolate from animal experiments in a deliberately pessimistic way [7, 66].

In one research study about 80 generations of mice were exposed at the rate of 2 Gy per generation without any detectable repercussion on the viability or fecundity of their descendants [59]. The absence of any detectable deleterious effect in this case may be due to mechanisms which eliminate most of the embryos carrying serious genetic defects at the beginning of pregnancy. This result is reassuring but is not proof of the harmlessness of radiation, as impairment of intellectual capacity cannot be demonstrated in studies on mice.

When one tries to estimate the risk due to irradiation, one must consider the dose received, not by an individual but by the whole population. In a human cell each gene is double; one is derived from the paternal chromosome and the other from the maternal chromosome. If they are identical they are called homozygotes, if not heterozygotes. A heterozygotic gene is effective in the first generation only if it is dominant. More usually a mutated gene is recessive and is not immediately manifest. In the course of procreation half the descendants will receive the normal gene and the other half the mutated gene which will thus be transmitted from generation to generation. In some circumstances even a heterozygotic recessive gene may have some limited influence; many authors think that recessive genes can alter the resistance, vigour and adaptability of an individual. Moreover a recessive gene can be expressed under different circumstances, either because it becomes homozygotic if the corresponding gene arising from the other parent contains the same mutation, or if the other gene is absent due to genetic recombination. A recessive gene becomes diluted in what is called the genome of the population, i.e. the whole genetic material of the individuals capable of reproduction. Normally in this genome there are a large number of recessive genes resulting from spontaneous mutations. Irradiation, like other mutagenic agents, e.g. chemicals, increases this genetic burden, but the result is the same whether an irradiated individual introduces 10 recessive genes into the genome or whether 10 persons introduce one. As far as genetic effects are concerned it is therefore necessary to consider the population dose, i.e. the sum of the doses received by the gonads of all the individuals composing the population (the genetically significant dose).

Several groups of experts have analyzed the enormous mass of information concerning genetic effects. The methods used to quantify genetic risks can be grouped under two headings [66]:

1. *The doubling dose method* which aims at expressing the risk in relation to the natural prevalence of genetic diseases in the general population. The doubling dose is the amount of radiation necessary to produce as many mutations as those occurring spontaneously in a generation. The rationale for the use of this method is that it permits one to express risks in tangible terms and that classes of genetic effects can be handled in the absence of information such as the number of genetic loci involved and their individual mutation rates. In 1962 the UNSCEAR report adopted 1 Gy as the best estimate of the doubling dose and this value is still being used although the lack of detectable effect in the descendants of the population at Hiroshima and Nagasaki suggests that the actual value might be much higher. The reason for adhering to the 1 Gy estimate is prudence in the absence of conclusive human data. Until human data become available there is no alternative but to use cautiously data obtained in other mammalian species. Table 12.7 shows the risks estimated with this method under conditions of continuous irradiation, that is with a continuous influx of new mutations until a new equilibrium is reached between those mutations that enter the gene pool and those that are eliminated.

Table 12.7 Estimates of risk of severe genetic disease per million live births in a population exposed to a genetically significant dose equivalent of 1 Sv per generation at low dose rate according to the doubling dose method.

Disease classification	Current incidence per million live births	Effect of 1 Sv per generation		
		First generation	Second generation	Equilibrium
Autosomal dominant and X-linked	10 000	1500	1300	10 000
Autosomal recessive	2500	5	5	1500
Chromosomal				
Due to structural anomalies	400	240	96	400
Due to numerical anomalies	3400	Probably very small		
Congenital anomalies	60 000	Not estimated†		
Other multifactorial diseases	600 000	Not estimated†		
Total estimated risk		1700	1400	12000

†The committee concluded that it was unable to provide meaningful risk estimates for these disorders. However, even with extreme assumptions (e.g. a 100% mutational component) the risk of severe hereditary harm in the first generation of offspring to the exposed individuals should not be higher than the present estimate of cancer risk.
According to [66], p. 31. Doubling dose assumed in these calculations is 1 SV.

2. *The direct method* which aims at expressing absolute risk in terms of expected increases in the prevalence of genetic disease. The risk estimates made with this method include: (a) the induction of genetic changes having dominant effects in the first generation (i.e. dominant mutations as well as recessive mutations, deletions and balanced reciprocal translocations with dominant effects). The estimates are based on dominant skeletal and cataract mutations in mice. (b) Unbalanced products of induced reciprocal translocations which may lead to congenitally malformed children. The estimates are based on

cytogenetic data from primates. The results are given in Table 12.8. The UNSCEAR committee estimated 10–20 per cGy per million live born as having genetic diseases caused by induced dominant mutations and about 10 extra cases of genetically abnormal children due to recessive mutations. Induced chromosomal rearrangement was estimated to cause between 1 and 15 cases after paternal irradiation and between 0 and 5 after maternal irradiation. Both methods give results of the same order of magnitude in spite of the different assumptions and reduction factors. To set these risks in context they must be compared with the natural frequency which is 107 per 1000 [7, 64, 66].

Table 12.8 Risk of induction of genetic damage in man per centigray of low-LET radiation at low dose rate, estimated using the direct method.

Risk	Expected frequency (per million) of genetically abnormal children in the first generation after irradiation of	
	Males	Females
Induced mutations having dominant effects	~ 10 – ~ 20	0 – ~ 9
Induced recessive mutations†	0	0
Unbalanced products of induced reciprocal translocation	~ 1 – ~ 15	0 – 5

†Although the risk is zero for the first generation about one extra case per million births would be expected in the following 10 generations (from partnership effect) and on certain assumptions, about 10 extra cases per million would be expected by the 10th generation (from effects due to identity by descent).
According to [66], p. 400.

As a first approximation it is generally assumed that all mutations are harmful, although this hypothesis is unduly pessimistic as many must be indifferent. Moreover, when estimating the hazard due to irradiation, either of an active population of 20–65 years or of the whole population, one must remember that irradiation of 60% of the subjects will have no genetic consequence as these individuals will bear no more children. To derive risk coefficients for genetic diseases in a population, one needs therefore to multiply the genetic risk estimates discussed earlier by 0·4.

Altogether the genetic risk of ionizing irradiation seems less serious than was at one time feared. However, it is best to remain prudent and to evaluate the risk with a pessimistic hypothesis, as is done by international committees of experts.

A recent report suggests that paternal irradiation may increase the incidence of leukaemia and non-Hodgkin's lymphoma in the children (Gardner *et al.* 1990). It concerns a case-control study of these diseases diagnosed between 1950 and 1985 in persons under 25 years of age born near Sellafield nuclear plant. A significant association was found with paternal employment at the plant and with the dose of external radiation received, particularly for a dose ≥ 100 mSv received before conception and ≥ 10 mSv during the last six months. There was no evidence that any other factor might have been responsible. This is the first report of an association between parental irradiation in humans and malignant disease in their offspring. If confirmed by other studies it will have an important impact on the philosophy of radiation protection (M. J. Gardner,

M. P. Snee, A. J. Hall, C. A. Powell, S. Downes, J. D. Terrell. Results of case-control study of leukaemia and lymphoma among young people near Sellafield nuclear plant in West Cumbria. *Br. Med. J.*, 1990, **300**: 423–429).

12.5 The biological basis of radiation protection: a comparison of risks

The object of radiation protection is to define how one can 'protect individuals, their descendants and the human race in its entirety' (ICRP) against the potential risks of ionizing radiation [31, 50]. 'It is likely that the level of safety needed to assure protection of all individuals of the human race will also be adequate to protect other species' (ICRP) as the human species is relatively radiosensitive. A policy for radiation protection therefore requires a quantitative analysis of these risks.

Comparison of the effects of different types of radiation

Radiations of different LET have different values of RBE. At a given dose, high-LET radiations cause more damage. The physical dose expressed in gray is therefore insufficient and to estimate the risk it is necessary to know the shape of the dose–effect relationship for the various types of radiation. However, although the RBE varies with dose and dose rate, in the daily practice of radiation protection it is not possible to use different values of this factor as a function of dose and dose rate. It is therefore necessary to choose fixed values for each type of radiation, based on the RBE in the range of doses and for the biological effects relevant in radiation protection. These conventional values of RBE are called *quality factors* (Q).

The product of the physical dose and the factor Q is called the *dose equivalent*. This quantity represents a biologically effective dose defined for the purposes of radiation protection. It is intended to provide a common quantitative scale for evaluation of the biological effects. In addition to the factor Q one could introduce into the dose equivalent other weighting factors taking account of the spatial distribution of dose in the organism, the dose rate, etc.; in practice, for the time being, no account is taken of these. The unit of dose equivalent is the Sievert (Sv); it is a unit of the international system (SI). The Sievert has replaced the rem which referred to the rad as the unit of dose. For photons $Q=1$, therefore $1\,Sv=1\,Gy$.

Expression of dose equivalent in Sievert (Sv) provides the same expression of potential risk for all types of radiation. This enables one to compare risks or to add the effects of different types of radiation.

Committed dose (or more precisely the committed dose equivalent). When radionuclides are incorporated in the body, the total dose depends on the period of time during which the radioactivity is present. The committed dose is the dose which will be received in an organ or tissue following the incorporation of one or more radionuclides, either until complete decay of the activity or, if the half-life is very long, during the whole life of the subject, assuming by convention that the expectation of life at the moment of contamination is 50 years. Depending on the distribution of incorporated radionuclides, either the whole body or several organs may be irradiated. In the latter case it is useful for evaluating risks to use the concept of effective dose.

The effective dose equivalent is obtained by multiplying the dose equivalent delivered to an organ (in Sv) by a 'risk factor' specific to that organ, taking account of the probability of induction of fatal cancer or severe genetic effects. The value of the weighting factor is chosen in such a way as to provide a virtual dose which would give the same risk for irradiation of the whole body (31 and Table 12.5). For example, irradiation of the breast to a dose of 10 mSv leads to the same carcinogenic risk as that of 1·5 mSv to the whole body. The effective dose equivalent was devised for adding long-term risks of partial irradiation. Its main application is the calculation of annual limits of incorporation of radioactive substances, taking account of their heterogeneous distribution in the body.

The collective dose equivalent of a population is the sum of the individual dose equivalents received by all the members of the population; it is expressed in man-Sievert. For example, if 1000 individuals each received a dose equivalent of 1 mSv the collective dose equivalent would be 1 man-Sv. This quantity is little used except for estimating the detriment to be expected from a particular scheme of radiation protection. One of the weaknesses of the concept is that it assumes implicitly that the dose–effect relationship is linear.

Natural background irradiation

Since the beginning of life on earth all living creatures have passed their lives in a bath of radiation. This has three origins: cosmic rays, natural radioelements present in the earth's surface and radioactivity incorporated in the body. There are large variations from one part of the earth to another (Table 12.9) and within each country, principally because of the nature of the local geology.

The dose from terrestrial γ-rays, due to radioactivity in the earth's surface, depends on the composition of the earth. It reaches more than 3 mSv year^{-1} in

Table 12.9 Estimates of per caput annual effective dose equivalent and of ranges, excluding extreme values, for the most important natural sources of radiation.

Source of irradiation	Annual effective dose eqivalent (mSv)	
	Mean	Typical range
External		
Cosmic rays	0·3	0·3–2
Terrestrial sources	0·4	0·2–1
Internal		
^{40}K	0·18	0·1–0·2
$^{238}U \rightarrow ^{226}Ra$	0·02	0·01–0·05
$^{222}Rn \rightarrow ^{214}Po$	1·1	0·3–5
$^{214}Po \rightarrow ^{210}Pb$	0·12	0·05–0·2
$^{232}Th \rightarrow ^{224}Ra$	0·02	0·01–0·05
$^{220}Rn \rightarrow ^{203}Tl$	0·16	0·05–0·5
^{14}C	0·02	0·02
Total (rounded)	2·4	1·5–6

From [66], p. 121.

regions where there is granite rich in uranium and thorium, for example in Colorado (USA) and Cornwall (UK). In some countries, for example in the province of Kerala on the south-west coast of India, it even reaches 30 mSv per year.

The dose due to cosmic radiation depends on altitude (it increases by a factor of 3 between sea level and 2000 m) because of screening by the atmosphere. It also varies, but to a lesser extent, with latitude (maximum at the poles, minimum at the equator).

One of the main sources of internal irradiation is potassium-40, a naturally occurring isotope of potassium which is an essential element in all organisms. Natural radioactivity is also ingested through food and drink.

Inhalation of radon-222 deposits radioactive decay products on the surface of the respiratory tract. These products emit α-particles giving short-range, high-LET radiation. The doses delivered have been underestimated until recently and are now a subject of great interest. Indoor exposure to radon varies widely from less than 1 mSv year^{-1} to over 20 mSv year^{-1}. In houses it depends on the entry rate from the soil and in apartments on the exhalation rate from the building materials. Materials based on granite or clay such as cement and plaster fabricated from gypsum produce radon. The concentration of radon depends on the ventilation. Sealing against draughts increases the concentration. In cold countries where there is little ventilation in the houses, the effective dose equivalent can reach $0 \cdot 1$ Sv year^{-1} or more.

It is difficult to estimate the risk attached to this type of irradiation. By extrapolating from the effect seen in miners exposed to radon, it has been estimated that exposure to radon in the UK might be responsible for 6% or more of the annual incidence of lung cancer [8]. However, the validity of extrapolating risk estimates to the general public from studies of miners is highly uncertain. There is no direct evidence of an increased risk of lung cancer in individuals living in houses with a high concentration of radon. Nevertheless an action level for radon exposure in the home has been recommended, $7 \cdot 5$ mSv year^{-1} in the USA and 20 mSv year^{-1} in the UK. Several hundred thousand houses exceed these limits. Thus the indoor radon exposure may constitute an unprecedented environmental health problem. However, there is still much debate about what control strategy to adopt [8, 10, 26, 54].

Except for radon the spatial distribution of natural exposure in the body is more or less uniform. It is delivered at a very low dose rate throughout the whole life-time.

Artificial radiation

Irradiation due to human activities varies between different countries. Among the artificial radiation sources, mention must be made of travel in aeroplanes (cosmic rays), watches with luminous dials, etc. (Table 12.10).

However, the most important source of artificial exposure is medicine: diagnostic radiology, nuclear medicine, and to a small extent radiotherapy and treatment at spas (certain mineral waters are relatively rich in radium or thorium). Many studies of irradiation due to radiodiagnosis show that it can be reduced by improving the techniques of examination [64–66].

Radioactive fall-out from nuclear weapon tests which were conducted during the 1950s and 1960s are still responsible for a small amount of irradiation. The doses corresponding to these various sources of radiation are shown in Table 12.10. Fall-out due to the accident at Chernobyl gave rise to a dose of about 0·05 mSv in Europe in 1987 and during the following years will result in a dose of about one-tenth of the dose due to fall-out from nuclear explosions in the atmosphere from 1952 to 1962. Tables 12.9 and 12.10 show that the most important problem from the point of view of public health is that of exposure to radon [8, 26, 54, 66].

Table 12.10 Sources of irradiation due to human activities†.

	Mean dose per year to the population (mSv)	Range in industrialized countries
Medical irradiation (mean dose to the population)		
Radiodiagnosis	0·50	0·3–0·7
Radiotherapy	0·01	
Nuclear medicine	0·1	
Fall-out from experimental atomic explosions (1952–63)	0·01	
Fall-out from Chernobyl	0·001	0·0001–0·003
Phosphate fertilizers	0·0001	
Air travel mean dose over the population (Paris–New York=0·03 mSv)	0·001	
Atomic power stations and discharges of radioactive effluent	0·0015	0·0006–0·002
Occupational exposure	0·005	0·002–0·01
Consumable goods (including watches with luminous dials)	0·008	
Total	1 mSv year^{-1}	

†The most important source of irradiation is radiodiagnosis [64, 66]. In industrialized countries this gives an average dose to the inhabitants close to that due to natural radiation. The other sources of radiation are much smaller. The use of atomic power stations (including the extraction of uranium, preparation of the fuel, and disposal of waste) causes only a relatively small amount of irradiation in France although it produces 70% of the electrical energy. The dose due to occupational exposure is referred to the whole population. Fall-out from Chernobyl varied with the distance from Russia and the meteorological conditions following the accident.
After [64].

The concept of dose limitation [31]

Originally the purpose of radiation protection was to keep the absorbed dose below the threshold at which an observable effect occurs in tissues considered critical (skin, eye, haemopoietic, gonads). The first recommendations of the International Commission on Radiological Protection (ICRP) in 1928 recommended a dose limit of about 50 cGy year^{-1}; it was based essentially on effects on the skin. After several reductions, based mainly on observations of haematological effects and also due to a growing wish to reduce risks to a minimum, this limit was fixed in 1958 at 50 mSv year^{-1} total body irradiation for occupationally exposed workers and 5 mSv year^{-1} for the general population. It has not been changed since. A further reduction is under consideration at present.

During the 1950s, when it was realized that one could not exclude the risk of carcinogenesis or mutagenesis at doses below the threshold for somatic effects, the significance of the maximum permissible dose changed. The purpose was no longer only to avoid tissue effects but also to keep the probability of carcinogenesis or mutation at a very low level, so that it would be 'negligible' for workers in relation to the other risks of professional life and for the general population in relation to those of daily life. This led to the concept of the maximum permissible dose (MPD), with the addition that it was desirable to keep the dose as low as reasonably achievable (ALARA) but that it was permissible to accept this dose when circumstances made it necessary. ICRP recommendations [31] are given in Table 12.11.

There is therefore a double problem. On the one hand scientific: What is the magnitude of the risk attached to low doses? On the other hand ethical: What risk is tolerable (value judgement)?

Table 12.11 Dose limits for ionizing radiation.

Category	Irradiation	Maximum accumulated dose
Workers category A§	Total body†	50 mSv year⁻¹
	Partial body	Per year
	Female breast	170 mSv
	Lens of eye	300 mSv
	Red marrow, Lung	400 mSv
	Other organs‡	500 mSv
Workers category B	Total body†	15 mSv year⁻¹
	Partial body	1/3 of the values for category A
General public	Total body†	5 mSv year⁻¹
	Partial body	1/10 of the values for category A

†Or haemopoietic organs and gonads.
‡Except haemopoietic, gonads and lens of eye.
§For workers of category A the limits are called 'maximum permissible doses' (MPD). The question of planned special exposures is not covered here.
After [31].
These values are likely to be revised in the next recommendation of the ICRP.

Scientific aspects

In scientific terms the preceding sections show that although it is difficult to estimate exactly the risk attached to low doses, one can nevertheless evaluate on the basis of pessimistic hypotheses an upper limit to the risk, with the understanding that the real risk is no doubt lower, almost zero in the case of a quadratic relationship. Account must also be taken of a reduction in risk at low dose rate. Table 12.5 gives the order of magnitude of the risks of carcinogenesis and mutation. Irradiation every year at the maximum permissible dose rate of $50 \, \text{mSv year}^{-1}$ ($5 \, \text{rem year}^{-1}$) continued for 50 years, clearly an unrealistic possibility, would lead to a total dose of $2 \cdot 5 \, \text{Sv}$ and a total cancer risk of less than 3×10^{-2}. Allowing for the latent period and the limited expectation of life after 50 years of work, this comes to about 10^{-3} per year. In fact the yearly dose actually received in most hospitals and nuclear power stations is of the order of

$2 \cdot 5$ mSv per year, giving a total accumulated risk of $1 \cdot 5 \times 10^{-3}$. About 20% of the population will die of cancer anyway, so the incidence of cancer would be increased to $20 \cdot 15\%$. Clearly these variations are much lower than those caused by different ways of life; for example the risk of cancer in a non-smoker is about 15% and in a subject who has smoked 15 cigarettes a day for 20 years about 23%. Also an increase from 20 to $20 \cdot 15\%$ would be impossible to detect by epidemiological studies.

The concept of collective dose is of limited validity. For example, if each member of a population of 1000 persons receives a dose of $0 \cdot 01$ Sv the collective dose will be 10 man-Sv. This idea of collective dose is of some use in evaluating the detriment connected with problems such as emission of radioactivity in air or water, but the concept lacks biological significance when the distribution of dosage in the population is heterogeneous. For example, the biological effect of 10 man-Sv would be very different if one subject alone had received this dose or if 10 000 people had received 1 mSv. In terms of carcinogenic or mutagenic risks, the notion of collective dose would be significant only if the dose–effect relationship were linear, giving a simple additivity of risks. As the curve is probably of the linear–quadratic type, the concept of collective dose does not express correctly the risk run by the population or, rather, it indicates its upper limit.

Ethical aspects

To make an ethical assessment it is necessary to use as reference the risks attached to other human activities (Table 12.12). For workers the aim is to limit the risk to that accepted in relatively safe industries and for the public to limit it to that habitually accepted in normal life, for example in public transport. For example, the risk of death caused by $0 \cdot 1$ mSv is equivalent to that involved in smoking 1 cigarette or a 100 h drive in a car. Occupational irradiation at 50 mSv year^{-1} is safer than the working life of railway or building workers (Table 12.13).

Table 12.12 Risks attached to human activities.

There is a one in a million risk of death from

650 km in an aeroplane
100 km in a motor car
Smoking one cigarette
2 h of passive smoking
$1 \cdot 5$ min of rock climbing
$1 \cdot 5$ weeks of work in a normal factory
1 h of sea fishing
$2 \cdot 5$ weeks on the contraceptive pill
Half a bottle of wine
Exposure to $0 \cdot 1$ mSv, i.e.
  (a) exposure at the MPD (workers) for half a day
  (b) 3 years of life close to a nuclear power station
  (c) mean dose received during three months from diagnostic radiology

After [49, 50].

Regulations

It is not the purpose of this book to discuss the regulatory aspects of radiation protection which are dealt with in numerous documents [31]. We will only recall the values of the dose limits recommended by the ICRP which are used in most

Table 12.13 Man life shortening in days

Type of activity	For 1 year of professional life	For 35 years of professional life
Deep-sea fishing	31·9	923
Coal mining	3·6	103
Oil refinery	2·6	74
Railway worker	2·2	63
Building worker	2·1	62
Industry (mean value)	0·5	13·5
Occupational irradiation at 50 mSv per year	1·3	32
Occupational irradiation at 5 mSv per year	0·1	3

After [51].

national and international regulations (Table 12.11). New (lower) dose limits are under discussion in some countries.

The population is divided into a number of categories:

1. Workers directly involved with ionizing radiation, called working condition A, habitually work in a controlled zone.† These are the people who are the most highly exposed to ionizing radiation.
2. Workers not directly involved with radiation, working condition B; they do not normally work in a controlled zone, although they may be exposed to radiation during their working life.
3. The general public: people who do not belong to either of the two previous categories. In this case, exposure to ionizing radiation is not connected with work but is a function of their geographical location, implying that exposure is permanent and not limited to working hours.‡ This category includes subjects of both sexes, of all ages, in good or poor health, not medically supervised. The annual limit of dose is 10 times lower than that for workers of category A, as this population is neither selected nor supervised. Also, the difference in the dose limits between workers and the general population rests on two considerations: (i) in the general population there are some people who are exceptionally radiosensitive, for whom the risks are increased: children and pregnant women; (ii) for genetic effects the total dose received by the whole population is more significant than individual doses. It is therefore proper to limit the former. If the proportion of radiation workers is small, the dose which they receive has little weight from a genetic

---

†One of the ways of ensuring safe working conditions is to limit access to areas where it is possible to receive doses greater than certain limits. Examples are hot laboratories in hospitals and rooms containing intense γ-ray sources. These areas are declared controlled zones if accumulated doses can exceed the limits for workers in category B (15 mSv year⁻¹ or 7·5 μSv h⁻¹ with 2000 working hours per year). Only workers in category A are authorized for regular work in these areas and the conditions of access are strictly controlled (authorized entry, wearing of personal dosemeters and sometimes special clothing, period of time spent in the area, measurement of contamination at the exit, etc.).

‡The general population can be exposed for 365 days year⁻¹ whereas workers are exposed during a maximum of 40 h week⁻¹, 48 weeks year⁻¹.

§In order to control the eventual 'genetic burden' the ICRP estimate that the general population should not be exposed to artificial non-medical irradiation exceeding on the average 1·7 mSv year⁻¹ for each member of the population of the world, i.e. 0·05 Sv in 30 years or one generation.

point of view, whereas a much smaller dose received by the whole population will have a much greater effect.§

Other factors for workers:

a. The limits are different depending on whether the whole body is irradiated (including the gonads and the haemopoietic organs) or only a part of the body: the extremities of the limbs, the skin and bony tissue, other organs. A certain number of particular cases must be considered.

b. Women of reproductive age: the dose must not exceed $0·013\,Sv$ in 3 consecutive months (instead of $0·03\,Sv$ per 3 months for male workers of category A).

c. Pregnant women: the annual dose must not exceed $0·015\,Sv$ and the dose during pregnancy (from the moment when it is known to delivery) $0·01\,Sv$.

d. Exceptional planned exposure. In exceptional circumstances it may be necessary that a worker should be exposed beyond the maximum dose for 3 months; however in no case should the dose exceed $0·12\,Sv$.

The attention paid to very long-term effects, even those which might occur after several generations, is a remarkable aspect of radiation protection when compared with the rules of protection against other noxious agents, physical or chemical. These very long-term effects are seldom considered for other agents.

The risks of occupational exposure are comparable with those encountered in other safe industries. *A fortiori*, the risks to the general public due to miscellaneous applications of ionizing radiation are small when compared with those of daily life.

Some administrators have systematically excluded pregnant women from controlled zones, particularly in diagnostic radiology. This is not justified on scientific considerations nor by the requirements of the regulations. If individual dosimetry for the previous 12 months shows that the dose received by the woman concerned during her work was less than $15\,mSv$, the regulations allow her to continue working.

Limits of incorporation of radionuclides

The annual limits of incorporation (ALI) are not, as in normal toxicology, a fraction of the quantity causing an observable reaction, but correspond to the activity which delivers the annual limit of dose equivalent.

If this dose equivalent is delivered by radionuclides of long half-life which are retained in the body over periods greater than a year, the committed dose equivalent is attributed to the year during which the radioactivity is incorporated. This is an acceptable convention: on the assumption that the individual concerned incorporates each year for 50 years the annual limit calculated in this way, the dose equivalent delivered each year is always lower than the annual limit of dose equivalent, which will be reached only at the 50th year.

The maximum permissible concentrations (MPC) in air and water can be calculated from these limits of incorporation. They are such that inhalation or ingestion, continued for a year, will lead to an incorporation lower than the limits mentioned above [31].

Let us take the example of iodine-131. The dose equivalent received by the thyroid per year must not exceed 500 mSv for workers and 50 mSv for the public, corresponding to an effective committed dose equivalent of 1·5 mSv for the public (W_T=0·03, Table 12.5). Knowing the volume of the thyroid, the annual limit of incorporation for the public is calculated to be 10^5 Bq¶ ($2·7\,\mu$Ci¶) by ingestion (drinking) and 2×10^5 Bq by inhalation. From the rate of fixation of iodine in the thyroid and the quantities of liquid and air ingested or inhaled every day, the MPC can be calculated. For the public this is 130 Bq l^{-1} (3·1 nCi l^{-1}) in water and 24 Bq per m^3 of air (648 pCi m^{-3}): an individual who drinks and eats only material containing this concentration of iodine-131 and who breathes air also with this concentration will receive in a year a dose below the maximum permissible limit, which is itself calculated with a safety factor. This MPC must not be applied to a temporary concentration. If one ingested drinks with a concentration 10 times the MPC for 4 weeks and a negligible concentration during the rest of the year, the total accumulated dose at the end of the year would remain less than the maximum permissible dose equivalent. For milk, a concentration of 400 Bq l^{-1} throughout the year, consumed at the rate of 0·5 l day^{-1}, would give a committed dose equivalent of 1 mSv year^{-1}. For an infant whose thyroid is much smaller, the same rate of consumption of milk would deliver a dose of 10 mSv.

After accidental release of radioactive iodine, stable iodide can be administered to avoid or reduce irradiation of the thyroid. Iodide given orally (particularly potassium iodide but also in the form of lugol or tincture of iodine diluted in milk) at a dose of 50–130 mg blocks the uptake of iodine by the thyroid about 15 min after administration, but does not expel radioactive iodine which was already fixed in the thyroid. For this reason, if there has been an accident, iodide should be given as quickly as possible to the personnel with the greatest risk of contamination. However, although stable iodide is not toxic when the correct dosage is used, it is difficult to organize this properly for an entire population. This preventive measure is therefore justified only if the concentration of radioactive iodine in food, drink or air is likely to exceed the MPC by a considerable factor for a period of time.

The MPC has been defined for the principal radionuclides. For a mixture of radionuclides or if the nature of the radioactivity is unknown, international and national regulations provide fixed values of MPC which depend on whether there are any α-emitting nuclides present [31].

Radiation accidents [19, 33]

Another way of assessing the effectiveness of radiation protection is to consider the accidents which have occurred since 1945. The most serious accident between 1945 and 1985 arose from fall-out from an experimental explosion at Bikini in March 1954. Due to a meteorological error (change in the direction of the wind) radioactive fall-out affected a Japanese fishing boat and the inhabitants of certain atolls in the Pacific. A total of 119 people needed medical attention and one died.

¶The *activity* of a radioactive source is defined by its rate of disintegration. The SI unit of activity is the becquerel (Bq), equal to 1 disintegration s^{-1}. The old unit was the Curie (Ci): 1 Ci=$3·7\times10^{10}$ Bq.

Among the millions of occupationally exposed workers (a million in the USA alone) the following accidents have been recorded:

(i)   12 accidents due to nuclear fission (called criticality accidents: 6 with experimental reactors, 4 in chemical operations, 2 in experiments on critical assemblies) have caused 9 deaths between 1945 and 1983 and 37 people required medical care.

(ii) 23 accidental exposures to X- or γ-rays, mostly connected with the manipulation of radioactive sources of cobalt or iridium which are the commonest sources used in industrial radiography (loss or theft of the source, error of manipulation, etc.). In total these accidents have caused 11 deaths and 35 serious exposures.

(iii) 156 serious localized exposures which required surgical intervention in 35 subjects.

(iv) 23 internal irradiations (accidental ingestion of radioelements) which mostly occurred in patients or laboratory personnel and caused 9 deaths and 29 cases of severe damage.

Thus in the 40 years before Chernobyl there were 29 fatal accidents due to ionizing radiation and 260 irradiations for which medical care was needed. It should be noted that none of these accidents occurred in atomic power stations. The only two serious accidents in atomic power stations in Western countries have been those at Windscale in October 1954 and Three Mile Island in March 1979. They did not give rise to any radiation greater than the maximum permissible doses for workers or public.

The accident at Chernobyl on April 26 1986 deserves special comment due to its severity, as it is closest to the type of major accident so often discussed [1, 9].

The reactor concerned was used for civil and military purposes (production of electricity and plutonium). It was a graphite-moderated reactor cooled by natural water which was used directly in the turbines, whereas in the reactors of Western power stations, in particular in PWR reactors, the primary coolant passes through a heat exchanger and transfers its heat to water which is used to operate the turbines. In the latter reactors an accident in the secondary circuit would therefore not lead to appreciable radioactive contamination; also Western reactors are enclosed in thick impervious containment structures which was not the case with the reactor at Chernobyl. This explains the seriousness of the loss of radioactivity, in contrast with the accident at Three Mile Island where the discharges were very small. Finally, when the liquid refrigerant was lost at Chernobyl the power of the reactor increased whereas Western reactors are designed in such a way that if there is loss of coolant the power is reduced.

The accident took place in several stages extending over about 10 days. For several hours the core of the reactor was in direct contact with the atmosphere, leading to the release of approximately 50 million Curies including several million Curies of iodine-131 and caesium-137. About 300 workers and firemen who fought the fire were heavily irradiated (about 1 Sv or more in a few hours); in addition they were wounded, burnt or contaminated. Two hundred received between 1 and 3 Gy, 100 more than 3 Gy, of whom 50 received more than 5 Gy (median dose 7·5 Gy). Thirty died as a result of the accident, either due to trauma [1], skin burn, bone marrow aplasia or a combination. Local residents of

Chernobyl were evacuated from a 30 km exclusion zone surrounding the reactor. Forty thousand persons received a mean dose of $0 \cdot 45$ Gy. Their follow-up will bring useful information. Radionuclides contributing most significantly to the dose were ^{131}I, [134]Cs and [137]Cs.

Except for the catastrophe at Chernobyl which occurred in a situation very different from that of Western power stations, few industries can show such a satisfactory record over such a long period. This underlines the usefulness of strict safety rules for nuclear reactors.

References

1. A. Baranov, R. P. Gale, A. Guskova *et al.*, Bone marrow transplantation after the Chernobyl Nuclear accident. *New England J. Med.*, 1989, **321**: 205–212.
2. V. Beral, H. Inskip, P. Fraser, M. Booth, D. Coleman, G. Rose. Mortality of employees of the United Kingdom Atomic Energy Authority, 1946–1979. *Br. Med. J.*, 1985, **291**: 440–447.
3. J. F. Bithell, A. M. Stewart. Prenatal irradiation and childhood malignancy: a review of British data from the Oxford Survey. *Br. J. Cancer*, 1975, **31**: 271–287.
4. J. D. Boice, M. Blettner, R. Kleinerman, *et al.*, Radiation dose and leukemia risk in patients treated for cancer of the cervix. *J. Natl. Cancer Inst.*, 1987, **79**: 1295–1311.
5. J. D. Boice, G. Engholm, R. A. Kleinerman *et al.*, Radiation dose and second cancer risk in patients treated for cancer of the cervix. *Radiat. Res.*, 1988, **116**: 3–55.
6. C. Borek. Radiation oncogenesis in culture. *Adv. Cancer Res.*, 1982, **37**: 159–232.
7. Committee on the Biological Effects of Ionizing Radiations. *The effects on population of exposure to low levels of ionizing radiation*: BEIR III. Washington, National Academy of Sciences, 1980.
8. Committee on the Biological Effects of Ionizing Radiations. *Health risks of radon and other internally deposited alpha-emitters*: BEIR IV. Washington, National Academy of Sciences, 1988.
9. R. E. Champlin, W. E. Kastenberg, R. P. Gale. Radiation accidents and nuclear energy: medical consequences and therapy. *Ann. Intern. Med.*, 1988, **109**: 730–744.
10. R. H. Clarke, T. R. E. Southwood: Risks from ionizing radiation. *Nature*, 1989, **338**: 197–198.
11. S. C. Darby, R. Doll, M. C. Pike. Mortality of employees of the United Kingdom Atomic Energy Authority, 1946–79. *Br. Med. J.*, 1985, **291**: 672.
12. S. C. Darby, R. Doll, S. K. Gill, P. G. Smith. Long-term mortality after a single treatment course with X-rays in patients treated for ankylosing spondylitis. *Br. J. Cancer*, 1987, **55**: 179–190.
13. N. E. Day. Radiation and multistage carcinogenesis, in: *Radiation carcinogenesis: epidemiology and biological significance* (J. D. Boice Jr., J. F. Fraumeni Jr., eds), pp. 437–443, Raven Press, New York, 1984.
14. J. Ferrera, J. Lipton, S. Hellman, S. Burakoff, P. Mauch. Engraftment following T-Cell depleted marrow transplantation. *Transplantation*, 1987, **43**: 461–467.
15. P. Fraser, M. Booth, V. Beral, H. Inskip, S. Firsht, S. Speak. Collection and validation of data in the United Kingdom Atomic Energy Authority mortality study. *Br. Med. J.*, 1985, **291**: 435–439.
16. R. J. M. Fry. Relevance of animal studies to the human experience, in: *Radiation carcinogenesis: epidemiology and biological significance* (J. D. Boice Jr., J. F. Fraumeni Jr., eds), pp. 337–346. Raven Press, New York, 1984.
17. R. P. Gale, Y. Reisner. The role of bone-marrow transplants after nuclear accidents. *Lancet*, 1988, **1**: 923–926.
18. F. B. Gibberd. Radiation and mental retardation. *Brit. Med. J.*, 1988 **297**: 153–154.
19. R. Gongora, H. Jammet. Radiolésions aiguës localisées. *Radioprotection*, 1983, **18**: 139–154.
20. D. T. Goodhead. Deductions from cellular studies of inactivation, mutagenesis, and transformation, in: *Radiation carcinogenesis: epidemiology and biological significance* (J. D. Boice Jr., J. F. Fraumeni Jr., eds), pp. 369–385. Raven Press, New York, 1984.
21. M. N. Gould. Radiation initiation of carcinogenesis in vivo: a rare or common cellular event, in: *Radiation carcinogenesis: epidemiology and biological significance* (J. D. Boice Jr., J. F. Fraumeni Jr., eds), pp. 347–358. Raven Press, New York, 1984.
22. E. J. Hall, T. K. Hei. Oncogenic transformation of cells in culture: Pragmatic comparisons of oncogenicity cellular and molecular mechanisms. *Int. J. Radiat. Oncol. Biol. Phys.*, 1986, **12**: 1909–1921.

23. A. Han, M. M. Elkind. Enhanced transformation of mouse 1OT ½ cells by 12-0-tetradecano-lyphorbol-13-acetate following exposure to X-rays or to fission-spectrum neutrons. *Cancer Res.*, 1982, **42**: 477–483.

24. A. Han, C. K. Hill, M. M. Elkind. Repair of cell killing and neoplastic transformation at reduced dose rates of 60Co γ-rays. *Cancer Res.*, 1980, **40**: 3328–3332.

25. E. R. Harvey, J. D. Boice, M. Honeyman, J. J. Flannery. Prenatal X-ray exposure and childhood cancer in twins. *New Eng. J. Med.*, 1985, **312**: 541–545.

26. R. M. Haynes. The distribution of domestic radon concentration and lung cancer mortality in England and Wales. *Radiation Protection Dosimetry*, 1988, **25**: 93–96.

27. M. Henry-Amar. Second malignancies after radiotherapy and chemotherapy for early stages of Hodgkin's disease (for the EORTC Radiotherapy-Chemotherapy Group). *J. Nat. Cancer Inst.*, 1983, **71**: 911–916.

28. C. K. Hill, B. A. Carnes, A. Han, M. M. Elkind. Neoplastic transformation is enhanced by multiple low doses of fission-spectrum neutrons, *Radiat. Res.*, 1985, **102**: 404–410.

29. L. F. Holm, K. E. Wiklund, G. E. Lundell, N. A. Bergman, G. Bjenkengren, E. S. Cederquist, U. B. C. Ericsson, L. G. Larsson, M. E. Lidberg, R. S. Lindberg, H. V. Wicklund, J. D. Boice. Thyroid cancer after diagnostic doses of iodine-131: a retrospective cohort study. *J. Natl. Cancer Inst.*, 1988, **80**: 1132–1138.

30. K. F. Hubner, S. A. Fry (eds). *The medical basis for radiation accident preparedness.* Elsevier–North Holland, New York, 1980.

31. ICRP: Publication 26, Recommendations of the International Commission on Radiological Protection. Annals of the I.C.R.P., *1, 3*, Pergamon Press, Oxford, 1977.

32. ICRP Publication 49, Developmental effects of irradiation on the brain of embryo and foetus. *Annals of the I.C.R.P.*, **16**: 4, Oxford: Pergamon Press.

33. H. P. Jammet. Problèmes posés par les irradiations accidentelles prolongées. *Bull. Acad. Nat. Med.*, 1979, **163**: 148–160.

34. H. Kato, W. J. Schull. Studies of the mortality of the A-bomb survivors. *Radiat. Res.*, 1982, **90**: 395–432.

35. A. R. Kennedy, J. Little. Evidence that a second event in X-ray induced oncogenic transformation *in vitro* occurs during cellular proliferation. *Radiat. Res.*, 1984, **99**: 228–248.

36. H. I. Kohn, R. J. M. Fry. Radiation carcinogenesis. *New Eng. J. Med.*, 1984, **310**: 504–511.

37. C. E. Land, J. D. Boice, R. E. Shore, J. E. Norman, M. Tokunaga. Breast cancer risk from low-dose exposures to ionizing radiation: results of parallel analysis of three exposed populations of women. *J. Nat. Cancer Inst.*, 1980, **65**: 353–376.

38. R. Latarjet, M. Tubiana. The risks of induced carcinogenesis after irradiation at small doses. The uncertainties which remain after the 1988 UNSCEAR report. *Int. J. Radiat. Oncol.*, 1989, **17**: 237–240.

39. C. C. Lusbaugh. On some recent progress in human radiobiology. In *Advances in Radiation Biology* (L. C. Augenstein, R. Mason, M. Zella, eds) 1969, 277–314. Academic Press, New York.

40. Medical Research Council's Committee on Effect of Ionizing Radiation. Lethality from acute and protracted radiation exposure in man. *Int. J. Radiat. Biol.*, 1984, **46**: 209–217.

41. R. H. Mole. Antenatal irradiation and childhood cancer: causation or coincidence. *Br. J. Cancer*, 1974, **30**: 1 99–208.

42. R. H. Mole. The LD 50 for uniform low LET irradiation of man. *Br. J. Radiol.*, 1984, **57**: 355–369.

43. R. H. Mole. Irradiation of embryo and fetus. *Br. J. Radiol.*, 1987, **60**: 17–31.

44. C. R. Muirhead, S. C. Darby. Modelling the relative and absolute risks of radiation-induced cancers. *J. R. Statist. Soc. A.*, 1987, **150**: part 2, 83–118.

45. National Council on Radiation Protection and Measurements (US). *Review of NCRP radiation dose limit for embryo and fetus in occupationally exposed women.* NCRP Report No. 53, 1977. *Medical radiation exposure of pregnant and potentially pregnant women.* NCRP Report No. 54, 1977.

46. National Council on Radiation Protection and Measurements. *Influence of dose and its distribution in time on dose–response relationships for low-LET radiations.* NCRP Report No. 64, 1980.

47. M. Otake, W. J. Schull. *In utero* exposure to A-bomb radiation and mental retardation. A reassessment. *Br. J. Radiol.*, 1984, **57**: 409–414.

48. M. C. Paterson, N. T. Bech-Hansen, P. J. Smith, J. J. Mulvihill. Radiogenic neoplasia, cellular radiosensitivity, and faulty DNA repair, in: *Radiation carcinogenesis: epidemiology and biological significance* (J. D. Boice Jr., J. F. Fraumeni Jr., eds), pp. 319–336. Raven Press, New York, 1984.

49. E. E. Pochin. Quantification of risk in medical procedures. *Proc. Roy. Soc. London*, 1981, **A 376**: 87–101.

50. E. E. Pochin. Radiation risks in perspective. *Br. J. Radiol.*, 1987, **60**: 42–50.

51. J. Reissland, V. Harris. A scale for measuring risks. *New Scientist*, 1979, **83**: 809–812.

52. R. E. Rowland, A. F. Stehney, H. F. Lucas. Dose–response relationship for radium-induced bone sarcomas. *Health Physics*, 1983, **44**, Suppl. 1: 15–31.
53. J. G. B. Russell. How dangerous are diagnostic X-rays? *Clinical Radiology*, 1984, **35**: 347–351.
54. J. M. Samet, A. V. Nero. Indoor radon and lung cancer. *New Eng. J. Med.*, 1989, **320**: 591–594.
55. W. J. Schull, M. Otake, J. V. Neel. Genetic effects of the atomic bomb; a reappraisal. *Science*, 1981, **213**: 1220–1227.
56. Y. Shimizu, H. Kato, W. J. Schull, D. Preston, S. Fujita, D. Pierce. Life span study report 11, part 1 – Comparison of risk coefficients for site specific cancer mortality based on the DS86 and T65DR shielded kerma and organ doses. *Technical report RERF TR12–87*, 1987.
57. Y. Shimizu, H. Kato, W. J. Schull. Life span study report 11, part 2 – Cancer mortality in the years 1950–1985 based on the recently revised doses (DS86). *Technical report RERF TR5–88*, 1988.
58. P. G. Smith, R. Doll. Mortality among patients with ankylosing spondylitis after a single treatment course with X-rays. *Br. Med. J.*, 1982, **284**: 449–460.
59. J. F. Spalding, M. R. Brooks, G. L. Tietjen. Comparative litter and reproduction characteristics of mouse populations for 82 generations of X-irradiated male progenitors. *Proc. Soc. Exp. Biol. Med.*, 1981, **166**: 237–240.
60. J. R. Totter, H. G. McPherson. Do childhood cancers result from prenatal X-rays? *Health Physics*, 1981, **40**: 511–524.
61. M. Tubiana, C. M. Lalanne. Évolution hématologique des malades soumis à une irradiation totale pour transplantation d'organes. *Ann. Radiol.*, 1963, **6**: 561–580.
62. R. L. Ullrich, J. B. Storer. Influence of γ irradiation on the development of neoplastic disease in mice. *Radiat. Res.*, 1979, **80**: 325–342.
63. United Nations Scientific Committee on the Effects of Atomic Radiation (UNSCEAR). *Sources and effects of ionizing radiation*, (UNE 77 IX 1). Report to the General Assembly, United Nations, New York, 1977.
64. United Nations Scientific Committee on the Effects of Atomic Radiation (UNSCEAR). *Ionizing radiation sources and biological effects*. United Nations, New York, 1982.
65. United Nations Scientific Committee on the Effects of Atomic Radiation (UNSCEAR). *Genetic and somatic effects of ionizing radiation*. Report to the General Assembly, with annexes. United Nations, New York, 1986.
66. United Nations Scientific Committee on the Effects of Atomic Radiation (UNSCEAR). *Sources, effects and risks of ionizing radiation*. Report to the General Assembly, with annexes. United Nations, New York, 1988.
67. A. Upton (ed.). *Radiation carcinogenesis*. Elsevier, New York, 1986.
68. D. W. van Bekkum, P. Bentvelzen. The concept of gene transfer–misrepair mechanisms of radiation carcinogenesis may challenge the linear extrapolation model of risk estimation for low radiation doses. *Health Phys.*, 1982, **43**: 231–237.
69. G. van Kaick, H. Muth, A. Kaul, H. Immich, D. Liebermann, D. Lorenz, W. J. Lorenz, H. Luhrs, K. E. Sheer, G. Wagner, H. Wegener Hand Wesh. Results of the German thorotrast study, in: *Radiation carcinogenesis: epidemiology and biological significance* (J. D. Boice Jr., J. F. Fraumeni Jr., eds), pp. 253–262. Raven Press, New York, 1984.
70. T. Wakabayashi, H. Kato, T. Ikeda, W. J. Schull. Studies of the mortality of A-bomb survivors. *Radiat. Res.*, 1983, **93**: 112–146.

Index